BODY IMAGE CARE
FOR CANCER PATIENTS

Body Image Care for Cancer Patients

PRINCIPLES AND PRACTICES

Edited by Michelle Cororve Fingeret, PhD, FAPOS
OWNER, FINGERET PSYCHOLOGY SERVICES
HOUSTON, TEXAS

Irene Teo, PhD
ASSISTANT PROFESSOR, DUKE-NUS MEDICAL SCHOOL
CLINICAL PSYCHOLOGIST, NATIONAL CANCER
CENTRE SINGAPORE
SINGAPORE

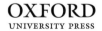

OXFORD
UNIVERSITY PRESS

OXFORD
UNIVERSITY PRESS

Oxford University Press is a department of the University of Oxford. It furthers
the University's objective of excellence in research, scholarship, and education
by publishing worldwide. Oxford is a registered trade mark of Oxford University
Press in the UK and certain other countries.

Published in the United States of America by Oxford University Press
198 Madison Avenue, New York, NY 10016, United States of America.

© Oxford University Press 2018

CIP data is on file at the Library of Congress
ISBN 978–0–19–065561–7

9 8 7 6 5 4 3 2 1

Printed by Sheridan Books, Inc., United States of America

CONTENTS

SECTION II CANCER-SPECIFIC SEQUELAE ASSOCIATED WITH BODY IMAGE DISTURBANCE

SECTION III SPECIAL POPULATIONS

CONCLUSION

CONTRIBUTORS

Ali Alias, BSc
McGill University
Montréal, Quebec, Canada

**Maria Antonietta Annunziata,
    PhD, PsyD**
Unit of Oncological Psychology
IRCCS Centro di Riferimento Oncologico
    di Aviano
Aviano, Italy

Lora L. Black, PhD
The Ohio State University
Columbus, Ohio

Kristen M. Carpenter, PhD
The Ohio State University
Columbus, Ohio

Alex Clarke, DClin, MSc, BSc (Hons)
Centre for Appearance Research
University of the West of England
Bristol, England, United Kingdom

Sarah M. DeSnyder, MD, FACS
Department of Breast Surgical Oncology
The University of Texas MD Anderson
    Cancer Center
Houston, Texas

Murray Drummond, PhD
Flinders University
Adelaide, South Australia, Australia

Michelle Cororve Fingeret, PhD, FAPOS
Owner, Fingeret Psychology Services
Houston, Texas

Brendan Gough, PhD
Leeds Beckett University
Leeds, England, United Kingdom

Justin Grayer, DClinPsy, BSc (Hons)
Adult Psychological Support Service
The Royal Marsden NHS Foundation Trust
London, England, United Kingdom

Esther Hansen, DClinPsy, BSc (Hons)
Department of Plastic and Reconstructive
    Surgery
Royal Free London NHS Foundation Trust
London, England, United Kingdom

Diana Harcourt, PhD, MSc, BSc (Hons)
Centre for Appearance Research
University of the West of England
Bristol, England, United Kingdom

Kristina Harper, MA
University of Houston—Clear Lake
Houston, Texas

Melissa Henry, PhD
Gerald Bronfman Department of Oncology
Faculty of Medicine
McGill University
Montréal, Quebec, Canada

Jimmie Holland, MD†
Department of Psychiatry and Behavioral
 Sciences
Memorial Sloan-Kettering Cancer Center
New York, New York

**Kate A. Hutcheson, PhD,
 CCC-SLP, BCS-S**
Department of Head and Neck Surgery
The University of Texas
M. D. Anderson Cancer Center
Houston, Texas

Hanne Konradsen, PhD, RN
Karolinska Intitutet
Department of Neurobiology
Care Sciences and Society
Huddinge, Sweden

Geok Ling Lee, PhD
Department of Social Work
National University of Singapore
Singapore

Vicky Lehmann, PhD
Department of Psychology
St. Jude Children's Research Hospital
Memphis, Tennessee

Jan S. Lewin, PhD, CCC-SLP, BCS-S
Department of Head and Neck Surgery
The University of Texas
M. D. Anderson Cancer Center
Houston, Texas

**Helena Lewis-Smith, PhD, MSc,
 BSc (Hons)**
Centre for Appearance Research
University of the West of England
Bristol, England, United Kingdom

Barbara Muzzatti, PhD, PsyD
Unit of Oncological Psychology
IRCCS Centro di Riferimento Oncologico
 di Aviano
Aviano, Italy

**Nicole Paraskeva, DHealthPsy, MSc,
 BSc (Hons)**
Centre for Appearance Research
University of the West of England
Bristol, England, United Kingdom

Jennifer Barsky Reese, PhD
Cancer Prevention and Control Program
Fox Chase Cancer Center
Philadelphia, Pennsylvania

Bethany Rhoten, PhD, RN
School of Nursing
Vanderbilt University
Nashville, Tennessee

Andy Roth, MD
Department of Psychiatry and Behavioral
 Sciences
Memorial Sloan-Kettering Cancer Center
New York, New York

**Mark V. Schaverien, MB, ChB, MD, MSc,
 Med FRCS (Plast)**
Department of Plastic Surgery
The University of Texas MD Anderson
 Cancer Center
Houston, Texas

Tammy A. Schuler, PhD
Association for Behavioral and Cognitive
 Therapies
New York, New York

†Deceased author.

Simona F. Shaitelman, MD, EdM
Department of Radiation Oncology
The University of Texas MD Anderson
  Cancer Center
Houston, Texas

Laura-Kate E. Shaw, PhD
Centre for Emotional Health
Macquarie University
Sydney, Australia

Kerry A. Sherman, PhD
Centre for Emotional Health
Macquarie University
Sydney, New South Wales, Australia

Irene Teo, PhD
Duke-NUS Medical School
National Cancer Centre Singapore
Singapore

Amanda L. Thompson, PhD
Director, Patient Support Services
Center for Cancer and Blood Disorders
Children's National Medical Center

Pediatrics and Psychiatry and Behavioral
  Science
George Washington University School of
  Medicine and Health Sciences
Washington, DC

Marrit A. Tuinman, PhD
Department of Health Psychology
University of Groningen
University Medical Center Groningen
Groningen, The Netherlands

Lori Wiener, PhD
Co-Director, Behavioral Health Core
Head, Psychosocial Support and Research
  Program
Pediatric Oncology Branch, Center for
  Cancer Research
National Institutes of Health
Bethesda, Maryland

INTRODUCTION

CHAPTER 1

THE INTERSECTION OF BODY IMAGE AND ONCOLOGY

Michelle Cororve Fingeret and Irene Teo

This book is wholly inspired by individuals with cancer who must adapt to various changes to their bodies as a result of their illness and its treatment. We have been fortunate and extremely blessed to be on the front lines delivering clinical care and conducting research together to address body image issues in the oncology setting. Working in this area since 2004, Fingeret has developed a comprehensive program of patient care activities, grant-funded clinical research, and professional education/training activities designed to enhance the care of patients struggling with changes to their appearance and bodily function from cancer and treatment-related side effects. Teo was among the first postdoctoral fellows trained to deliver specialized body image care in the oncology setting as part of this program and now disseminates her research and clinical expertise in this area across the globe in Singapore. We feel the time is ripe for us to make a seminal contribution to the field of body image and cancer by facilitating the publication of the first academic textbook on this topic. We have brought together a passionate and extremely accomplished group of co-authors from around the world to offer their collective wisdom on best practices and principles of body image care for patients with cancer that is rooted in empirical research. We intend for this book to be relevant to a multidisciplinary audience of healthcare professionals and for it to be useful in training and other educational settings.

As we set out to train the next generation of researchers and clinicians in the fields of body image and oncology, we must recognize that these professionals will not know of a world where these arenas are distinct and separate. We have come to recognize and appreciate the space where these fields intersect and know we have crossed the frontier where specialized training in body image and oncology is valued. We would not be here without the efforts of individuals such as Thomas Cash, Thomas Pruzinsky, and David Sarwer, whose outstanding research and scientific contributions to the field of body image pushed it beyond the study of eating disorders and into an array of medical contexts. The study of the psychology of appearance and disfigurement has also significantly shaped scientific inquiry and clinical interventions addressing body image difficulties of cancer patients, largely led by Nicola Rumsey and Diana Harcourt at the Centre for Appearance Research and James Partridge of Changing Faces. Moreover, it is the groundbreaking work of Jimmie Holland, who founded the field of psycho-oncology that ultimately enabled medical professionals to appreciate the importance of addressing adverse psychological and social sequelae of cancer treatments. Indeed, the seminal Institute of Medicine report, *Cancer Care for the Whole Patient*, released in 2008 provided a roadmap for the field of psychosocial oncology, recommending that psychosocial services become an integral part of quality cancer care.

Body image is a critical psychosocial issue for patients with cancer as the disease and its treatment can result in profound changes to one's appearance and/or bodily functioning. Regardless of whether these changes are temporary or long-lasting, a rapidly growing body of scientific research identifies the deleterious psychological impact that various types of appearance alterations, sensory changes, and functional impairments can have on patients and families throughout the cancer treatment trajectory. It is important to consider the wide range of bodily changes a patient with cancer may undergo prior to, during the process of, and following treatment which can include, but is not limited to, hair loss, scarring/disfigurement, skin discoloration, lymphedema, weight gain/loss, sexual dysfunction, infertility, pain, fatigue, limb loss, dysarthria, dysphagia, placement of stoma, and use of prosthesis. We explore the impact of these and many other types of bodily changes related to cancer and its treatment throughout this book to elucidate a better understanding of the body image experiences of patients with cancer.

Among the adverse psychological effects of body image changes include debilitating levels of social anxiety and clinical depression as well as worsened relationships with partners and impaired sexuality. Body image issues have been examined in a wide array of cancer patients, including but not limited to those with breast, cervical, colorectal, head and neck, hematological, ovarian, prostate, renal, skin, and testicular cancers. As body image research expands to incorporate many different cancer populations, there is a need to appraise the landscape to identify common themes and findings, take stock of what has been learned, and determine where researchers and clinicians should go from here. It is crucial to appraise existing approaches to the assessment and treatment of body image difficulties being utilized in the oncology setting in order to determine whether certain methods merit widespread attention and dissemination.

As the field of body image and cancer evolves, it fulfills an important promise of being interdisciplinary. Oncologists, psychologists, psychiatrists, nurses, physician assistants, social workers, physical therapists, occupational therapists, speech and language pathologists, and other allied healthcare professionals play a vital role in the development and delivery of psychosocial interventions to address body image issues. We consider the unique ways these professional disciplines are directly involved in the delivery of body image care.

- Oncologists, nurses, physician assistants, and all other primary members of a patient's medical team are responsible for the diagnosis and treatment of the patient's cancer as well as the management of treatment-related side effects. The primary medical team plays a pivotal role in helping educate patients about their illness and what to expect from treatment, which includes addressing concerns about body changes that are likely to occur or have occurred. They must be able to identify a patient's body image distress, provide care and support related to body image concerns during clinical encounters, and recognize when to make a referral to other healthcare providers to address body image disturbance.

- Speech and language pathologists and rehabilitation specialists (who provide physical and occupational therapy) represent a larger group of healthcare providers involved in the delivery of medical care that addresses treatment-related side effects which significantly disrupt a patient's body image. Chief among these side effects are impairments related to pain, lymphedema, limb loss, speech and language impairments, and vision and/or hearing loss. Other medical professionals delivering services to address bone health, bowel management, dental care, fatigue, nausea, neuropathy, nutrition, physical deconditioning, sexual dysfunction, and skin care issues can also be considered within this group. These individuals deliver specialized body image care in that they directly treat and work to ameliorate body image suffering of patients. Similar to the primary medical team members, they must be able to provide care and support related to body image concerns and recognize when to make a referral to other providers to address body image disturbance.

- Mental health specialists include psychologists, psychiatrists, social workers, psychiatric nurses, and counselors. These healthcare professionals provide specialized care in psychosocial oncology and are needed to address difficulties patients and families have coping with body image changes due to cancer and its treatment from an emotional and social perspective. There is a range of training and expertise within each of these professional disciplines related to the provision of psychosocial care which relate, for instance, to the ability to deliver certain types of interventions or to prescribe psychotropic medication. However, these specialists can be relied upon to promote optimal psychological and social adjustment as patients come to terms with body image changes from cancer and its treatment. Mental health specialists also play a vital role in training other members of the medical team on how to more effectively communicate with and support patients with body image distress during routine clinical encounters.

PURPOSE AND STRUCTURE OF THE BOOK

The purpose of this book is to introduce the first comprehensive text to delineate principles and practices of body image care for cancer patients that can be utilized by healthcare professionals across various disciplines to enhance care delivery and continue to fuel scientific advancements in the field. This textbook covers issues at the forefront of clinical care for defining, assessing, and treating body image disturbance in cancer patients through a synthesis of scientific findings. The chapters in this book are organized into three sections: Fundamentals of Body Image and Cancer, Cancer-Specific Sequelae Associated with Body Image Disturbance, and Special Populations. All the chapters are structured to ensure that implications for research and clinical practice are clearly delineated.

FUNDAMENTALS OF BODY IMAGE AND CANCER

The first section, Fundamentals of Body Image and Cancer, broadly covers theoretical foundations of body image (Chapter 2), assessment tools and intervention strategies used in the oncology setting (Chapters 3 and 4), and body image considerations related to cancer type and treatment trajectory (Chapters 5 and 6).

In Chapter 2, Rhoten reviews conceptual foundations of body image dating back to the 1920s and presents neurological, psychoanalytic, nursing, and psychological perspectives on the construct of body image. Furthermore, conceptualizations of body image within oncology are extensively discussed, and theoretical models of body image developed for specific types of cancer are highlighted.

In Chapter 3, Annunziata, Muzzatti, and Fingeret delineate pertinent considerations when assessing body image in an oncology setting. Key aspects of body image relating to cancer patients are defined and discussed. Particular attention is given to reviewing an array of body image instruments relevant for cancer patients and describing key content areas when conducting a clinical assessment of body image concerns for this patient population.

In Chapter 4, Lewis-Smith, Harcourt, and Clarke describe various psychological approaches to support people whose appearance and/or body image has changed as a result of cancer. They utilize a stepped care framework to consider the diverse psychosocial needs of individuals with appearance concerns and attend to empirical evidence supporting the development and delivery of body image interventions.

Chapter 5 provides an overview of research on body image challenges experienced by patients and survivors across breast and other sexual organ–related, gastrointestinal, head and neck, skin, brain, sarcoma, ocular, and systemic cancers. Lehmann and Tuinmann frame this discussion utilizing a visibility-stability model to facilitate understanding of disease-specific effects of cancer treatment on body image. They further highlight the central importance of changes to functioning as a key aspect of body image.

Chapter 6 considers body image–related challenges throughout the cancer treatment trajectory from cancer detection and diagnosis through active treatment and into cancer survivorship. Sherman and Shaw provide an overview of research on the manner in which active treatment can adversely impact a patient's body image. They further highlight the manner in which body image concerns can serve as a barrier to cancer detection and can arise from risk-reducing or prophylactic treatment to minimize hereditary cancer risk, two important areas of body image literature which are often overlooked.

CANCER-SPECIFIC SEQUELAE ASSOCIATED WITH BODY IMAGE DISTURBANCE

Section II, Cancer-Specific Sequelae Associated with Body Image Disturbance, reviews scientific literature and provides recommendations for treatment of body image issues associated with specific disease- and treatment-related side effects. This section begins with an overview of findings involving appearance alterations (Chapter 7) and functional loss (Chapter 8) stemming from cancer. Remaining chapters in the section address specific symptoms of sexual dysfunction, lymphedema, and speech and swallowing impairment (Chapters 9, 10, and 11, respectively).

In Chapter 7, Paraskeva, Clarke, and Harcourt draw from collective literature in areas of disfigurement, altered appearance, and visible differences to demonstrate the psychological impact of appearance changes involving weight, scarring from surgery, alopecia, ascites, and lymphedema. They further present a comprehensive framework of psychological adjustment to living with visible differences that has been extensively studied and is directly applicable to patients with cancer.

Henry and Alias shed light on body image implications of functional loss following cancer in Chapter 8, with a particular focus on limb and sensory loss. They provide a conceptual framework of functioning and how it relates to body image using the World Health Organization's International Classification of Functioning, Disability and Health model. This is one of few chapters in the book that effectively draws upon literature in pediatric and adult oncology populations and thereby offers more broadly based clinical applications.

Chapter 9 considers the relationship between body image and sexuality and offers a review of evidence-based assessment and intervention techniques for sexual problems and fertility issues among cancer patients and survivors. Carpenter and Black address issues related to sexual dysfunction in men and women, including problems with desire, arousal, orgasm, and sexual pain. Special considerations for pediatric cancer survivors are covered as well.

In Chapter 10, DeSnyder, Shaitelman, and Schaverien focus on the profound effects that lymphedema affecting the upper extremity, one or both of the lower extremities, the trunk, or the head and neck region can have on a patient's body image. They define lymphedema, describe the stages of lymphedema, identify risk factors, and describe available treatments to manage this dreaded side effect. Further attention is given to delineating guidelines for educating patients about risk-reducing behaviors and evidence-based precautions.

The final chapter in this section covers speech and swallowing impairment, as these body image changes may result in long-term disabling outcomes for patients and can be profoundly distressing. Lewin, Fingeret, and Hutcheson highlight the importance of a strong collegial collaboration among all members of the multidisciplinary team to facilitate functional restoration and optimal psychosocial adjustment. They review basic processes involved in speech and swallowing, functional assessment and rehabilitation techniques, and considerations for assessment and treatment of body image concerns within this patient population.

SPECIAL POPULATIONS

The final section of the book is devoted to special populations and reviews topics in body image care of cancer patients that are rarely addressed but are of great clinical importance. The section begins with a focus on exploring body image issues across the lifespan first in children and adolescents with cancer (Chapter 12) and then in geriatric oncology patient populations (Chapter 13). Attention then turns to examining body image among men (Chapter 14) and couples (Chapter 15). The section concludes with a focus on examining body image within various cultural contexts, specifically Western and Asian cultures (Chapters 16 and 17, respectively).

In Chapter 12, Thompson and Wiener provide an overview of existing research about body image in children and adolescents with cancer. They delineate the impact of cancer on the developing body image of children and adolescents and identify risk factors for the development of poor body image during and after treatment. Further attention is given to discussing principles of clinical care for addressing body image issues among the young and describing varied strategies for minimizing the impact of body changes.

In Chapter 13, Schuler, Roth, and Holland discuss the impact of cancer on body image concerns across the latter part of the lifespan. They describe complex interactions between cancer and body image in older men and women (aged 65 years and above), which warrants attention as more than half of all cancers occur in patients of this age group. They offer a range of global recommendations for the treatment of body image distress in older patients.

Drummond and Gough highlight broad issues men face with respect to body image in Chapter 14. They review relevant research on men's body image and masculinities as well as illness-induced body dissatisfaction among men. They provide specific examples of male body image issues within the context of prostate cancer, which is the leading gender-specific cancer among men.

Hansen, Reese, and Grayer describe clinical and research-based interventions focused on helping couples cope with body image distress associated with cancer in Chapter 15. They present an overview of observational research as well as couple-based intervention studies addressing body image cancer. Using a relational framework, they also provide detailed guidance on approaches for assessment, case conceptualization, and management of body image distress for couples.

In Chapter 16, Harper and Konradsen provide a broad overview of a Western cultural perspective on appearance and body image. They review key Western cultural tenets relevant to our understanding of body image and apply these to the oncology setting. Similarly, Chapter 17 provides a broad overview of an Asian cultural perspective on body image and cancer. Lee and Teo review key Confucian concepts and how these influence the body image experiences of patients with cancer. They also review relevant research findings on body image and psychosocial oncology conducted in Asia. Taken together, these final chapters offer an important reminder of the need to consider cross-cultural issues when developing studies, interpreting research findings, or delivering clinical care.

CONCLUDING REMARKS

At the heart of this book is the desire to educate multidisciplinary healthcare professionals about the delivery of high-quality body image care for patients with cancer and to promote further research in this arena. Thus practical approaches to intervention and case examples are incorporated across all chapters to ensure that healthcare providers are able to directly apply the principles of body image care to enhance their daily work with patients in the oncology setting. We conclude this book with a synthesis of findings across major themes of the book. Finally, we provide our vision for an ideal future where no patient suffers from unmet psychosocial needs related to body image as a result of cancer and its treatment. It is our hope that this book will make a major contribution to clinical care and research that will greatly benefit patients and their families.

SECTION I

FUNDAMENTALS OF BODY IMAGE AND CANCER

CHAPTER 2

THEORETICAL FOUNDATIONS OF BODY IMAGE

Bethany Rhoten

INTRODUCTION

During the past century, our understanding of body image has changed as scholars have continued to refine (a) what is meant by the term "body image," (b) the contextual nature of body image, (c) how body image affects our interactions with others, and (d) our understanding of how body image is related to other psychological constructs (e.g., shame, emotional distress, quality of life). Although body image in the context of disordered eating has traditionally received the majority of the field's focus, the body image of individuals with cancer as well as other chronic medical conditions and injuries has begun to receive more focus from clinicians and researchers. The purpose of this chapter is to review the theoretical foundations of body image that shape our understanding of body image in individuals with cancer. By understanding the origin and history of body image conceptualization, researchers and clinicians in cancer care can build upon the existing knowledge base to develop appropriate and timely assessments of body image, train oncology healthcare providers to include body image in holistic survivorship care, and design interventions that appropriately address the body image needs of this population.

Neurological, psychoanalytic, psychological, nursing, contextual, fear-avoidance, information-processing, feminist, evolutionary, genetic, and positivist viewpoints have all influenced the conceptualization of body image. Furthermore, many disease-specific conceptualizations, particularly in the context of oncology, have shaped how we understand the body image of individuals with cancer. Although Webster's currently defines body image as "a subjective picture of one's own physical appearance established both by self-observation and by noting the reactions of others," this description cannot encompass the evolved complexity of its current meaning as a fluid, multidimensional construct.[1]

While body image may mean one thing for a healthy adult, it has a vastly different meaning for individuals suffering from eating disorders where individuals' perception of their bodies may be distorted. Thinking about body image in the context of oncology where patients are experiencing an array of physiological, appearance, and functional changes adds further complexity. Until the late 1900s body image research largely concentrated on the study of perceptual dimensions of the bodily experience, such as body size estimation.[2] Although perception of physical appearance has traditionally been central to our understanding of body image, other factors are crucial in fully understanding and describing an individual's experience. Furthermore, the factors that influence an individual's perception have been further elucidated as researchers and clinicians have focused on understanding a variety of body image perspectives.

Another complex issue in the conceptualization of body image is that it falls along a continuum between body image disturbance and positive body image. Thus, body image may not fit neatly into one category or another; rather, it is an individualized phenomenon. We know that both personal and external factors contribute to an individual's body image. Furthermore, the absence of body image disturbance may not necessarily mean that an individual has a positive body image. Where an individual falls along the body image continuum in addition to the importance an individual places on issues related to body image may shift as his or her experiences and circumstances change.

Both the way we think about body image generally and how we think about body image specifically in the oncology setting have changed and continue to change. Individuals with cancer may not necessarily experience body image disturbance linked to misperception of body size or shape. Rather, they must adjust to varying degrees of disfigurement as well as physical disability that impacts their day-to-day activities, their interaction with others, and their psychological health. We must now think about body image changes in patients with cancer as an expected outcome for which specific attention must be paid. We no longer think about body image in patients with cancer the same way we do about patients with eating disorders. Body image disturbance in the context of cancer may not be viewed, necessarily, as pathological.

This chapter describes the theoretical foundations of studying and examining body image. We examine both historical and contemporary influences as we review the work of Head, Schilder, Cash, Pruzinsky, Price, Slade, Newell, Dropkin, Rhoten, Fingeret, and White, who have contributed to our theoretical understanding of body image. More specifically, we explore the conceptual shifts that have allowed us to transition from describing the body image of people with cancer using theories developed to describe otherwise healthy adolescents and adults to theories that are tailored and conceptually appropriate for this population and their cancer-related experiences. We begin by examining the history of shifting perspectives of body image conceptualization. Then we discuss the conceptualization of body image within the context of specific types of cancer and cancer as a whole. Key concepts, their definitions, and usage are summarized in Table 2.1. We conclude the chapter by discussing implications for research and practice.

Concept	Definition	Usage
Body schema	Describes the integration of body perceptions; created unconsciously, serving as a frame of reference for body movements and postures	Head (1920)
Body image	Picture of our own body that we form in our mind; composed of conscious and unconscious experiences	Schilder (1950)
	Emphasizes perceptions, thoughts, and feelings about the body and bodily experience; multifaceted; intertwined with feelings about the self; socially determined; transactional; not entirely fixed or static	Cash & Pruzinsky (1990)
	Composed of body reality (the body as it really exists), body ideal (ideal picture in one's head of how one should look and perform), and body presentation (how the body is presented to the outside environment); influenced by self-image (mental picture of how the self is perceived by others) and environment (symbolic, internal, and external)	Price (1990)
	Loose mental representation of the body's shape, form, and size; influenced by history of sensory input to body experience, history of weight change/fluctuation, cultural and social norms, individual attitudes to weight and shape, cognitive and affective variables, individual psychopathology, and biological variables	Slade (1994)
	Multidimensional experience resulting from investment in appearance and the match or mismatch between objective reality and ideal self	White (2000)[a]
	Influenced by historical and developmental influences (cultural socialization, interpersonal experiences, physical characteristics, personality attributes) as well as proximal events and processes (appearance-schematic processing, activating events, internal dialogues, body image emotions, self-regulatory strategies and behaviors)	Cash & Pruzinsky (2002)
	Multifaceted; entails perceptions, thoughts, and feelings about the entire body; determined by importance placed on physical appearance and body integrity	Fingeret (2010)[a]
	Formed via historical implications (demographic, psychological, medical factors), disease/treatment factors (tumor characteristics, cancer treatment, reconstruction), and external evaluation of outcomes	Fingeret (2013)[a]
Body image reintegration	Occurs as individual copes with his or her body alteration through optimizing the use of residual structures and function, restoration of self-expression, and reestablishment of sociality	Dropkin (1989)[a]

(continued)

Concept	Definition	Usage
Body image disturbance	Resulting from avoidance of changed body and appearance	Newell (1999)
	Resulting from disfigurement and alterations in function; influenced by personal, social, and environmental factors; patient acceptance leads to body image reintegration	Rhoten (2013)[a]
	Composed of a self-perception of change in appearance and displeasure with the change or perceived change in appearance, a decline in an area of function, and psychological distress regarding changes in appearance and/or function	Rhoten (2016)[a]

[a] Oncology-focused.

HISTORY OF BODY IMAGE CONCEPTUALIZATION PERSPECTIVES

The conceptualization of body image progressed throughout the 20th and 21st centuries as scientists and philosophers shifted from viewing body image as a function of an individual's psychosomatic development and perception to incorporating the influence of external factors.

HENRY HEAD: NEUROLOGICAL PERSPECTIVE, 1920

The roots of body image research are in clinical neurology and focused on perceptual inaccuracies. Some of the first known body image–related inquiries concerned individuals who had suffered brain damage resulting in a distorted perception of the body. The brain was thought to be central in maintaining a normal pattern of body experience while psychological factors were thought to play a negligible role in any distortion.[3] Studies of individuals focused particularly on which regions and specific structures of the brain were responsible for bodily function and perception.[3] Thus, there was no expectation that an individual's perception of his or her body was a coping response to stress rather than the result of actual brain damage or other neuropathology.[3]

British neurologist Henry Head first used the term "body schema" to describe the integration of body perceptions. Head asserted that body schemas were created unconsciously yet served as a frame of reference for body movements and postures. As an individual moved throughout his or her world, he or she would unconsciously assemble a body schema upon which any new movements or postures would be judged.[3] Body schema was thought to be a pragmatic representation of the body's spatial properties, which included the length of limbs and limb segments, their arrangements, the configuration of the segments in space, and the shape of the body surface.[4–8] Although the term "body schema" became popular, it was unclear exactly how it influenced an individual's judgement of his or her body.[3] This conceptualization of an unconscious body schema formed the basis for future studies of body image.

PAUL SCHLIDER: NEUROLOGICAL & PSYCHOANALYTICAL PERSPECTIVE, 1950

Australian neurologist Paul Schilder was the first to significantly shift the understanding of a neurologically focused "body schema" toward a fluid conceptualization of "body image" that incorporated psychoanalytic and sociological elements. He proposed that both conscious and unconscious experiences in addition to any existing pathological elements influenced an individual's experience of body image. Schilder first used the phrase "body image" in his book *The Image and Appearance of the Human Body* to mean the picture of our own body that we form in our mind, or the way in which the body appears to oneself.[9] He was heavily influenced by a psychoanalytic perspective.[3] Schilder was particularly interested in the misperception of reality and its contribution to the manifestation of body image distortions, and he spent a significant amount of time studying patients with schizophrenia and other psychopathological disorders. He believed that body image was influenced by internal physiological, libidinous, and sociological elements. These elements influenced an individual's perception which ultimately resulted in an individual's body image. Perception of one's own body was thought to be the central part of an individual's body image. This conceptualization of body image allowed scientists to expand their understanding of why an individual might feel hostility toward him- or herself or why someone with an amputated leg might still feel that the leg was present.

CASH AND PRUZINSKY: PSYCHOLOGICAL PERSPECTIVE, 1990

The study of body image received increasing attention in the late 1900s. Psychologists Thomas Cash and Thomas Pruzinsky published an edited book, *Body Images: Development, Deviance, and Change,* in 1990.[10] This work highlighted the multidimensional nature of body image and the need for a multidisciplinary approach to studying of body image, primarily in the context of eating disorders.

Cash and Pruzinsky identified the following seven integrative themes that encompassed a variety of perspectives: (a) body images refer to perceptions, thoughts, and feelings about the body and bodily experience; (b) body images are multifaceted; (c) body image experiences are intertwined with feelings about the self; (d) body images are socially determined; (e) body images are not entirely fixed or static; (f) body images influence information processing; and (g) body images influence behavior.[11] The study of body image began to include not only a perceptual component but also an individualized attitudinal component.

Although the objective appearance of the body was still considered important, an individual's perception of his or her body and subsequent attitudes toward it, particularly its attractiveness and its competence, were thought to significantly influence body image. In addition to body size, body proportionality was also thought to influence the perception of one's body. Cash and Pruzinsky importantly highlighted that body image was transactional within an individual's environment. Perhaps most significantly, the study of body image changed from narrowly viewing body image as a static trait to being more broadly seen as an experiential state that could change over a person's life. Individuals could have differing body image trajectories depending on their personal characteristics, historical experiences, and interactions with the world around them.[11]

PRICE: NURSING PERSPECTIVE—BODY IMAGE CARE MODEL, 1990

Price noticed the increasingly common diagnosis of "altered body image" in the care plans of patients who faced radical surgeries and other disfiguring medical conditions. He developed the Body Image Care Model in response to the apparent need for nurses to engage in body image care for these patients.[12] This model was meant to serve as a reference for nurses in considering the body image needs of patients and to guide the delivery of individualized care.

Price described the following ten assumptions that underpin his model:[12]

1. Human beings possess a dynamic personal image of their body, and this comprises three central components: body reality, body ideal, and body presentation.
2. Change in body image is brought about through a changing environment. The environment is both real/tangible, symbolic, internal and external to the human body.
3. Body image is adjusted regularly in health as well as in illness or injury. This adjustment is a response to puberty, maturation, aging, and other anticipated environmental events.
4. Human beings interact with their environment. Part of this interaction is designed to sustain a satisfying body image.
5. The means by which body image is sustained in the face of a changing environment is through adjustment of the three central body image components, through the use of coping strategies and calling upon a social support network.
6. When the components of body image are satisfactorily balanced, this contributes to a sense of well-being and may be termed body image health. Failure of any one body image component may result in an altered body image.
7. Body image is affected by environment and in turn contributes, either positively or negatively, to personal self-image.
8. Self-image is also negotiated in society, with the individual developing a sense of self-worth. Body image is important in this negotiation.
9. There is an individually determined, limited range of environmental change in which a satisfactory "normal" body image can be sustained. When this is exceeded, altered body image results.

10. In these circumstances the individual will need additional professional nursing care to assist him or her in achieving a state of body image equilibrium. Price asserted that the balance and tension of body reality, body ideal, and body presentation in the context of and interacting with one's coping strategies, social support network, self-image, and environment were necessary to maintain a satisfactory personal body image (Figure 2.1).[12]

Unlike previous theorists, Price provided concrete descriptions of the components of body image and the elements important to caring for an individual's body image. He defined *body reality* as the body as it really exists, constrained by the effects of human genetics and the wear and tear of life in the external environment; malignancies are one source of abrupt change to body reality.[12] Price's definition of *body ideal* was close to Schilder's definition of body image; it is the picture in a person's head of how he or she would like the body to look and to perform. He noted that although body reality rarely meets an individual's standard of body ideal, these two concepts are balanced by an individual's *body presentation*; this is how the body is presented to the outside environment: the way a person dresses, grooms, walks, talks, and chooses to present him- or herself.[12] Price defined social support networks as providing the milieu in which a normal body image is first formed and an altered body image is reintegrated into society. *Self-image* was thought to be the mental picture of how the self, including but encompassing more than the physical body, was perceived by others.[12] Price's *environment* was a four-part concept in this model consisting of the real environment, the symbolic environment, the internal environment, and the external environment.

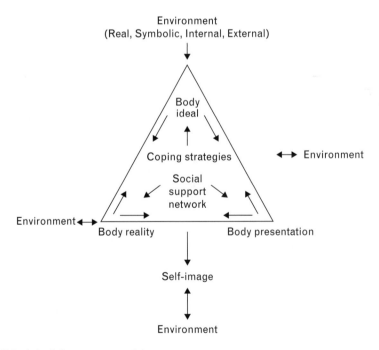

FIGURE 2.1: Price's body image care model.

Price B. A model for body image care. Journal of Advanced Nursing. *1990; 15:585–593. Reprinted by permission.*

The Body Image Care Model was one of the first conceptual models to describe explicit linkages among various aspects of body image and its related concepts. Price addressed malignancies as a possible source of change to body reality and thus suggested that cancer could affect the balance of an individual's body image.

SLADE: CONTEXTUAL PERSPECTIVE, 1994

By now, many scientists and clinicians agreed about the important role of perception in determining an individual's body image. Slade expanded the conceptualization of body image by incorporating, more significantly, an attitudinal component. The assumptions that underpinned Slade's Model of Body Image were (a) people have a mental representation of their bodies which is not fixed but rather takes a finite range; (b) given no particular emotional or attitudinal bias, the average judgement will be in the middle of the range; and (c) given a strong concern about personal body size, individuals will veer toward the outer extremities of the finite range, thus demonstrating body image disturbance.[13]

Slade suggested that body image was a "loose mental representation of the body's shape, form, and size" that is influenced by at least seven factors: (a) history of sensory input to body experience, (b) history of weight change/fluctuation, (c) cultural and social norms, (d) individual attitudes toward weight and shape, (e) cognitive and affective variables, (f) individual psychopathology, and (g) biological variables (Figure 2.2).[13]

This progressive, multidimensional model of body image included not only the influence of individual factors but also the influence of diverse contextual factors on an individual's body image. It explained the influence of individual and sociocultural factors on both the attitudinal and perceptual components of body image. It also encompassed the influence

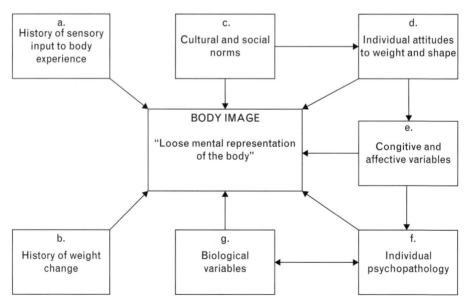

FIGURE 2.2: Slade's model of the factors influencing development and manifestation of body image.

Slade P. What is body image. Behaviour Research and Therapy. *1994;32(5):497–502. Reprinted by permission.*

of media on body image.[14,15] By this point, the study of body image had progressed to encompass factors external to the individual's own mind and experience. The effect of time on an individual and on society was also seen as an important influencer of body image. An individual's experience over time could influence his or her body image. This perspective is important as we move toward thinking about body image in the oncology setting.

NEWELL: FEAR AVOIDANCE PERSPECTIVE, 1999

Until the early 1990s there was little focus given to the body image experiences of disfigured individuals.[16] Most prior conceptual models had been developed based on the pathology of eating disorders. Clinicians and researchers began to take interest in individuals' differing reactions to disfigurement. Research had shown that the degree of disfigurement did not necessarily correspond to the degree of psychological distress or body image disturbance.[17] Newell developed the Fear-Avoidance Model of Psycho-Social Difficulties following Disfigurement.[18] This model was based on a cognitive-behavioral approach to body image disturbance and Lethem's Fear-Avoidance Model of Exaggerated Pain Perception (Figure 2.3).[19,20]

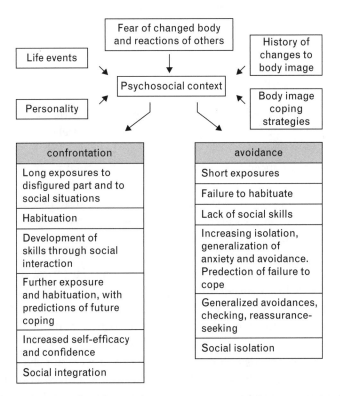

FIGURE 2.3: Newell's fear-avoidance model of psychosocial difficulties following disfigurement.

Newell R. Altered body image: a fear-avoidance model of psycho-social difficulties following disfigurement. Journal of Advanced Nursing. *1999;30(5):1230–1238. Reprinted by permission.*

Newell's model asserted that certain aspects of a person's life created the social context which mediates his or her response along the continuum of confrontation and avoidance: (a) life events, (b) personality, (c) history of changes to body image, (d) body image coping strategies, and (e) fear of changed body and the reaction of others to it.[18] The model suggested that fear was likely to lessen with continued exposure and to increase with avoidance, the reactions of others being held constant.[18] Thus, individuals who avoid their changed appearance will experience body image disturbance while, conversely, those who confront their changed appearance will not have a disturbed body image. Newell describes a progression of behaviors associated with confrontation: (a) long exposure to the disfigured part and to social situations; (b) habituation; (c) development of skills through social interaction; (d) further exposure and habituation, with predictions of future coping; (e) increased self-efficacy and confidence; and (f) social integration.[18] Conversely, other behaviors indicate progressive avoidance: (a) short exposure; (b) Failure to habituate; (c) lack of social skills; (d) increasing isolation, generalization of anxiety and avoidance, predicting failure to cope; (e) generalized avoidance, checking, reassurance-seeking; and (f) social isolation.[18]

In summary, avoiding one's changed appearance leads to social isolation, and confronting one's changed appearance leads to social integration. Newell's model was one of the first to be targeted toward the study of individuals with a changed appearance rather than those with perceptual inaccuracies (e.g., individuals with eating disorders). This model is particularly of use in studying body image in the context of oncology, as many individuals who undergo cancer treatment may notice both temporary and permanent changes to their appearance.

CASH AND PRUZINSKY, 2002

Cash and Pruzinsky published *Body Image: A Handbook of Theory, Research and Clinical Practice* in order to provide for contemporary views and comprehensive coverage of body image with clinical perspectives for practice and constructive ideas for future research.[21] Eight sections covered conceptual foundations, developmental perspectives, assessment, individual and cultural differences, body image disorders, medical contexts, medical and surgical interventions, and psychosocial interventions.[22] They described a variety of conceptual foundations for body image but focused primarily on a cognitive-behavioral view.[23–27]

The contemporary cognitive-behavioral perspective on body image emphasized the role of historical and developmental influences as well as proximal events and processes on an individual's body image investment and evaluation.[24] Historical and developmental influences included cultural socialization, interpersonal experiences, physical characteristics, and personality attributes.[24] Proximal events and processes included appearance-schematic processing, activating events, internal dialogues, body image emotions, and adjustive, self-regulatory strategies and behaviors (Figure 2.4).[24]

Although the specific needs of individuals with cancer were not elucidated in their review of body image conceptualization, this handbook importantly discussed body image in a diverse array of populations and contexts in subsequent chapters. Particularly innovative was its focus on body image in a variety of medical contexts including oncology. The detailed contribution of clinicians and researchers to the study of body image in the oncology

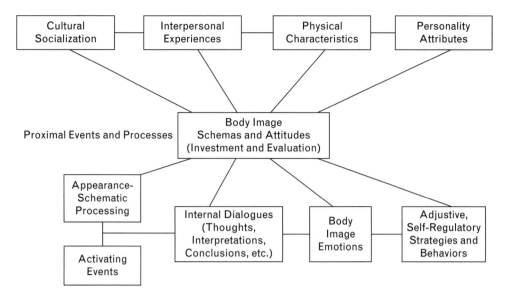

FIGURE 2.4: Cash's cognitive-behavioral model of body image development and experiences.

Cash T. Cognitive-behavioral perspectives on body image. In: Cash T, Pruzinski T, eds. Body Image: A Handbook of Theory, Research, and Clinical Practice. *New York: Guilford Press; 2002: 38–46. Reprinted by permission.*

setting is detailed in a subsequent section of this chapter. Cash and Pruzinsky suggested that body image be conceptualized and studied in ways that transcended eating disorders, and they maintained that weight-related and appearance concerns comprised only a limited portion of the applicability of body image research.[27] They also encouraged the incorporation of "objective" appearance variables other than body mass into research studies.[27] They recommended that future studies examine body image investment as a variable of significant importance. Finally, they recommended a paradigm shift whereby research would recognize the importance of studying the experience of "positive body image" in order to elucidate the role of resilience and protective factors in an individual's body image.[27]

CASH AND SMOLAK, 2012

Cash and Smolak presented an updated handbook with more contemporary consideration of body image. Cash's chapter on the cognitive-behavioral perspective of body image remains largely unchanged from the previous edition, with the exception of the removal of the focus on "schemas." Body image attitude replaced the outdated concept of body image schemas.[28]

Smolak and Cash make several conceptual recommendations in the conclusion of this volume. They suggest that body image theorizing needs to progress toward examining healthy body image and the promoting protective factors.[29] They also propose that body image theorizing focused on appearance should perhaps be shifted toward function, competence, and gender roles, particularly outside the context of disordered eating.[29] These recommendations have significant implications for studying body image specifically in the context of oncology. The following sections review (a) body image theorizing that has occurred in people with specific types of cancer and (b) body image theorizing within the context of cancer as a whole.

CONCEPTUALIZATIONS OF BODY IMAGE WITHIN ONCOLOGY

Cancer and its treatment often causes unwelcome changes in physical appearance and bodily functioning. Although the aforementioned conceptualizations of body image have been useful for understanding the weight-related body image disturbance in the context of disordered eating, it is important to understand the broader role body image plays in the experience of a person who has cancer. While the previous models all emphasize misperception of body size and shape as a key part of body image disturbance, patients with cancer may not have misperceptions. A patient's body may look different than it did prior to cancer treatment, and this potentially disturbing difference is not inherently pathological. Although an individual's body image experience is subjective, it encompasses physical function as well as appearance concerns, particularly for individuals with cancer. Thus, an oncology-specific conceptualization of body image was needed. These oncology-specific models also incorporate the issue of physical function as part of an individual's body image.

CONCEPTUALIZATION OF BODY IMAGE WITHIN SPECIFIC TYPES OF CANCER

Body image specifically in the context of head and neck cancer has been the focus of body image theorizing. This is most likely due to the highly disfiguring nature of treatment and associated physical dysfunction.

DROPKIN, 1989

Dropkin's Model of Body Image Reintegration with Head and Neck Surgery: Coping with Postoperative Disfigurement/Dysfunction was developed in order to allow nurses to predict behaviors that indicated body image reintegration in the postoperative period following head and neck cancer surgery. Body image reintegration was thought to encompass optimizing the use of residual structure and function, restoration of self-expression, and reestablishment of sociality thus indicating that an individual had learned to cope with his or her body alterations after head and neck cancer surgery (Figure 2.5).

Dropkin's model was based on Lazarus and Folkman's Cognitive-Transactional Theory of Stress, in which stress, defined as a surgical procedure resulting in body alteration, was viewed as a dynamic unfolding process rather than a static unitary event that exceeded an individual's coping resources.[30–32] The Dropkin model depicted body image as being influenced by an individual's appraisal of his or her surgical procedure/body alteration.[32]

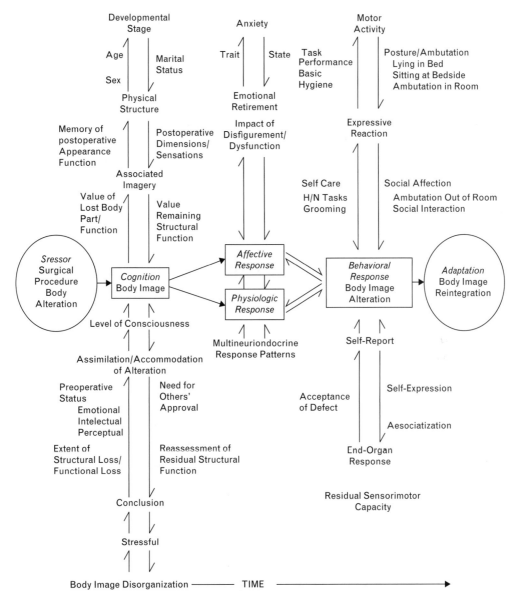

FIGURE 2.5: Dropkin's model of body image reintegration with head and neck surgery: coping with postoperative disfigurement/dysfunction.

Dropkin M. Coping with disfigurement and dysfunction after head and neck cancer surgery: a conceptual framework. Seminars in Oncology Nursing. *1989;5(3):213–219. Reprinted by permission.*

How an individual processed his or her body alteration was influenced by a number of factors including developmental stage, physical structure, associated imagery, level of consciousness, and assimilation/accommodation of alteration.[32] Individuals were thought to have employed both problem-focused and emotion-focused coping in response to head and neck cancer surgery.[32] Problem-focused coping was used in response to situations appraised as being changeable. Emotion-focused coping was used in response to situations appraised as being unchangeable. Evidence of these two types of coping indicated that a person was attempting to progress toward reintegration.[32]

Dropkin focused on postoperative days 4 to 6 as the pivotal period in terms of body image reintegration.[32] Her model specified that performance of self-care tasks, social interaction, and self-report during that critical time period indicated that a person was confronting his or her changed body, adequately coping during the postoperative period, and thus progressing toward the goal of body image reintegration.[32]

RHOTEN, 2013

Although Dropkin's model focused on the immediate postoperative period, patients with head and neck cancer may have body image disturbance long after treatment. In response to the need for conceptualization of body image along the treatment and recovery continuum, Rhoten developed a conceptual framework of body image specific to patients with head and neck cancer.[33] Rhoten and colleagues proposed that head and neck cancer and its treatment results in two main tumor/treatment-related physical effects: (a) disfigurement and (b) alterations in function (dysfunction). The framework demonstrates that patients may have dysfunction and/or disfigurement at any point along the trajectory of their diagnostic and treatment course rather than only postoperatively. Personal, social, and environmental factors were thought to moderate the effect of dysfunction and disfigurement on body image in both a positive and negative direction, depending on the individual. Thus, some patients may accept changes in physical appearance and function over time, leading to "reintegration," while others may not. Rhoten's framework also proposed that body image was not considered static but rather an evolving phenomenon over the course of a patient's life. Body image reintegration was thought to be important for patients with head and neck cancer in order to maximize self-image, social reintegration, and psychological well-being (Figure 2.6).

FINGERET, 2013

Fingeret and colleagues' work enveloped biological, social, and psychosocial factors to show how their complex interactions influenced body image in women undergoing breast reconstruction.[34] They subsequently developed a conceptual framework that illustrated the interactions among and dimensions of important patient-reported outcomes including patient satisfaction, body image, and quality of life. Their work proposed that historical implications (demographic, psychological, and medical factors), disease/treatment factors (tumor characteristics, cancer treatment, and reconstruction), and external evaluation of outcomes (surgeon's view of outcome, significant others' views on outcome, and objective measures of treatment outcome) are essential to the formulation and evolution of body image.[34] Fingeret and colleagues integrated literature from psychology, psychosocial oncology, nursing, public health, plastic surgery, and general medicine to holistically describe these interrelated but distinct concepts in order to guide future research design for this population. Although patient satisfaction, body image, and quality of life

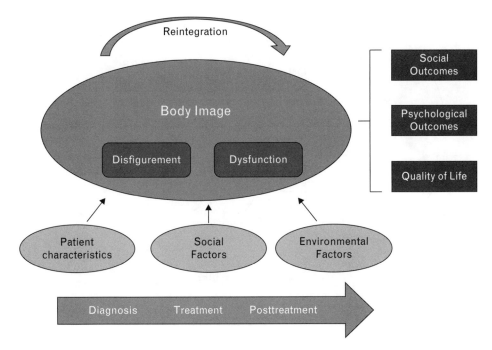

FIGURE 2.6: Rhoten's conceptual framework of body image in head and neck cancer patients.

Rhoten B, Murphy B, Ridner S. Body image in patients with head and neck cancer: a review of the literature. Oral Oncology. *2013;49:753–760. Reprinted by permission.*

overlapped conceptually, each was proposed to contain distinct dimensions. Patient satisfaction dimensions included satisfaction related to breast aesthetics, overall treatment, and the process of care; body image included a patient's perceptions, cognitions, behaviors, and emotions; and quality of life included physical, psychological, social, and sexual well-being.[34] Fingeret and colleagues' conceptualization demonstrates the trend in body image conceptualization toward integration of a more holistic, yet highly applicable view for patients with cancer (Figure 2.7).

BROADER ONCOLOGY-SPECIFIC CONCEPTUALIZATIONS OF BODY IMAGE

WHITE, 2000

White noted that body image problems among cancer patients were inconsistently described and lacked a unified conceptualization.[35] Although many conceptualizations of body image had been useful for understanding the weight-related body image of adolescents and adults in the context of disordered eating, these conceptualizations did not adequately capture the experience of a person with cancer. Cancer-related appearance change had not received the depth of examination given to that of primarily weight-related appearance change.

He noticed that as psychologists began studying body image, an interest in the subjective elements of body image was added to complement the early emphasis on neurological

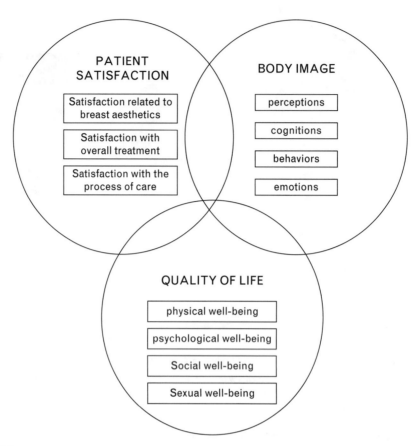

FIGURE 2.7: Fingeret's model of patient satisfaction, body image and quality of life for women undergoing breast reconstruction.

Fingeret M, Nipomnick S, Crosby M, Reece G. Developing a theoretical framework to illustrate associations among patient satisfaction, body image, and quality of life for women undergoing breast reconstruction. Cancer Treatment Reviews, *2013;39(6):673–681. Reprinted by permission.*

and perceptual elements.[35] White felt that a cognitive-behavioral approach to studying body image was particularly appropriate in context of oncology as cognitive-behavioral models were based on the premise that individuals are constantly processing information and that the nature and results of this processing can be used to understand psychological dimensions of human experience. Thus, White drew on the available literature to conceptualize body image through a heuristic cognitive-behavioral model of important body image dimensions (Figure 2.8).[35]

White noted that researchers did not often clearly distinguish the specific dimension of body image they were interested in understanding.[35] First, there may or may not be a congruence between objective reality regarding appearance and the subjective perception of the extent and nature of appearance or cancer-related appearance change (see area 1 on Figure 2.8). Perceived appearance change may be processed in terms of individuals' beliefs about themselves and their appearance. It is proposed that the most important interrelated construct here is the body image schema (area 3) and that the content of this will determine both the degree to which a person has an investment in the changed body

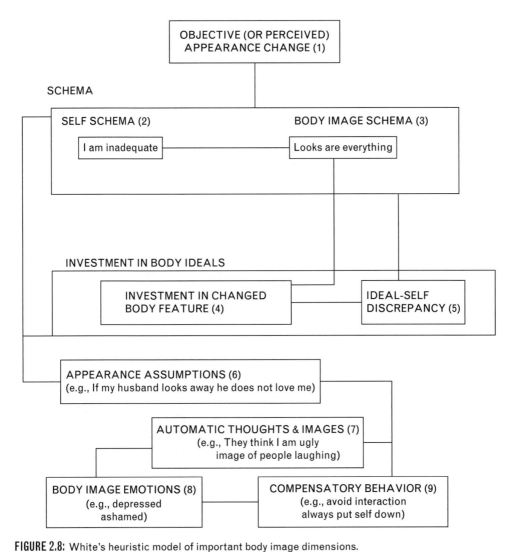

FIGURE 2.8: White's heuristic model of important body image dimensions.

White C. Body image dimensions and cancer: a heuristic cognitive behavioural model. Psycho-Oncology. *2000;9:183–192. Reprinted by permission.*

feature or features (area 4) and the presence of an actual self: ideal self-discrepancy (area 5). The investment in discrete physical attributes is important in determining the nature of the relationship between these components of the model and subsequent information processing. It is assumed that these components (areas 2, 3, 4, and 5) will determine the precise nature of the cross-situational assumptions (area 6), which are important in determining situation-specific automatic thoughts and images (area 7), which in turn determine the predominant emotional consequences (area 8) and compensatory behaviors (area 9). In summary, cancer patients with a perceived or actual appearance change, accompanied by the presence of a threat to their ideal selves (resulting from the content of their self and body image schemata), will experience negative appearance-related assumptions, thoughts, images, emotions, and behaviors if this ideal self-discrepancy relates to a physical attribute in which they have significant personal investment.[35] White advocated for the use of cancer-specific body image models to influence how clinicians and clinical staff referred to patients.[35] He argued that by delineating the multidimensional aspects of body image in the context of cancer, researchers would be better able to conduct research studies.[35]

FINGERET, 2010

Fingeret expanded the conceptualization of body image concerns in the context of cancer by describing them as existing on a continuum ranging from patients who are completely unconcerned about their bodily changes to patients with severe levels of body image concerns.[36] Importantly, at the center of the continuum are patients who experience an average or normative amount of body image concerns. Although individuals at the center of the continuum may experience some difficulties in adjusting to their body image changes, they have realistic expectations for their cosmetic and functional outcomes. This model suggests those who place more importance on their physical appearance and value their body's integrity may experience more struggles related to the perceived or real appearance and functional alterations to their body postprocedure.[36] Because many patients with cancer undergo substantial changes to their bodily aesthetics and functioning, body image disturbance in this population should not be considered pathological.[36] Fingeret emphasizes the limitations of previous oncological research that used overly simplified and conflicting definitions to describe body image. She maintained that body image was a multifaceted construct that entailed the perceptions, thoughts, and feelings about the body as a whole. Thus, it could not be evaluated in its entirety with a solitary approach. Fingeret suggested a method for healthcare providers to address body image changes with patients. This approach focused on healthcare providers ensuring patients that body image changes are common, addressing patient concerns, and recognizing the consequences of body image changes to patients (Figure 2.9).[36]

RHOTEN, 2016

Although most theories of body image focus on both positive and negative influencing factors, Rhoten focused on the negative experience of body image disturbance, specifically in adults with cancer. She was motivated to conduct a concept analysis by the need for a standardized language surrounding body image disturbance in the context of adults with cancer. Her work emphasized the role that cancer and its treatment play in promoting body image disturbance.

Rhoten's concept analysis of body image disturbance in adults treated for cancer identified three defining attributes: (a) a self-perception of change in appearance and displeasure with the change or perceived change in appearance, (b) a decline in an area of function, and (c) psychological distress regarding changes in appearance and/or function.[37] Thus, body image disturbance could manifest itself via depressive symptoms, social anxiety, social avoidance, and social isolation.[37] The presence of one or more of these referents might indicate that an individual needed further body image assessment.

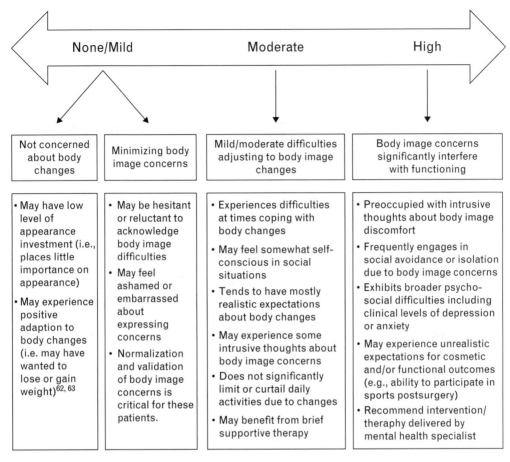

FIGURE 2.9: Fingeret's model of body image concerns among patients with cancer.

Fingeret, M. Body image and disfigurement. In MD Anderson Manual of Psychosocial Oncology. New York, NY: McGraw-Hill; 2010: 271–288. Reprinted with permission.

Through her concept analysis using Walker and Avant's method, Rhoten sought to reduce the conflation of body image disturbance with disfigurement.[37] As previously mentioned, not all individuals who experienced disfigurement would experience body image disturbance. Body image disturbance in patients treated for cancer did not hinge solely on a changed appearance but rather the individual's reaction to perception of a changed appearance and decline in function.[37] Because of varying reactions to a changed appearance and changed level of function, individuals in this population who experienced body image disturbance could become socially isolated from their peers and family members, thus making employment and normal socialization impossible.[37]

IMPLICATIONS FOR RESEARCH

There are numerous implications for scientists aiming to further our understanding of body image in the context of oncology. A primary consideration of undertaking this area of research is the need to approach body image, particularly in the oncology setting, as a multidimensional experience that is influenced by a myriad of internal and external factors. Next, it is important that the study of body image be framed within an oncology-focused conceptualization. Although attitudinal aspects of body image have previously dominated body image conceptualization, it is important to include cancer-specific factors that may influence body image in future conceptual models. As evidence is gathered in a diverse group of oncology populations, it should be integrated into our conceptual understanding of this phenomenon. Conceptualization of body image in the context of oncology should be continually refined as we receive feedback from patients, clinicians, and other scientists.

It has been established that the body image experiences of patients in the oncology setting differ in some respects from the experience of those with disordered eating. In addition to an individual's perception of his or her appearance, functional decline and psychological distress regarding one's appearance must also be considered by researchers. The contribution of these issues to one's overall body image has yet to be thoroughly described or quantified. There are still many gaps in our understanding of cancer-specific issues that may influence body image. Furthermore, different types of cancer and treatment may have varying impacts on body image.

Although we know that disfigurement does not always predict body image disturbance, cancers that cause more disfigurement in addition to functional difficulties may lead to more body image disturbance. It will be important to predict which patients are more likely to experience body image disturbance in conjunction with their cancer diagnosis and treatment trajectory. Another gap in our conceptual understanding of body image in the context of cancer is the timing and trajectory of body image disturbance. By identifying which patients are more likely to experience body image disturbance and when they are most likely to experience it, scientists can develop appropriate and timely targeted interventions.

There is a significant need for conceptually driven oncology-specific intervention development to alleviate and minimize body image disturbance in this population. Although many body image interventions focus on correcting perceptual inaccuracies and reframing one's attitude toward one's body, targeted oncology-specific interventions should also address practical issues that patients experience. Multidimensional interventions should address troublesome social situations patients may face (i.e., someone staring at them in a store). Cancer site-specific strategies for patients to reintegrate their new appearance and function should be included. For example, a patient who undergoes a colectomy may have different functional body image concerns than a patient who undergoes head and neck cancer surgery. In both examples, a patient has undergone cancer treatment that may contribute to body image disturbance. The functional challenges following treatment and the strategies to mitigate their impact on body image, however, may be quite different.

The ultimate goal of body image research in the oncology setting should be to develop novel interventions that help patients adjust to their changed body in such a way that they are able to navigate their feelings about their body and appearance, successfully interact with others, and avoid social isolation. Although patients may not look or feel the way they did before their cancer diagnosis, it is important for them to adjust to their "new" life in a way that does not cause continued harm from their cancer experience.

IMPLICATIONS FOR CLINICAL PRACTICE

A variety of clinical implications stem from this review of the theoretical foundations of body image in the context of cancer. First, clinicians must be aware of how cancer and its treatment can uniquely influence body image. Short- and long-term body image disturbance may be caused by both the physical and emotional experience of cancer and its treatment. Although temporary appearance changes like hair and weight loss may be disturbing, many individuals who complete cancer treatment are left with other long-term appearance and function-related changes that may cause protracted body image disturbance.

It is important to identify individuals who may be more likely to experience body image disturbance in response to their disease. Individuals who have a history of body image problems may be more likely to have body image problems during and after cancer treatment. As researchers identify risk factors for body image disturbance and oncology-specific interventions are developed, it will be important for oncology clinicians to screen their patients for body image disturbance.

Additionally, clinicians need to be aware of how body image disturbance can manifest in this population. Avoidance of social interaction or isolation from pre-cancer social networks may indicate that a patient needs to be evaluated for body image disturbance. Individuals who experience body image disturbance should be referred to specialized providers who can help them navigate this phenomenon and its potentially negative effects. These individuals should receive interventions at the earliest possible time to enhance protective factors against body image disturbance.

REFERENCES

1. Webster's Dictionary Online. Definition of body image. Retrieved from http://www.merriam-webster.com/medical/body+image. Accessed May 2014.

2. Thompson J. *Body Image Disturbance: Assessment and Treatment*. New York: Pergamon Press; 1990.

3. Fisher S. The evolution of psychological concepts about the body. In: Cash T, Pruzinsky T, eds. *Body Images: Development, Deviance, and Change*. New York: Guilford Press; 1990:3–18.

4. Head H. *Studies in Neurology, Vol 2*. London: Oxford University Press; 1920.

5. Haggard P, Wolpert D. Disorders of body schema. In: Haggard P, Wolpert D. *High-Order Motor Disorders: From Neuranatomy and Neurobiology to Clinical Neurology*. London: Oxford University Press; 2005:261–271.

6. Holmes N, Spence C. The body schema and the multisensory representation(s) of peripersonal space. *Cogn Process*. 2004;5(2):94–105.

7. Macaluso E, Maravita A. The representation of space near the body through touch and vision. *Neuropsychologia*. 2010;48(3):782–795.

8. Maravita A, Spence C, Driver J. Multisensory integration and the body schema: close to hand and within reach. *Curr Biol*. 2003;13(13):R531–R539.

9. Schilder P. *The Image and Appearance of the Human Body*. New York: International Universities Press; 1950.

10. Cash T, Pruzinsky T, eds. *Body Images: Development, Deviance, and Change*. New York: Guilford Press; 1990.

11. Pruzinsky T, Cash T. Integrative themes in body-image development, deviance, and change. In: Cash T, Pruzinsky T, eds. *Body Images: Development, Deviance, and Change.* New York: Guilford Press; 1990:337–347.

12. Price B. A model for body-image care. *J Adv Nurs.* 1990;15:585–593.

13. Slade P. What is body image. *Behav Res Therapy.* 1994;32(5):497–502.

14. Hamilton K, Waller G. Media influences on body size estimation in anorexia and bulimia: an experimental study. *Br J Psychiatry.* 1993;162:837–840.

15. Waller G, Hamilton K, Shaw J. Media influences on body size estimation in eating disordered and comparison subjects. *Br Rev Bulimia Anorexia Nervosa.* 1992;6:81–87.

16. MacGregor F. Facial disfigurement: problems and management of social interaction and implications for mental health. *Aesthet Plast Surg.* 1990;14:249–257.

17. Reich J. The surgery of appearance: psychological and related aspects. *Med J Australia.*1969;2:5–13.

18. Newell R. Altered body image: a fear-avoidance model of psycho-social difficulties following disfigurement. *J Adv Nurs.* 1999;30(5):1230–1238.

19. Newell R. Body image disturbance: cognitive-behavioral formulation and intervention. *J Adv Nurs.*1991;16:1400–1405.

20. Lethem J, Slade P, Troup J, Bentley G. Outline of a fear-avoidance model of exaggerated pain perception: I. *Behav Res Therapy.* 1983;21(4):401–408.

21. Grilo C. Book review: Body Image: A Handbook of Theory, Research, and Clinical Practice. *N Engl J Med.* 2003;348:1415–1416.

22. Cash T, Pruzinsky T, eds. *Body Image: A Handbook of Theory, Research, and Clinical Practice.* New York: Guilford Press; 2002.

23. Krueger D. Psychodynamic perspectives on body image. In: Cash T, Pruzinsky T, eds. *Body Image: A Handbook of Theory, Research, and Clinical Practice.* New York: Guilford Press; 2002:30–37.

24. Cash T. Cognitive-behavioral perspectives on body image. In: Cash T, Pruzinsky T, eds. *Body Image: A Handbook of Theory, Research, and Clinical Practice.* New York: Guilford Press; 2002:38–46.

25. Williamson D, Stewart T, White M, York-Crowe E. An information-processing perspective on body image. In: Cash T, Pruzinsky T, eds. *Body Image: A Handbook of Theory, Research, and Clinical Practice.* New York: Guilford Press; 2002:47–54.

26. McKinley N. Feminist perspectives and objectified body consciousness. In: Cash T, Pruzinsky T, eds. *Body Image: A Handbook of Theory, Research, and Clinical Practice.* New York: Guilford Press; 2002:55–62.

27. Cash T, Pruzinsky T. Future challenges for body image theory, research, and clinical practice. In: Cash T, Pruzinsky T, eds. *Body Image: A Handbook of Theory, Research, and Clinical Practice.* New York: Guilford Press; 2002:509–516.

28. Cash T. Cognitive-behavioral perspectives on body image. In: Cash T, Smolak L, eds. *Body Image: A Handbook of Science, Practice, and Prevention,* 2nd ed. New York: Guilford Press; 2012:39–47.

29. Smolak L, Cash T. Future challenges for body image science, practice, and prevention. In: Cash T, Smolak L, eds. *Body Image: A Handbook of Science, Practice, and Prevention,* 2nd ed. New York: Guilford Press; 2012:471–478.

30. Lazarus R. *Psychological Stress and the Coping Process.* New York: McGraw-Hill; 1966.

31. Lazarus R, Folkman S. *Stress, Appraisal and Coping.* New York: Springer; 1984.

32. Dropkin M. Coping with disfigurement and dysfunction after head and neck cancer surgery: a conceptual framework. *Sem Oncol Nurs.* 1989;5(3):213–219.

33. Rhoten B, Murphy B, Ridner S. Body image in patients with head and neck cancer: a review of the literature. *Oral Oncol.* 2013;49:753–760.

34. Fingeret M, Nipomnick S, Crosby M, Reece G. Developing a theoretical framework to illustrate associations among patient satisfaction, body image and quality of life for women undergoing breast reconstruction. *Cancer Treat Rev.* 2013;39(6):673–681.

35. White C. Body image dimensions and cancer: a heuristic cognitive behavioural model. *Psychooncology;* 2000;9:183–192.

36. Fingeret M. Body image and disfigurement. In *MD Anderson Manual of Psychosocial Oncology.* New York: McGraw-Hill; 2010:271–288.

37. Rhoten B. Body image disturbance in adults treated for cancer—a concept analysis. *J Adv Nurs.* 2016;72(5):1001–1011.

CHAPTER 3

BODY IMAGE ASSESSMENT IN THE ONCOLOGY SETTING

*Maria Antonietta Annunziata, Barbara Muzzatti,
and Michelle Cororve Fingeret*

Body image assessment in oncology settings relates to both clinical practice and research. The chapter begins with a historical overview of body image assessment, including a description of key aspects and various perspectives on the construct of body image. Next, we recall the main issues linked to assessment in psychology and general reasons for recommending body image assessment in cancer patients. Tools for assessing body image in adult cancer patients are then described, together with a discussion of their performance in both research and clinical contexts. Assessment of body image in pediatric cancer patients is covered elsewhere in this book (see Chapter 12).

BRIEF HISTORICAL OVERVIEW OF BODY IMAGE ASSESSMENT

Until the 19th century when the study of humanity (including its organic nature, functioning, and health) was fragmented into different sciences and disciplines separated by fields of study with autonomous investigative methods, reflections on the body belonged to philosophy. For instance, in the fourth century BC, Plato wrote that people are bound to their bodies like an oyster to its shell, thus highlighting how the subjective experience is strictly integrated with the body.[1] Merleau-Ponty, in the first half of the 20th century, introduced the "Leib," in opposition to the "Körper" (the Cartesian tradition); the Leib, as a whole body, had its own subjectivity and was placed in the world.[2]

In 1911, Head and Holmes explicitly introduced the theoretical concept of "body schema," which was already present in previous writings.[3] It is made up of two complementary concepts: the "body schema," which is an unconscious representation of the relative position and space of one's body segments, and the "body image," which involves more explicit and conscious knowledge of the external form and morphological characteristics of one's body.[3]

Cash and Smolak[4] retraced the study of body image over the 20th century and the first decade of this century, recognizing some milestones in the evolution of the assessment of this construct. They highlight Schilder's work in 1935 which sought to integrate the concept of body schema by combining a neurological approach with the study of body image, including psychological and sociocultural aspects. They also describe Fisher's work, in the second half of the 20th century, which considered the structure and development of boundaries of body image, as well as its strength and permeability, from a psychodynamic perspective. In the last decade of the 20th century, Cash and Thompson contributed to the delineation of a multidimensional definition of body image, initiated a methodological debate on its measurement and treatment, and enlarged its field of application to include eating disorders, disabilities, and disfigurement. Cash and Smolak[4] define body image as complex and multidimensional. They further argue that it is influenced by gender, ethnicity, culture, and age and is shaped by the state of the body and the state of the mind. They ultimately propose that body image assessment should be multifaceted in nature.

KEY ASPECTS OF BODY IMAGE

In 1999, Thompson et al.[5] argued that body image classification is "tricky," because different aspects of this construct have been described with interchangeable terms that may generate confusion. At that time, over 16 terms were identified as being used to refer to body image (e.g., weight satisfaction, size perception accuracy, body satisfaction, appearance satisfaction, appearance evaluation, appearance orientation, body esteem, body schema, body distortion). Since then, much research has been conducted to further delineate and define unique aspects of body image and to consider ways to approach its investigation.

For the purpose of this chapter, we consider key aspects of body image that relate to individuals being treated in an oncology setting. As such, we look beyond aspects of body image more traditionally investigated in eating disorders such as perceptions of body size/weight and instead direct our attention to body image terminology more directly associated with the experiences of cancer and its treatment.

Although there are undoubtedly other body image terms that can be considered within this context, we believe that the following 12 concepts bear particular relevance to body image assessment in the oncology setting: body image cognitive distortions, body image coping strategies, body image distress/dysphoria, body image disturbance, body image evaluation, body image ideals, body image investment, body image satisfaction/dissatisfaction, body image state, body integrity, body stigma, and body vulnerability. These terms

TABLE 3.1: Key Aspects of Body Image Relevant to the Oncology Setting

Body Image Term	Definition
Body image cognitive distortions	Cognitive biases or distortions in the processing or interpretation of appearance-related information or events central to body image functioning[6]
Body image coping strategies	Cognitive and behavioral activities that persons use to manage threats or challenges to their body image[7]
Body image distress/dysphoria	Involves the degree to which one experiences negative body image emotions in different contexts or activities[8]
Body image disturbance	A wide-ranging construct that encompasses many aspects of negative body image including body image dissatisfaction, distress (or dysphoria), and dysfunction (or impairment)[9]
Body image evaluation	Refers to one's satisfaction or dissatisfaction with his or her body and his or her evaluative beliefs about it[10]
Body image ideals	Involves discrepancies that exist between self-perceived and idealized/desired physical attributes[11]
Body image investment	Beliefs about the importance and influence of one's appearance in life, including the centrality of appearance to one's sense of self[10]
Body image satisfaction/dissatisfaction	The degree to which one is satisfied or dissatisfied with his or her appearance or body shape[5]
Body image state	The personal evaluation of appearance or other aspects of body image in this particular moment of one's life[12]
Body integrity	Investment in the idea that one's worth is depending on his or her body being intact and that compromising the physical integrity of the body results in a decreased sense of self-worth[13]
Body stigma	Feelings of a need to keep the body hidden[14]
Body vulnerability	Feelings of susceptibility of the body to an illness[14]

may not be fully mutually distinct from one another, as in the case of body image distress/dysphoria, body image disturbance, and body image dissatisfaction, although nuances may be present. These terms are further defined in Table 3.1 with their references.

Evaluating body image means, at the outset, deciding which aspect(s) of the body image construct are to be taken into consideration. Among factors that can influence the selection of a body image construct include the degree to which one is interested in assessing cognitions, feelings, and/or behaviors related to body image. One must determine whether the focus of the assessment is to be on the body as a whole or on an individual body part. Further considerations include whether to utilize a situation-specific approach (i.e., focusing on a particular context) versus a general-dispositional approach (broadening the focus to general situations rather than specific contexts), which has implications regarding the use of a generic tool or a disease-specific instrument. The assessment may be focused on evaluating change over time or on the present time point only. In any case, it is important to place the body image evaluation within the broader context of conducting a psychological assessment, which will be further discussed later.

PSYCHOLOGICAL ASSESSMENT: OVERVIEW AND APPLICATIONS IN AN ONCOLOGY SETTING

Psychological assessment is a complex and diverse process that requires a thorough understanding of the means and procedures available, a reasoned and rigorous application of the methods chosen, and a careful interpretation of the results obtained.[15–18] Psychological assessment is a very extensive theoretical field: however, it is useful to know some of its basic principles as well as fundamental problematic issues that can arise. In this section, we offer an overview to introduce the reader to basic topics of psychological assessment (see also Box 3.1).

The first question inherent in the measurement of a psychological construct relates to how the psychological construct of interest is defined and operationalized (as discussed earlier). It is vital to consider that the theoretical model of any given construct influences its recording method. Whether one is evaluating a psychological construct such as "depression," "anxiety," or in this case "body image," knowledge of the literature relating to the construct of interest facilitates decisions regarding how to proceed with assessment.

The second important issue is the purpose of the evaluation process, which can be broadly grouped into two main categories: (a) clinical motivation (e.g., enhancing the body image outcomes [usually individually] of a patient) or (b) research motivation which involves, for example, systematic investigation of a research question to understand or enhance body image outcomes for a specified population. Ultimately, this classification system can serve as a useful criterion for initial selection of the type of tool or approach.

Methodologies for psychological assessment employed in an oncology setting typically include but are not limited to clinical interview, behavioral observation, self-report

---

BOX 3.1 PSYCHOLOGICAL ASSESSMENT PROCESS: THE KEY STEPS

1. Define the psychological construct of interest.
2. Determine the purpose of the evaluation process.
   2.1. Take into consideration user's characteristics, contextual variables, and organizational practices.
   2.2. Know the psychometrics and administering properties of different procedures/tools.
3. Choose the most suitable method/tool.
4. Perform the assessment (consider possible biases).
5. Code, compare (with norms if available), and interpret obtained data.
6. Provide feedback and plan next steps.

questionnaires, or standardized tests (alone or in combination). At the initial stages of the assessment process, contextual variables (e.g., the availability of an adequate setting) must be taken into consideration as well as organizational practices (including time available, economic resources, training/expertise of the evaluator).

Each methodology and tool can be evaluated with respect to validity, reliability and responsiveness[15-18] and are subject to bias, which should not be overlooked. The concepts of validity, reliability, and responsiveness are further defined and described in Table 3.2. It must be considered that beyond the assessment methodology itself, each patient will emit responses that are influenced by unconscious, cognitive, emotional, social, or motivational factors.[19,20] For example, the validity of a patient's responses could be affected by the nature of the stimulus used in the assessment (e.g., length of phrasing, use of negatives) or because of contextual reasons (e.g., a noisy or disturbed setting). High levels of emotional reactivity (e.g., state anxiety[21]), which are likely to be present when a patient has just received a cancer diagnosis, is commencing cancer treatment, or has been told of worsening prognosis, can itself influence a person's responses. Similarly, salient events (personal or collective) can induce responses based on the use of heuristics (representativeness, availability, anchoring, affection) that can compromise responses.[19,20,22] Social desirability (the tendency to respond in such a way as to be socially appropriate and in line with the majority) and acquiescence (the tendency to answer yes to all stimuli regardless of their content) are other possible biases that may affect an assessment.[19,20] Additionally, the motivation (intrinsic or extrinsic; genuine or fraudulent, as in the case in which a person is subjected to a psychological assessment to obtain advantages such as a reduction of workload, or economic or social securities) can also distort the results of an assessment.

TABLE 3.2: Critical Properties of Psychological Assessment Tools

Property	Definition
Validity	
Construct	Determination of the underlying factorial structure of the tool
Convergent	Correspondence of the tool to other already validated measures that assess the same construct
Discriminant	Tool's ability to discriminate between different participants groups
Criterion	Tool's ability to distinguish cases from non-cases
Cross-cultural	Applicability of the tool to other cultural/linguistic contexts
Linguistic equivalence	Establishment of the equivalent value of the tool's version in a language other than the original one
Feasibility	Tool's acceptance by compilers
Proportion of positive responses	Tool's ability to capture the presence of all the aspects of the construct being considered
Reliability	
Internal consistency	Measure of the homogeneity of items composing the tool
Temporal stability	Indication whether the obtained scores remain constant over time
Responsiveness	
Responsiveness	Measure of tool ability in detecting changes

After choosing the most appropriate evaluation methodology, the individual performing the assessment should then choose the assessment tool and adhere to standardized instructions for administration (if applicable). Interpreting the results may involve direct comparison with normative data. This step suggests questioning the comparability of the data obtained with normative data and considering issues of cross-cultural validity. Only if the entire process is followed with awareness and objectivity will it ultimately lead to relevant information from a clinical point of view and/or statistical significance, so as to be informative and functional for the purpose for which the assessment was undertaken.

Within an oncology setting, psychological assessment is warranted from the time a patient is diagnosed. Readers are referred elsewhere for a discussion of broad-based assessment tools to evaluate distress, depression, anxiety, and other aspects of emotional well-being in cancer patients.[23] The remainder of this chapter is more specifically focused on delineating an approach to the assessment of body image issues of cancer patients within both research and clinical contexts.

As described in detail throughout this book, the disease of cancer and its treatments affect the body in various ways, directly or in the form of side effects, including long-term or late side effects. A patient's body image, therefore, may fluctuate throughout the cancer treatment trajectory (from diagnosis to long-term survival or progression) and can be affected by the temporary or permanent nature of body-related changes, the sudden or gradual onset of these changes, or the visibility of changes to the self and others. Body image concerns can also come about due to functional loss, particularly when an organ is tied to sexuality or one's identity/profession (e.g., lesions in the vocal cords in a singer/ performer).

Body image is widely recognized as a critical psychosocial issue for cancer patients, with concerns about appearance and body changes varying based upon clinical features of the disease and side effects of treatment broadly affecting functioning and quality of life (see also Annunziata, Giovannini, & Muzzatti;[24] Fingeret, Teo, & Epner;[25] Rhoten;[26] Paterson, Lengacher, Donovan, Kip, & Tofthagen;[27] Lehmann, Hagedoorn, & Tuinman[28]). Body image concerns can also interfere with the course of disease and treatment, influencing therapeutic adherence and determining therapeutic decisions. A negative body image, as well as the inability to accept bodily changes resulting from disease, can adversely impact social functioning (intimate, interpersonal relationship), general functioning, and quality of life.

BODY IMAGE ASSESSMENT WITHIN A RESEARCH CONTEXT

Next, we provide an overview of tools for evaluating body image concerns of cancer patients that may be of particular value within a research context. These tools are comprised of self-report questionnaires, with published reports of their psychometric properties, that fall into one of three broad categories: (a) disease-specific body image instruments developed for cancer patients, (b) broad-based quality of life instruments used in oncology research that have a body image component, and (c) general body image instruments that have relevance for use with cancer patients.

DISEASE-SPECIFIC BODY IMAGE INSTRUMENTS

Several reviews have been published summarizing the available literature on body image measures developed specifically for use in an oncology setting.[24, 29–31] Between 1993 and 2017, we have witnessed growth, albeit slow, in the development of cancer-specific body image assessment tools. Among the most comprehensive reviews on this topic conducted to date was published in March 2017. Muzzatti and Annunziata[31] performed a computer-based literature search in PubMed, Psychology and Behavioral Sciences Collection, and Scopus databases. The search strategy cross-referenced cancer (or oncology or neoplasm) and body image and assessment (or questionnaire, or scale, or inventory, or measure, or psychometrics). This research was completed by a database search by tool name and a manual search of the reference lists of the selected papers. From the 657 initial records found, 23 papers met the selection criteria referring to eight body image tools, which were extensively described by the authors. Seven of the tools identified were developed specifically for cancer patients.

Table 3.3 provides a brief overview of the seven cancer-specific body image tools identified by Muzzatti and Annunziata[31] for adult cancer patients. Of these tools, the Body Image Scale (BIS)[36] is the most widely used and has the distinct advantage of being brief (10 items) and the only cancer-specific body image tool that is deemed applicable for patients with any cancer site and any form of cancer treatment. Items for the BIS were initially developed within the European Organization for Research and Treatment Center (EORTC) Quality of Life study group and have subsequently been used in numerous multicenter randomized clinical trials for breast cancer patients.[36] The broad-ranging appeal of this instrument is recognized as it has been translated and studied with Portuguese, Korean, Thai, Dutch, Spanish, and Turkish patient populations.

Five of the measures described in Table 3.3 were developed primarily for use with breast cancer patients. These include the Body Image After Breast Cancer Questionnaire (BIBCQ),[14] Body Image and Relationship Scale (BIRS),[33] Breast Impact of Treatment Scale (BITS),[46] Measure of Body Apperception (MBA),[13] and Sexual Adjustment and Body Image Scale (SABIS).[50] These measures vary in length, aspects of body image being assessed, and extent to which psychometric properties have been established. All of these measures have been translated and subsequently evaluated for use with other cultures, thereby further expanding the reach of body image assessment tools. The BIBCQ and BIRS are relatively longer than the other breast cancer body image measures and as such cover a broader array of body image aspects to assess the long-term impact of breast cancer on body image. The BITS conceptualizes body change stress in a similar manner to traumatic-like stress symptoms. As such this instrument assesses for re-experiencing, avoidance, numbing, and arousal symptoms that may arise from breast cancer and/or breast surgeries. The SABIS evaluates sexual functioning in addition to body image and contrasts prior body image and sexual adjustment as compared with postsurgical adjustment to body image and sexuality changes. The MBA is a brief measure that focuses specifically on evaluating body image

TABLE 3.3: Specific Body Image Instruments Developed for Cancer Patients

Name of Instrument	Brief Description	Population	Summary of Tested Psychometric Properties[31]
Body Image After Breast Cancer Questionnaire[14,32]	45 items, evaluates body vulnerability, body stigma, limitations, body concerns, transparency, arm concerns	Breast cancer patients; Chinese version has also been developed	Has established: convergent, discriminant, and cross-cultural validity, internal consistency, and temporal stability
Body Image and Relationship Scale[33–35]	32 items; evaluates attitudes toward appearance, health, physical strength, sexual relationships, and social functioning after treatment	Breast cancer patients; Swedish and Brazilian versions available	Has established: convergent and cross-cultural validity
Body Image Scale[36–44]	10 items; designed to evaluate satisfaction/ dissatisfaction with appearance changes resulting from cancer and its treatment	Considered applicable for patients with any cancer site and any form of cancer therapy; Portuguese, Korean, Thai, Dutch, Spanish, and Turkish versions available	Has established: convergent, discriminant and cross-cultural validity; internal consistency and temporal stability
Body Image Screener for Cancer Reconstruction[45]	4 items; designed as a brief screening tool which can be used as part of routine clinical practice	Cancer patients undergoing reconstructive surgery	Has established criterion validity
Breast Impact of Treatment Scale[46,47]	13 items; evaluates body change stress following breast cancer surgery	Breast cancer patients; Malay version available	Has established: convergent, discriminant, and cross-cultural validity; internal consistency and temporal stability
Measure of Body Apperception[13,48,49]	8 items; evaluates body image investment; concerns about appearance and bodily integrity	Breast cancer patients; Spanish version available; adapted version for head and neck cancer patients available	Has established: convergent and cross-cultural validity; internal consistency
Sexual Adjustment and Body Image Scale[50–52]	14 items; evaluates body image and sexual adjustment; evaluates prior and post body image, prior sexual adjustment, impact on sexual functioning and sexual importance of breasts	Breast cancer patients; Turkish version available; adapted version for patients with gynecological cancers available	Has established: convergent, discriminant, and cross-cultural validity; internal consistency and temporal stability

investment and concerns about bodily integrity. This measure is now being adapted and tested with patient populations other than breast cancer, specifically head and neck cancer patients.[49]

The BICR[45] has undergone limited testing but was designed to be a brief body image screening tool that could be incorporated as part of clinical practice. This four-item measure was developed with cancer patients undergoing reconstructive surgery for the purpose of assisting medical professionals with identifying patients experiencing body image distress who may benefit from a referral for specialized psychosocial care. Items are related to concerns about recent changes to appearance, worry about future appearance changes from reconstructive surgery, time spent thinking about appearance, and time spent avoiding activities due to appearance concerns. This tool has already been administered to patients with an array of cancer types. While this tool has undergone minimal testing, it is the only body image assessment instrument with data on criterion validity available as a cut-off score was able to differentiate patients interested in receiving body image counseling from those who were not interested.

QUALITY OF LIFE INSTRUMENTS WITH A BODY IMAGE COMPONENT

Because body image is a fundamental psychosocial concern for cancer patients, it is unsurprising that quality of life instruments which broadly assess social, emotional, and functional well-being of patients often incorporate items on body image. It is beyond the scope of this chapter to provide a comprehensive overview of quality of life tools used in the oncology setting. However, there are quality of life assessment instruments employed in the oncology setting that have been widely used to study body image as a secondary outcome. The two most prominently used tools, which have both undergone extensive validation, are the FACIT Measurement system and European Organization for Research and Treatment of Cancer Quality of Life Questionnaire (EORTC QOLC-30).

The FACIT measurement system comprises a large range of questionnaires that measure health-related quality of life for people with chronic illnesses.[53] It is designed such that a general measure can be administered to all cancer patients, the Functional Assessment of Cancer Therapy–General, which has core scales of physical well-being, social/family well-being, emotional well-being, and functional well-being. In addition to this general scale; most researchers will also administer a cancer-specific subscale which comprises additional items relevant to that cancer type. It is within these additional items that body image–related content can often be found (e.g., FACT-B for patients with breast cancer, FACT-BI for patients with bladder cancer, FACT-C for patients with colorectal cancer, FACT-HN, for patients with head and neck cancer).

The EORTC QLQ-30[54,55] is an integrated system for assessing health-related quality of life of cancer patients participating in international trials. The EORTC QLQ-30 comprises both multi-item scales and single-item measures capturing functioning, symptoms, and global health status. Similar to the FACIT system, there are modules for different patient populations. It is within these modules that have disease-specific symptoms where body image items are included (i.e., breast cancer module, ovarian cancer module).

Other selected quality of life questionnaires used in the oncology setting that have been studied in relation to body image are the University of Washington–Quality of Life Questionnaire (UW-QOL) and the Breast-Q©. These two instruments focus on evaluating quality of life for specific cancer types, and both have been extensively validated and translated across numerous languages. The UW-QOL has 15 items and is designed to measure health-related quality of life in patients who receive treatment for head and neck cancer.[56] The Breast-Q© is a multiscale, multimodule patient-reported outcome instrument that is designed to measure health-related quality of life and patient satisfaction in women who undergo breast surgery. Within an oncology setting it can be used to quantify the impact of breast conservation therapy as well as breast reconstruction, pre- and postoperatively, on health-related quality of life and patient satisfaction.[5]

GENERAL BODY IMAGE INSTRUMENTS— RELEVANT FOR USE WITH CANCER PATIENTS

In contrast to the limited number of body image instruments developed for cancer patients, there are a wealth of such instruments designed for other patient groups or for the general population that can be of value in an oncology setting. Cash is widely known for his work in developing self-report questionnaires to assess various facets of body image in the general population,[6–11,58–65] and dominates the literature in this arena. His work has fueled others to evaluate these questionnaires with medical populations beyond eating disorders. Moreover, a number of body image instruments have been developed by others, some of which were specifically designed for medical populations. We present 15 body image instruments that relate specifically to the body image concepts discussed in Table 3.1 and have relevance for use in an oncology setting. These instruments are described briefly, and readers are referred elsewhere for further details on associated psychometric properties.[30,58] Table 3.4 provides a list of these body image instruments and the associated body image concepts they assess.

Cash has developed 10 body image instruments that have potential relevance for use in body image oncology research or clinical practice. These include the Appearance Schemas Inventory–Revised, Assessment of Body Image Cognitive Distortions, Body Exposure During Sexual Activities Questionnaire, Body Image Coping Strategies Inventory (BICSI), Body Image Disturbance Questionnaire, Body Image Ideals Questionnaire, Body Image States Scale, Body Image Quality of Life Inventory, Multidimensional Body Self-Relations Questionnaire, Situational Inventory of Body Image Dysphoria (see Table 3.4 for instrument references). Detailed information on these instruments including how to access and purchase them are provided elsewhere.[58]

Among the questionnaires developed by Cash, the Appearance Schemas Inventory–Revised (ASI-R) has been evaluated specifically for use with breast cancer patients. Chua et al.[72] investigated the ASI-R factorial structure by means of both exploratory and confirmatory factor analysis in a sample of breast cancer patients undergoing breast reconstruction to determine the usefulness of the measure with this patient group. They found a different factor structure than reported in the validation study conducted with college students. Their findings suggest the more suitable factor model for breast cancer participants corresponds to

Body Image Instruments Developed by Cash and Colleagues

Body Image Instrument	Body Image Concepts Assessed	Additional Details
Appearance Schemas Inventory–Revised[59]	Body image investment	20 items; evaluates the importance, meaning, and influence of appearance in one's life
Assessment of Body Image Cognitive Distortions[6]	Body image cognitive distortions	18 items; evaluates cognitive errors or distortions related to body image thoughts in different situations
Body Exposure During Sexual Activities Questionnaire[60]	Body image distress/dysphoria	28 items; measure of body image experiences in the specific, situational context of sexual relations
Body Image Coping Strategies Inventory[7]	Body image coping strategies	29 items; assesses appearance fixing, avoidance, positive rational acceptance
Body Image Disturbance Questionnaire[61]	Body image disturbance, body image distress/dysphoria	7 items; assesses appearance-related concerns, preoccupation with these concerns, emotional distress, impairment in social, occupational or role functioning, behavioral avoidance
Body Image Ideals Questionnaire[11]	Body image satisfaction; body image ideals	11 items; measures degree of discrepancy of self-perceived and idealized physical attributes; considers valence or importance of each physical ideal to the person
Body Image States Scale[62]	Body image state, body image evaluation	6 items; measures evaluation and affect about physical appearance at a particular point in time
Body Image Quality of Life Inventory[63]	Body image evaluation	19 items; measures negative to positive impact of body image on various areas of life and psychosocial functioning
Multidimensional Body Self-Relations Questionnaire[64]	Body image satisfaction, body image investment, body image evaluation	69 items; consists of 10 subscales, evaluation and orientation in relation to appearance, fitness, health/illness, weight preoccupation, body area satisfaction
Situational Inventory of Body Image Dysphoria[65]	Body image distress/dysphoria	48 items or 20-item short-form; assesses frequency of negative body image emotions across specific situational contexts

Other Body Image Instruments

Body Image Instrument	Body Image Concepts Assessed	Additional Details
Adapted Satisfaction with Appearance Scale[66]	Body image distress/dysphoria	15 items, assesses subjective body image distress and perceived social impact of body image dissatisfaction; has been adapted for various illnesses

(continued)

Body Esteem Scale[67]	Body image distress/ dysphoria; body image evaluation	35 items; evaluates degree to which one has positive or negative feelings about various parts or aspects of the body; relates to physical conditioning, attractiveness, body strength and weight concerns
Body Satisfaction Scale[68]	Body image satisfaction	16 items; assessing satisfaction with body parts half involving the head, half involving the body
Derriford Appearance Scale[a,69,70]	Body image distress/ dysphoria; body image disturbance	59-item or 24-item forms; evaluates distress and difficulties experienced in living with problems of appearance; developed for medical and nonmedical populations
Fear of Negative Appearance Evaluation Scale[71]	Body image distress/ dysphoria	6 items; assesses apprehension about appearance evaluation by others

[a] Cash, T.F. (2004a). *Body-image assessments: Manuals and questionnaires.* Available from the author's website http://www.body-images.com.

three moderately correlated and reliable factors: appearance self-evaluation (eight items), appearance power/control (five items), and appearance standards and behaviors (seven items).

There are several additional body image instruments, not developed by Cash and colleagues, which merit consideration for use in oncology research or practice. These include the Adapted Satisfaction with Appearance scale, Body Esteem Scale, Body Satisfaction Scale, Derriford Appearance Scale (DAS), and Fear of Negative Appearance Evaluation Scale (see Table 3.4 with references included). The most widely used body image instrument in research on disfigurement of individuals living with visible differences is the DAS. This scale has undergone extensive psychometric evaluation and normative data are available from the UK population. Versions of the DAS are also available in Spanish, French, Swedish, Japanese, and Korean.[73] Work is ongoing on Dutch, Danish, and Portuguese translations. Another scale worth specific mention is the Adapted Satisfaction with Appearance Scale (ASWAP). This body image instrument is of interest as it was initially developed for use with burn survivors, has subsequently been adapted for patients with scleroderma, and has more recently been further evaluated for use with head and neck cancer patients.[74] The ASWAP evaluates non-weight related body image disturbance as well as social discomfort related to changes in appearance caused by illness.

Research Example

In 2016, Teo and colleagues conducted research to delineate salient dimensions of body image concerns in cancer patients preparing for head and neck reconstruction.[74] A sample of 140 patients completed self-report questionnaires evaluating numerous aspects of body image which include body image dissatisfaction, body image disturbance, perceived social impact of body image changes, body image investment, body image coping, head and neck function, and head and neck appearance concerns. Participants were administered the BIS, BIDQ, ASWAP, ASI-R, BICSI, FACT-HN, and Head and Neck Survey.[74] *Using Bayesian nonparametric factor analyses, two fundamental areas of body image concerns emerged: appearance distress and functional difficulties. These findings have important implications for the assessment and treatment of body image distress related to appearance, perceived social consequences of altered appearance, and functional difficulties (i.e., speech and swallowing impairment) as major areas of body image concerns for head and neck cancer patients. These areas all warrant attention as part of clinical assessment for this patient population.*

BODY IMAGE ASSESSMENT WITHIN A CLINICAL CONTEXT

Within a clinical context, the motivation for conducting a body image assessment involves gaining a clear understanding of the nature and extent of a patient's body image concerns and the manner in which these concerns are affecting the functioning of that individual. In this section we review fundamental elements of conducting a clinical assessment and particular considerations for content areas to include within a clinical interview focused on assessing body image in an oncology setting. This is presented alongside a conceptual framework for ways to approach conversations about body image with cancer patients.

FUNDAMENTAL ELEMENTS OF CONDUCTING A CLINICAL ASSESSMENT

A cornerstone of any clinical assessment process involves (a) behavioral observations and (b) the clinical interview. Behavioral observations are a key source of information and refer to outward appearance, actions, gestures, and posture as well as other aspects of verbal or nonverbal behavior that can be discerned during an interaction. Clinicians must generally attend to the patient's mood, affect, quality of thought process, level of eye contact, and attention span. When assessing body image outcomes, however, additional behavioral observations that are of particular relevance include (a) grooming behaviors (Does the patient's appearance/demeanor give off the impression of being highly invested in appearance or alternatively avoiding grooming altogether?) (b) covering/hiding/camouflaging of an appearance defect (Does the patient attempt to conceal a physical defect with bandages or clothing? Is the bandage necessary for healing? Does the patient position his or her body in such a way as to hide or obscure certain body parts from being seen?) (c) noticeable changes to a patient's body functioning and how the patient compensates (Does the patient have altered/impaired speech or hearing, difficulties with gait, partial/complete loss of limb?).

The clinical interview process can be more or less structured depending on the purpose, timing, and setting of the interview. For example, a more formal structured interview process is warranted within the context of a clinical research study or if systematic outcomes are being collected and evaluated as part of a clinical program. A semistructured interview may be more efficient and better suited for hospital or community practice settings to allow for greater flexibility in how the interview is being conducted. Initial focus should be given to obtaining a comprehensive psychosocial history along with a patient's disease/treatment history. Specific inquiry regarding whether the patient has a history of eating disorders and/or cosmetic surgery is warranted considering their relevance to body image functioning. The clinician can then concentrate on assessing the nature and extent of any current body image concerns the patient is experiencing along with concerns about future changes to appearance and/or body functioning. Table 3.5 provides further details on key content areas worth considering when evaluating current and/or future body image concerns. These recommendations are offered based on our clinical experience with this patient population.

A clinical assessment may also be supplemented by the use of self-report questionnaires, which can include body image tools presented in Tables 3.3 and 3.4 along with other assessment tools to evaluate depression, anxiety, or other clinically relevant mental health outcomes.[23] As discussed earlier, the BICR has demonstrated some value for use as a screening tool to facilitate referral for body image counseling. Other body image tools may be used within the context of a clinical assessment to identify specific thought patterns or behaviors in need of intervention (e.g., ABCD, SIBD).

TABLE 3.5: Content Areas for Clinical Assessment of Body Image Outcomes

	Current Body Image Concerns	Concerns about Future Changes
Description of which body part(s) affected	X	X
Description of how body has changed	X	
Expected/unexpected nature of body changes	X	
Expectations for future changes to the body		X
Difficulties with viewing affected body part(s)	X	
Preoccupation with body image changes (time spent thinking about these changes)	X	X
Distress related to body image changes (describe emotions, their intensity)	X	X
Avoidance of activities due to body image concerns (occupational, social, other)	X	X
Grooming behaviors/rituals (or avoidance of grooming)	X	X
Reassurance seeking behaviors related to body image	X	X
Importance/meaning of affected body part(s)	X	X
Concerns about sexuality/intimacy	X	X

APPROACHING CONVERSATIONS ABOUT BODY IMAGE WITH PATIENTS

Fingeret has developed a conceptual framework for approaching conversations about body image in the oncology setting that can serve as a foundation for a clinical assessment. This framework, referred to as *the Three C's*, is described in detail elsewhere[30] and referenced throughout this book. Although the Three C's was developed primarily to facilitate conversations about body image between healthcare professionals and patients during a routine medical encounter, the basic principles of this approach apply to clinicians conducting a thorough body image assessment. The Three C's involves reminding patients that it is very *common* to experience body image difficulties as a result of cancer and its treatment, to inquire in an open-ended manner about the nature and extent of the *concerns* they have about body image, and to further explore the *consequences* or impact of body image concerns on their day-to-day functioning.

We offer some practical suggestions about ways to incorporate the Three C's model within a clinical assessment. If one has specialty training or experience in addressing body image challenges of cancer patients or more generally in the area of psychosocial oncology, it can be useful at the outset of a clinical assessment to identify oneself as a "body image specialist" or a "psychosocial oncology specialist." This important step helps set the stage for the clinical assessment and can initially reduce shame or stigma of seeing a mental health professional. Consider the following introductory scripts for beginning a consultation/assessment session.

> *"Hello Ms. Smith. My name is X and I am a body image specialist. What that means is that I help patients with cancer learn to cope with body image changes they experience as a result of cancer and its treatment. My training and background is in the area of [psychology, psychiatry, social work, nursing], and I provide counseling to patients to help them address concerns about body image and develop greater body image acceptance. It is normal for patients with cancer to experience concerns about changes to their body and appearance. These concerns can arise at any time during cancer treatment. Some patients worry about how their body and appearance will change from the time they are diagnosed with cancer. For other patients, body image difficulties may not arise until they are going through or even after they have completed treatment. This is very common and to be expected. What, if any, concerns are you having about the way your body looks, feels or functions?"*
>
> *OR*
>
> *"Hello, Ms. Smith. My name is X and I am psychosocial oncology specialist. What that means is that I help patients with cancer learn to cope with psychological and social challenges they experience as a result of cancer and its treatment. My training and background is in the area of [psychology, psychiatry, social work, nursing], and I provide counseling to patients and families to help them address emotional concerns they have about their cancer experience. Many patients experience concerns about changes to their body image as a result of cancer and its treatment."*

Beyond the introductory statement and framing one's work as specializing in body image or psychosocial oncology, these sample scripts serve to normalize and validate body image concerns of patients. Normalizing body image concerns is a critical component of this framework to reduce shame, embarrassment, or stigma. The assessment can then proceed to obtain necessary information from the patient regarding the nature and extent of his/her body image concerns.

Case Example: Rebecca

Rebecca, age 38, was recently diagnosed with early stage breast cancer and has plans to undergo a bilateral mastectomy with implant-based reconstruction. She was referred to psychology services because of "her extreme sadness and seeming inconsolability" surrounding her cancer diagnosis. Rebecca arrives to the consultation session appearing stylish in a designer suit and elegant hairstyle. She works as an attorney and travels extensively for her job, representing clients of major corporations. Rebecca explains that she is extremely concerned about future changes to her breasts from surgery. She states that her breasts are her "best feature." She is single and convinced that no man will ever find her attractive again. She is worried about how her clothes will fit her following surgery and is unconvinced she will be able to tolerate looking at the scars on her breast. She noted that she spends several hours a day thinking about or searching for photos on the Internet of breast reconstruction outcomes. She finds many of these photos depressing and traumatic. She is seeking help to identify creams or procedures that may later be used to minimize or eliminate breast scars. Rebecca's initial assessment suggests that she is experiencing considerable body image distress related to her breast cancer and its treatment. It is recommended that she engage in several counseling sessions ahead of surgery to help her with managing her anticipatory anxiety surrounding future body image changes and to help her develop realistic expectations for treatment outcome. Postoperative counseling is also recommended to assist with grieving the loss of her breast, to facilitate initial mirror viewing following surgical treatment, and to help her with body image acceptance following cancer treatment.

Case Example: Tim

Tim, age 59, has recently undergone a left thumb amputation due to sarcoma. He was referred for body image counseling by his treatment team because he is having difficulty adhering to his physical therapy regiment and is making suboptimal progress with his rehabilitation. The patient arrives with a bandage that covers his left thumb area and wraps up over his wrist and partway up his arm. His eye contact is poor and his mood appears depressed and anxious. He explains that he has been unable to view his defect and scars that extend partway up his arm. He keeps this area covered at all times. He indicated that he has isolated himself from his family and avoids leaving his home. He denies suicidal thoughts, indicating that he is very spiritual and believes strongly in God. His body image concerns are considered severe, and it is recommended that intense therapy be provided using gradual exposure to help the patient manage his extreme body image distress.

Case Example: Teresa

Teresa, age 55, has been receiving chemotherapy for several months for a lymphoma. She has previously declined the proposal to talk about her emotional well-being with a member of the treatment team because she "feels calm" and does not feel "the need," but she willingly agrees to participate in screening and multidimensional assessment programs when asked. Thus, during one of her clinic visits, she completes a battery of psychological assessments, which includes the BIS. Her composite score of 18 on this scale is significantly higher than the average score of 13.67 (range 9–17) as found in this patient population.[36]

Teresa is provided with feedback of her assessment results. It is explained to her that having body image concerns is normal and to be expected when undergoing cancer treatment. Her BIS scores indicate that she is experiencing particular struggles with feeling self-conscious about her appearance changes, being dissatisfied with her appearance, and feeling that her body is less whole due to effects of cancer and its treatment. It is believed that it may benefit her greatly to talk with a body image specialist about these concerns. Teresa agrees to be seen by the psychologist on staff for further assessment of these concerns. She feels relieved that she is being offered a supportive space where fears and concerns about her appearance as well as the appeal and functionality of her body can be specifically addressed.

CONCLUSIONS

Over the past three decades, we have seen meaningful growth in measurement tools and approaches to facilitate the assessment of body image within an oncology setting. This includes the development and adaptation of body image measures across different cultures and for disease sites other than breast cancer. As the field proliferates undoubtedly there will be further body image concepts identified and body image instruments introduced. These concepts and tools must be rigorously evaluated to determine their validity and usefulness in clinical practice or research.

Within a clinical context, the sensitive and personal nature of discussing body image for cancer patients cannot be overlooked. Many patients are likely to be reticent to admit their body image concerns because they feel ashamed or guilty for worrying about their appearance when they are undergoing and surviving cancer treatment. They often express embarrassment related to feeling "vain." Much can be done to help normalize and validate these issues for patients, thereby enabling them to feel more comfortable and safe to talk about them.

ACKNOWLEDGMENTS

The authors wish to thank Ms. Anna Vallerugo, MA, for her editorial assistance.

REFERENCES

1. Cioffi F, Luppi G, Vigorelli A, Zanette E, Bianchi A. *Il discorso filosofico—1; L'età antica e medievale* [The philosophical speech—1; the antique and middle age]. Milano-Torino: Pearson Italia; 2011.

2. Cioffi F, Luppi G, Vigorelli A, Bianchi A, O'Brien S. *Il discorso filosofico 3 b—Novecento e oltre* [The philosophical speech—3b; the twenty century and after]. Milano-Torino: Pearson Italia; 2011.

3. Cacciari C, Papagno C. (Eds.). *Psicologia generale e neuroscienze cognitive; Manuale per le professioni medico-sanitarie* [General psychology and cognitive neurosciences; handbook for medical/health professions]. Il Mulino, Bologna; 2006.

4. Cash TF, Smolak L (Eds.). *Body Image: A Handbook of Science, Practice, and Prevention*. New York: Guilford Press; 2011.

5. Thompson JK, Heinberg LJ, Altabe M, Tantleff-Dunn S. *Exacting Beauty: Theory, Assessment, and Treatment of Body Image Disturbance*. Washington, DC: American Psychological Association; 1999.

6. Jakatdar TA, Cash TF, Engle EK. Body-image thought processes: the development and initial validation of the Assessment of Body-Image Cognitive Distortions. *Body Image*. 2006;3:325–333.

7. Cash TF, Santos ME, Williams EF. Coping with body image threats and challenges: validation of the Body Image Coping Strategies Inventory. *J Psychosom Res*. 2005;58:191–199.

8. Cash TF. The Situational Inventory of Body-Image Dysphoria: psychometric evidence and development of a short form. *Int J Eat Disord*. 2002;32(3):362–366.

9. Cash TF, Grasso K. The norms and stability of new measures of the multidimensional body image construct. *Body Image*. 2005;2;199–203.

10. Cash TF. Cognitive-behavioral perspectives on body image. In TF Cash, L Smolak, eds., *Body Image: A Handbook of Science, Practice, and Prevention*. New York: Guilford Press; 2011:39–47.

11. Cash TF, Szymanski ML. The development and validation of the Body-Image Ideals Questionnaire. *J Personality Assess*. 1995;64(3):466–477.

12. Menzel JE, Krawczyk R, Thompson J. Attitudinal assessment of body image for adolescents and adults. In: Cash TF, Smolak L, eds. *Body Image: A Handbook of Science, Practice, and Prevention*. New York: Guilford Press; 2011:154–169.

13. Carver CS, Pozo-Kaderman C, Price AA, et al. Concern about aspects of body image and adjustment to early stage breast cancer. *Psychosom Med*. 1998;60(2):168–174.

14. Baxter NN, Goodwin PJ, Mcleod RS, Dion R, Devins G, Combardier C. Reliability and validity of the Body Image after Breast Cancer Questionnaire. *Breast J*. 2006;12(3):221–232.

15. Kadzin AE. Research Design in Clinical Psychology. New York: Prentice Hall; 1992.

16. McBurney DH, White TL. *Research Methods*. Belmont, CA: Wadsworth; 2007.

17. Muzzatti B. *Salute e qualità della vita; Il benessere globale dell'individuo* [Health and quality of life; The comprehensive well-being of the person]. Rome: Carocci; 2012.

18. LoBiondo-Wood G, Haber H. *Metodologia della ricerca infermieristica* (5th ed.) [Research methods in nursing]. Milano: McGraw-Hill; 2004

19. Zammuner VL. *Tecniche dell'intervista e del questionario* [Techniques for the interview and for the questionnaire]. Bologna: Il Mulino; 1998.

20. Castelli L. *Psicologia sociale cognitiva; Un'introduzione* [Cognitive social psychology: an introduction]. Bari: Laterza; 2004.

21. Spielberger CD. *State-Trait Anxiety Inventory (Form Y)*. Palo Alto, CA: Mind Garden; 1983.

22. Motterlini M, Crupi V. *Decisioni mediche: un punto di vista cognitive* [Medical decisions: a cognitive perspective]. Milano: Raffaello Cortina; 2005.

23. Pirl WF. Instruments in psycho-oncology. In: Holland JC, Breitbart WS, Jacobsen PB, Lederberg MS, Lozalzo MJ, McCorkle R, eds. *Psycho-Oncology*, 2nd ed. New York: Oxford University Press; 2010.

24. Annunziata MA, Giovannini L, Muzzatti B. Assessing the body image: relevance, application and instruments for oncological settings. *Support Care Cancer*. 2012;20(5):901–907.

25. Fingeret MC, Teo I, Epner DE. Managing body image difficulties of adult cancer patients, lessons from available research. *Cancer*. 2014;120(5):633–641.

26. Rhoten BA. Body image disturbance in adults treated for cancer—a concept analysis. *J Advance Nurs*. 2016;72(5):1001–1011.

27. Paterson CL, Lengacher CA, Donovan CA, Kip KA, Tofthagen CS. Body image in younger breast cancer survivors, a systematic review. *Cancer Nurs*. 2016;39:e39–e58.

28. Lehmann V, Hagedoorn M, Tuinman MA. Body image in cancer survivors: a systematic review of case-control studies. *J Cancer Surviv*. 2015;9:339–348.

29. Hopwood P. The assessment of body image in cancer patients. *Eur J Cancer*. 1993;29A(2):276–291

30. Fingeret MC. Body image and disfigurement. In: Anderson MD, ed. *Manual of Psychosocial Oncology*. New York: McGraw-Hill; 2010:271–286.

31. Muzzatti B. Annunziata MA. Body image assessment in oncology: an update review. *Support Care Cancer*. 2017;25(3):1019–1029.

32. Zhang J, Zhu X, Tang L, et al. [Psychometric features of the body image after breast cancer questionnaire-Chinese version in women with breast cancer]. *Zhong Nan Da Xue Xue Bao Yi Xue Ban*. 2014;39(1):73–77.

33. Hormes JM, Lytle LA, Gross CR, Ahmed RL, Troxel AB, Schmitz KH. The Body Image and Relationships Scale: Development and validation of a measure of body image in female breast cancer survivors. *J Clin Oncol*. 2008;26:1269–1274.

34. Larsson YH, Speck R, Schmitz KH, Johansson K, Gyllenstend AL. The Body Image and Relationship Scale: A Swedish translation, cultural adaptation, and reliability and validity testing. *Eur J Physiother*. 2014;14(2):67–75.

35. Vieira EM, dos Santos MA, Santos DB, et al. [Validation of Body Image Relationship Scale for women with breast cancer]. *Rev Bras Ginecol Obstet*. 2015;37(10):473–479. doi: 10.1590/SO100-720320150005354.

36. Hopwood P, Fletcher I, Lee A, Al Ghazal S. A body image scale for use with cancer patients. *Eur J Cancer*. 2001;37:189–197.

37. Moreira H, Silva S, Marques A, Canavarro MC. The Portuguese version of the Body Image Scale (BIS)—psychometric properties in a sample of breast cancer patients. *Eur J Oncol Nurs*. 2010;14(2):111–118.

38. Khang D, Rim HD, Woo J. The Korean version of the Body Image Scale—reliability and validity in a sample of breast cancer patients. *Psychiatry Investig*. 2013;10(1):26–33.

39. Songtish D, Hirunwiwatkul P. Development and validation of the Body Image Scale among Thai breast cancer patients. *J Med Assoc Thai*. 2013;96(Suppl. 1):S30–S39.

40. van Verschuer VM, Vrijland WW, Klem TM. Reliability and validity of the Dutch-translated Body Image Scale. *Qual Life Res*. 2015;24(7):1629–1633.

41. Gómez-Campelo P, Bragado-Álvarez C, Hernández-Lloreda MJ, Sánchez-Bernardos ML. The Spanish version of the Body Image Scale (S-BIS): psychometric properties in a sample of breast and gynaecological cancer patients. *Support Care Cancer*. 2015;23(2):473–481.

42. Karayurt Ö, Edeer AD, Süler G, et al. Psychometric properties of the Body Image Scale in Turkish ostomy patients. *Int J Nurs Knowl*. 2015;26(3):127–134.

43. Whistance RN, Gilbert R, Fayers P, et al. Assessment of body image in patients undergoing surgery for colorectal cancer. *Int J Colorectal Dis*. 2010;25(3):369–374.

44. Stead ML, Fountain J, Napp V, Garry R, Brown JM. Psychometric properties of the Body Image Scale in women with benign gynaecological conditions. *Eur J Obstet Gynecol Reprod Biol*. 2004;114(2):215–220.

45. Fingeret MC, Nipomnick S, Guindani M, Baumann D, Hanasono M, Crosby M. Body image screening for cancer patients undergoing reconstructive surgery. *Psychoonocology*. 2014;23(8):898–905.

46. Frierson GM, Thiel DL, Andersen BL. Body change stress for women with breast cancer: the Breast-Impact of Treatment Scale. *Ann Behav Med*. 2006;32:77–81.

47. Zainal NZ, Shuib N, Bustam AZ, Sabki ZA, Guan NC. Reliability and validity of the Malay Version of the Breast-Impact of Treatment Scale (MVBITS) in breast cancer women undergoing chemotherapy. *Asian Pac J Cancer Prev*. 2013;14(1):463–468.

48. Perczek R, Carver CS, Price AA, Pozo-Kaderman C. Coping, mood, and aspects of personality in Spanish translation and evidence of convergence with English versions. *J Pers Assess*. 2000;74(1):63–87.

49. Jean-Pierre P, Fundakowski C, Perez E, et al. Latent structure and reliability analysis of the measure of body apperception: cross-validation for head and neck cancer patients. *Support Care Cancer.* 2013;21(2):591–598.

50. Dalton EJ, Rasmussen VN, Classen CC, et al. Sexual Adjustment and Body Image Scale (SABIS): a new measure for breast cancer patients. *Breast J.* 2009;15:287–290.

51. Özalp E, Karslıoğlu EH, Aydemir Ö, et al. Validating the Sexual Adjustment and Body Image Scale (SABIS) with breast cancer patients. *Sex Disabil.* 2015;33(2):253–267.

52. Ferguson SE, Urowitz S, Massey C, et al. Confirmatory factor analysis of the Sexual Adjustment and Body Image Scale in women with gynecologic cancer. *Cancer.* 2012;118(12):3095–104.

53. FACIT.org, http://www.facit.org/FACITOrg.

54. EORTC, http://groups.eortc.be/qol/.

55. Aaronson NK, Ahmedzai S, Bergman B, et al. The European Organisation for Research and Treatment of Cancer QLQ-30: A quality of life instrument for use in international clinical trials in oncology. *J Natl Cancer Inst.* 1993;85:365–376.

56. Rodgers SN, Lowe D. The University of Washington Quality of Life Scale. In: Michalos AC, ed. *Encyclopedia of Quality of Life and Well-Being Research.* Amsterdam: Springer Netherlands; 2014:6821–6824.

57. Breast-Q, www.qportfolio.org/breastq; Cohen WA, Mundy LR, Ballard TN, Klassen A, Cano SJ, Browne J, Pusic AL. The Breast-Q in Surgical Research: A review of the literature 2009–2015. *J Plastic Reconstr Aesthet Surg.* 2016;69(2):149–162.

58. Body image assessments, http://www.body-images.com/assessments/

59. Cash TF, Melnyk SE, Hrabosky JI. The assessment of body image investment: an extensive revision of the Appearance Schemas Inventory. *Int J Eat Disord.* 2004;35:305–316.

60. Cash TF, Maikkula CL, Yamamiya Y. "Baring the body in the bedroom": body image, sexual self-schemas, and sexual functioning among college women and men. *Electr J Hum Sex.* 2004; http://www.ejhs.org/volume7/bodyimage.html

61. Cash TF, Phillips KA, Santos MT, Hrabosky JJ. Measuring "negative body image": validation of the Body Image Disturbance Questionnaire in a non-clinical population. *Body Image.* 2004;2:199–203.

62. Cash TF, Fleming EC, Alindogan J, Steadman L, Whitehead A. Beyond body image as a trait: the development and validation of the Body Image States Scale. *Eat Disord.* 2002;10:103–113.

63. Cash TF, Jakatdar TA, Williams EF. The Body-Image Quality of Life Inventory: further validation with college men and women. *Body Image.* 2004;1:279–287.

64. Brown TA, Cash TF, Mikulka PJ. Attitudinal body-image assessment: factor analysis of the Body-Self Relations Questionnaire. *J Personal Assess.* 1990;55:135–144.

65. Cash TF. The Situational Inventory of Body-Image Dysphoria: psychometric evidence and development of a short form. *Int J Eat Disord.* 2002;32:362–366.

66. Heinberg LJ, Kudel I, White B, Kwan A, Medley K, Wigley F, Haythornthwaite J. Assessing body image in patients with systemic sclerosis (scleroderma): validation of the Adapted Satisfaction with Appearance Scale. *Body Image.* 2004;4:79–86.

67. Franzoi SL, Shields SA. The Body Esteem Scale: multidimensional structure and sex differences in a college population. *J Personal Assess.* 1984;48:173–178.

68. Slade PD, Dewey ME, Newton T, Brodie D, Kiemle G. Development and preliminary validation of the Body Satisfaction Scale (BSS). *Psychol Health.* 1990;4:213–220.

69. Carr T, Harris D, James C. The Derriford Appearance Scale (DAS-59): a new scale to measure individual responses to living with problems of appearance. *Br J Health Psychol.* 2000;5:201–215.

70. Carr T, Moss T, Harris D. The DAS24: a short form of the Derriford Appearance Scale DAS59 to measure individual responses to living with problems of appearance. *Br J Health Psychol.* 2005;10(Pt. 2):285–298.

71. Lundgren JD, Anderson DA, Thompson JK. Fear of negative appearance evaluation: development and evaluation of a new construct for risk factor work in the field of eating disorders. *Eat Behav.* 2004;5:75–84.

72. Chua AS, DeSantis SM, Teo I, Fingeret MC. Body image investment in breast cancer patients undergoing reconstruction: taking a closer look at the Appearance Schemas Inventory–Revised. *Body Image.* 2015;13:33–37.

73. Derriford Appearance Scales, http://www.derriford.info/.

74. Teo I, Fronczyk KM, Guindani M, Vannucci M, Ulfers SS, Hanasono MH, Fingeret MC. Salient body image concerns of patients with cancer undergoing head and neck reconstruction. *Head Neck.* 2016;38(7):1035–1042.

INTERVENTIONS TO SUPPORT PATIENTS AFFECTED BY AN ALTERED APPEARANCE

Helena Lewis-Smith, Diana Harcourt, and Alex Clarke

INTRODUCTION

Changes to appearance as a consequence of cancer and its treatment can be a constant re-minder to patients of their diagnosis and an indicator of their condition to other people. These changes may be temporary (such as pallor associated with severe anemia and hair loss during chemotherapy) or persist after treatment (e.g., scarring). Medical and sur-gical advances in recent years have increased the range of treatment options, and, in some instances, procedures that aim to "improve" appearance and restore form and function are now available (e.g., numerous surgical options to recreate a breast shape after mastectomy). However, these developments in treatment are not a panacea for the appearance-related dis-tress that many patients experience. There is, therefore, a need for psychosocial support and body image interventions alongside medical and surgical treatment.

As we have seen previously in this text (see Chapter 7), many individuals who have been diagnosed with cancer find themselves preoccupied by the changes to their appearance and/or functional aspects of their body image because of the challenge to their own identity and the scrutiny and unsolicited interest provoked in other people when appearance changes are visible to them. Often their concerns are dismissed by other people as inconsequential (*"you'll get used to it"*) or the legitimacy of their concerns is challenged (*"just be thankful that the cancer has been successfully treated"*) or they are unaware that effective interventions to support people affected by appearance-related concerns are available. (*"there's nothing we can do about that: it's all up to you now"*). However, over recent years, considerable progress has been made in better understanding how appearance-related concerns and body image issues arise, under what circumstances they can be problematic, and the ways in which psychological intervention can be helpful.

Systematic reviews of interventions to support adults and young people affected by an altered appearance or visible difference of any kind, including those resulting from cancer, have highlighted the dominance of cognitive-behavioral therapy (CBT) and social interaction skills training in this field to date.[1–4] In addition, a systematic review of 24 body image interventions specific to women treated for breast cancer identified 7 that had significantly improved body image either in the short term or at follow-up,[5] several of which centered around physical-activity.[6–8] However, these systematic reviews have all highlighted methodological limitations, including small sample sizes, questionable suitability of control/comparison groups and outcome measures, and limited use of randomized controlled trials (RCTs), which have made it difficult to draw definitive conclusions about the effectiveness of the interventions under consideration.

In this chapter we consider the use of psychosocial approaches to support people whose appearance and/or body image has changed as a result of cancer and reflect on the challenges facing health professionals and researchers who are looking to provide evidence-based care. We also refer to interventions that seek to support patients making decisions about reconstructive surgery that aims to restore their appearance, since these procedures have been referred to as "body image surgery." We have not included physical activity approaches since they are not typically delivered by mental health specialists. Further, some previous evaluative studies have identified possible adverse consequences from physical activity, in relation to injury and worsening of fatigue, both during and following active treatment for cancer.[9,10]

When contemplating how to organize this chapter, we considered a number of viable approaches. Using a biomedical approach would involve considering different types of cancer individually and possible interventions to address the specific psychosocial difficulties associated with each one. This would have the advantage of allowing varying functional difficulties to be considered; it is important to acknowledge that for some diagnoses, such as those affecting the head and neck, changes in appearance are closely allied to changes in function such as speech and eating. However, whilst this biomedical approach would be valid, it would be unduly lengthy and repetitive since many of the appearance-related issues facing cancer patients (e.g., managing other people's reactions to an altered appearance) are common, irrespective of their specific diagnosis. In contrast, a generic approach such as that proposed by the British Psychological Society's Division of Clinical Psychology Faculty for Oncology and Palliative Care recommends that all cancer patients, irrespective of specific diagnosis, could benefit from support and treatment for common issues including anxiety, depression, coping with functional change, uncertainly of prognosis, and treatment decisions.[11] Again, this could be a useful structure, but both of these approaches have been well described elsewhere and would limit the opportunity to focus specifically on altered appearance in depth. Importantly, previous research suggests that targeting risk factors specific to body image is more effective than targeting general stress-vulnerability factors,[12] and the largest study to date of factors and processes predicting adjustment to visible difference[13] also concluded that interventions aimed at appearance-specific constructs will be more effective and beneficial than general psychosocial interventions.

We have therefore chosen to focus this chapter on appearance-specific interventions and to structure it in terms of the stepped care framework developed by members of the Centre for Appearance Research (CAR) at the University of the West of England, Bristol, in the UK.[14] Figure 4.1 illustrates the CAR framework, edited to demonstrate both generic and cancer-specific interventions. Stepped care models such as this, where interventions become more intense as one moves up the framework, are common in other areas including support for depression or eating disorders (Bower & Gilbody, 2005). The UK's National Institute of Clinical Excellence (NICE) offers stepped care models for mental health, such as general anxiety disorder or panic disorders, with all suspected presentations of the condition at step 1 (with recommended interventions at this level including information and assessment), through levels of ascending severity to the most severe presentations at level 4 (highly specialized interventions). NICE guidelines propose that an individual start at the lowest step possible (with the least intrusive interventions) and progress through each step sequentially, if needed. In contrast, the CAR framework suggests that people may begin at any level on the pyramid and move fluidly through the other levels as required.

Whilst an established framework such as the NICE stepped care model could have been used in the current context, we recognize the benefits of a more targeted, appearance-specific approach and therefore use the CAR framework to illustrate a range of appearance-specific interventions deemed suitable for a variety of cancer diagnoses, highlighting whether these are cancer-specific or for people with visible differences more broadly. We believe this framework will be a useful starting point for clinicians working with cancer patients, since it considers the differing needs of individuals with appearance concerns.

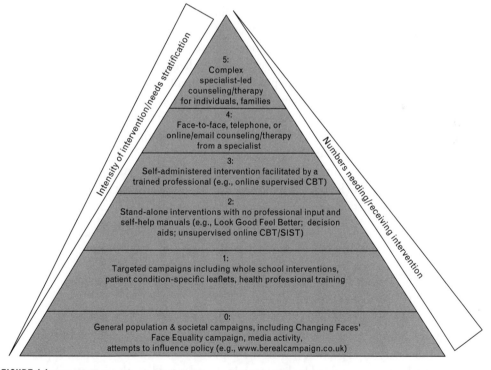

FIGURE 4.1: The CAR framework of appearance-related interventions.

From Rumsey N, Harcourt D. Where do we go from here? In: Rumsey N, Harcourt D, eds. The Oxford Handbook of the Psychology of Appearance. *Oxford: Oxford University Press, 2012: 679.*

THE CAR FRAMEWORK OF APPEARANCE-RELATED INTERVENTIONS

The CAR framework is a stepped model of care summarizing interventions for populations of people experiencing distress due to an altered appearance or visible difference of any kind. In other words, it is not cancer-specific. It is worth stressing that our use of this framework does not imply that everyone who experiences an altered appearance as a result of cancer will require all the interventions at every level of the framework; some people are not unduly worried by the changes to how they look and may see these as a manageable "price to be paid" for treatment of their cancer. In other words, people with low appearance investment, and those considered to demonstrate positive growth from the experience, may not be particularly troubled or distressed by changes to their appearance.

The triangular shape of the framework is a useful descriptor since the numbers of people represented is smaller at the apex whilst the expertise and training of those delivering the interventions here is greater (i.e., far fewer people are likely to require specialist one-to-one interventions delivered by a highly trained psychosocial specialist [level 5] compared with the numbers who could benefit from targeted information available in clinics [level 1]). Level 0 interventions in the framework are intended to inform the general population. Level 1 interventions are targeted to a specific patient group; such interventions can be useful for patients with lower levels of appearance distress and may offer benefits more broadly to a given population. Interventions at levels 2 and above are designed for those who experience body image distress or worry or ruminate about their altered looks and body image and whose day-to-day lives are negatively impacted as a result (the psychosocial impact of an altered appearance is considered at length in Chapter 7). This framework can be used to summarize ways of supporting people to overcome challenges associated with appearance and body image issues and to promote positive adjustment, acceptance by others, and diversity of appearance. Social interaction skills and CBT are evident at all levels, and whilst there is good evidence for the effectiveness of these generally and specifically with people experiencing body image distress,[1,15–17] large-scale trials comparing different approaches in an oncology setting are still needed.

We next consider interventions at each level of the CAR framework, starting with the most general, lowest level (level 0) and moving up the triangle to the most intense, which warrant specialist support for patients with complex needs.

LEVEL 0—GENERAL POPULATION AND SOCIETAL CAMPAIGNS

Societal interventions (level 0 on the framework) aim to promote understanding and acceptance of diversity in appearance, with the expectation that people whose appearance has altered might be less troubled by how they look and would receive less attention about it from others if society was more accepting and placed less importance on appearance and idealized images of beauty. Both traditional (TV, press, radio) and social media have a significant role to play at this level. The depiction in the media and elsewhere of people who have been diagnosed with and treated for cancer often involves images that rely on visible changes to appearance (typically hair loss) in order to indicate the presence of the disease, but this can raise some dilemmas. For example, charities that seek to support people affected by cancer and/or fund research in this field often use images of women and young people with chemotherapy-induced alopecia when seeking to raise funds for their cause. Whilst this may prove financially fruitful, some may argue that such images can also reinforce the view that an altered appearance due to cancer treatment is a fundamentally negative experience and an indicator of a person's diagnosis. This might be the case for many patients, yet many others manage the challenge of hair loss and other appearance changes very well and resent being identified and labeled by virtue of their appearance.

The UK charity Changing Faces campaigns to promote acceptance of diversity of appearance and to challenge negative attitudes toward people who look in any way different from "the norm." The charity's activities aimed at the general public are examples of level 0 interventions. For example, campaigns that have involved posters displayed on the London underground included a woman who had acquired a facial disfigurement as a result of cancer treatment, alongside text that encouraged the viewer to treat her in same way as they would any other person (e.g., the message read *"I know you're dying to ask what happened to me, but don't make it your first question . . . You'll also realise, like all my friends do, that once you've got to know me, you won't see my disfigurement anymore"*) with the aim of changing attitudes and promoting positive acceptance rather than stigmatizing behaviors such as avoidance. These posters were particularly powerful since they were displayed where there would usually be adverts for beauty products and clothing, with digitally enhanced images that could be heralded as examples of the unattainable beauty ideals typically promoted by the media. These idealized images will never be achievable for most people, including those whose appearance has shifted even further from these ideals because of the impact of cancer treatment. More recently, the charity's "Face Equality" campaign has aimed to work with the media to try to inform the public about, and change negative attitudes toward, people with a visible difference of any sort.[18]

Breast Cancer Care, the largest UK-based charity specifically set up to support people affected by the disease, ran a body image campaign which included a video of women talking about their experiences of body image after breast cancer.[19] This resource, available through the charity's website (www.breastcancercare.org.uk/body), is a level 0 intervention since it can influence the general public's views and understanding of the impact of appearance changes for those affected.

Social activism campaigns, defined as intentional actions aiming to bring about social change, are further examples of level 0 interventions. These often employ social media as a powerful tool to deliver and promote messages and change. For example, in 2014, images of an Australian woman, Beth Whaanga, made international headlines for revealing the impact that hysterectomy, mastectomy, and breast reconstruction scars, as well as weight changes and hair loss, had had on her body since she was diagnosed with breast cancer. The reactions and comments about these images were both positive and negative, with some people expressing their discomfort with seeing changes to appearance that were being graphically revealed but are usually hidden from public view. The subsequent campaign (https://www.facebook.com/underthereddress) aims to achieve respect for people with cancer, awareness of what they are going through, and positive body image amongst those affected, under the slogan *"scars aren't ugly, they mean you're alive."*

Whilst interventions at level 0 can aim to change societal attitudes, evaluating their impact and effectiveness can be challenging and many have not been the focus of rigorous research. This is needed, to ensure that there are no unexpected consequences of these interventions. For example, a small focus group study of reactions to some of the Changing Faces posters found that some people felt they were being somewhat accused of negative attitudes and behaviors that they did not consider themselves to have.[20]

There is clearly a place for interventions at the general population/societal level, but even if they were to change some people's attitudes, they would be unlikely to remedy all the concerns that cancer patients have. Interventions offering support at an individual or patient group level are still needed.

LEVEL 1—INFORMATION PROVISION THROUGH TARGETED CAMPAIGNS

Interventions at this level are targeted toward specific populations (such as patient groups) rather than particular individuals on the basis of their specific assessed need. These should be easy for patients to access and for health professionals to provide or direct patients toward and may be sufficient for patients who have a low level of need. Examples of interventions at this level include condition-specific leaflets and websites providing information, advice, and techniques. However, like any intervention involving information provision, it is important that they are reviewed regularly and kept up-to-date.

At this level, it is relevant to incorporate support for body image and appearance changes as part of routine care for all cancer patients and encouraging an ethos of care in which these are given the recognition they deserve. This includes ways of identifying those in need of support (considered later in this chapter), providing presurgical information about how appearance or functioning might be altered by treatment, and ensuring that all patients are prepared for significant events such as seeing the results of surgery that has changed how they look, rather than letting this occur in an ad hoc, unsupported manner. However, despite the number and variety of resources at this level, there is a lack of evidence to support their effectiveness in reducing patients' appearance-related distress.

Online resources offering easy access to other patients' experiences fit this category of intervention. In some instances, patients' experiences are the primary focus of the resource. For example, the website Healthtalk Online provides information about a range of health issues through videos and audio recordings of people's real-life experiences, including those associated with changes to appearance due to different types of cancer and treatment (http://www.healthtalk.org/peoples-experiences/cancer). Elsewhere they are included as a single component within broader resources, such as those aiming to support patients through treatment decision-making. For example, the online breast reconstruction decision aid BRECONDA[21] includes video clips of women talking about how they made their choice about surgery. Research has examined both the benefits and possible negative impact on patients of hearing about other people's first-hand experiences and of contributing experiences themselves.[22] For example, patients may find valuable information which can serve to alleviate fears and inform treatment decisions and coping strategies. However, if the experiences are biased, inaccurate, or atypical, the information may be distorted and potentially lead to patients making worse decisions. Similarly, whilst hearing about others' experiences and contributing their own can help patients feel connected to and supported by others who are facing similar difficulties, this may also evoke feelings of anxiety or despair, or perhaps even guilt or inadequacy if others appear to be coping better.

Web-based resources provided by cancer charities also offer self-help psycho-educational material concerning treatment-related appearance changes. UK-based Macmillan Cancer Support provides information and practical advice regarding cancer treatment and camouflage, in addition to psychological strategies to help manage appearance-related anxiety, unhelpful thinking, and the reactions of others. Similarly, Breast Cancer Care (www.breastcancercare.org.uk) provides a downloadable "Moving Forward" pack containing information on a wide range of issues which may arise following treatment. It includes three pages specifically addressing body image concerns and signposting women to other parts of the pack which discuss the use of a prosthesis and clothing. While these online self-help sources of psycho-educational body image guidance may be helpful, to our knowledge, neither have undergone rigorous evaluation. Regarding similar interventions for other cancer groups, a pilot test was conducted of a psychoeducational booklet for patients undergoing treatment for oral cancer.[23] A multidisciplinary group of health professionals developed the booklet, which was reviewed by patients themselves before pilot testing. It contained information about the cancer and treatment, in addition to effective coping strategies, including ways to help manage appearance concerns, particularly when in social situations. The booklet was found to be acceptable, and significant improvements in body image were identified among the intervention group three months later compared with a control group.

Activities and resources aimed at targeting an entire school system, rather than at patient groups, are further examples of interventions at this level. For example, young people who are treated for cancer are likely to be away from school for a considerable period of time. Returning to school can be a worrying time, particularly for those whose appearance has altered considerably as a result of the treatment they have undergone. This can be particularly difficult for those in adolescence, a time in life where appearance is typically very (if not *the most*) important issue for young people.[24] Advising all staff at the school (including, e.g., catering staff, school nurses, caretakers, and not only the child's teacher) on how to support the child appropriately, how to respond to other children's questions, how to deal with bullying and teasing, and how to facilitate students' successful reintegration without drawing further attention to their altered appearance or reinforce negative stereotypes are examples of whole school, level 1 interventions (see, e.g., the resources for use in primary and secondary schools available through the charity Changing Faces https://www.changingfaces.org.uk/resources/education). Alongside these whole school interventions, re-entry programs that support young people who have undergone treatment in developing skills to help them deal with the questions and attention they may attract when they return to school[25] could be useful in this instance. This example of a level 1 and higher level intervention being used in combination to support a young person both individually and by educating and supporting those around him or her is an interesting illustration of the need to consider the impact of cancer on body image from a range of perspectives and in terms of a mixed economy of intervention. However, the limited research demonstrating effectiveness of interventions at this level has been highlighted previously.[12,26]

LEVEL 2—SELF-ADMINISTERED INTERVENTIONS WITHOUT SPECIALIST INPUT

Level 2 on the CAR framework includes stand-alone, self-administered interventions that do not involve "specialist" (i.e., a fully trained, highly skilled practitioner working across the whole area of body image) input in their delivery. Interventions at this level target individuals for whom brief psycho-educational material will not suffice but who are not in need of individualized intervention to address their body image concerns. Such individuals may require support in form of support groups led by other patients that are educational or supportive in nature or self-help manuals, such as *The Body Image Workbook*,[27] which are written by specialists but are self-administered. Whilst potentially helpful, interventions of this nature do not tend to be evaluated for their effects.

Other interventions at this level which have undergone evaluation include behavioral camouflage-based interventions. Many patients who have lost, or fear losing, their hair during chemotherapy choose to wear a wig in an attempt to restore their "normal" appearance and sense of self,[28] avoid the reactions of other people, and save themselves and others any awkwardness or discomfort about their appearance. Interventions aiming to support patients affected by hair loss, for example through workshops delivering advice and techniques on using makeup, wigs, hats, and headscarves, are widely available and therefore often easily accessible for many patients. For example, the Look Good Feel Better intervention (www.lookgoodfeelbetter.org) aims to improve self-esteem and quality of life of people undergoing cancer treatment. Workshops are delivered by beauty professionals who volunteer to teach small groups of people how to use makeup, wigs, and skin and nail products in an attempt to disguise any changes to appearance (including the loss of eyelashes and eyebrows) to improve how they feel about their appearance and reduce feelings of stigmatization. A significant improvement in self-image, social interaction, and anxiety was reported after attending a single workshop[29] but was no longer evident two weeks later. Further, an intervention which taught a sample of patients with oral cancer (over 90% of which were men) to apply camouflage makeup was found to improve satisfaction with two items on the Body Areas Satisfaction Scale (the face and body weight) three months later.[30] Similarly, HeadStrong is a volunteer-led service provided by Breast Cancer Care in the UK offering advice on scalp care and the use of hats and headscarves to disguise hair loss as an alternative to wigs. A small qualitative study found that women valued the opportunity to learn a range of techniques to cover their alopecia and described the sessions as being helpful but not necessarily meeting all their needs.[31] In particular, they still felt a need for emotional support to help them manage their feelings about hair loss.

Methods such as these that rely on camouflage-based techniques can be useful additions to a varied toolbox of interventions for any patient, so that patients can feel confident in using an array of strategies depending on the particular circumstances and issues they are facing. However, camouflage-based approaches can become problematic if a person is overreliant on them to the extent that he or she is unable to continue with normal day-to-day activities without them. Furthermore, relying on covering up or disguising changes to appearance means that an individual is faced with the challenge of how and when to "reveal" his or her altered appearance, which may become a particularly stressful issue, for example in the context of establishing new intimate relationships.

Recently, researchers explored the use of an expressive writing exercise (a widely used therapeutic approach with a long track record of effectiveness with other patient and non-patient groups), incorporating principles of mindfulness (which has been shown in previous studies to benefit people with body image concerns) and compassion-focused therapy (including self-kindness, mindful awareness, and a sense of common humanity) as an intervention for women treated for breast cancer.[32] The authors reported improved body image attitudes amongst women who were given self-compassionate–focused prompts to write about their thoughts and feelings about their bodies, compared with those who wrote about their bodies without any structured guidance. This study shows the potential for an easily accessible, self-administered paper-based intervention of this sort, which could be adapted for testing with other cancer patient groups.

LEVEL 3—SELF-ADMINISTERED INTERVENTIONS FACILITATED BY A TRAINED PROFESSIONAL

Interventions categorized as level 3 involve the input of a trained professional (i.e., health professionals from differing backgrounds who have mental health training), alongside self-administered support, and can be delivered one-to-one or in a group format. Interventions at level 3 target patients who experience a degree of body image concerns which cannot be addressed by behavioral camouflage approaches or self-help materials alone but who do not require the support of a fully trained practitioner with expertise in body image issues.

As one example of a level 3 intervention, a two-day social interaction skills workshop for people with a variety of visible differences was shown to improve self-reports of social avoidance and distress and confidence in meeting strangers and new people. Participants exchanged and practiced ideas for managing common experiences such as staring and negative comments, planned a series of graded exposure tasks, and shared progress at a follow up session (for more detail see Robinson et al.).[17] These improvements were sustained at six-week and six-month follow-up. This study included participants with visible differences that were a result of cancer treatment, although the small sample size precluded an analysis of the benefits of the intervention for different patient groups, and the lack of a control group is a further limitation. However, the significance of this study should not be overlooked since it informed the development and evaluation of future interventions in this field. Similarly, a specialist nurse-delivered social rehabilitation program for head and neck cancer patients was found to decrease social embarrassment and consequently improve social functioning.[33] However, this study was limited by its small sample and absence of a control group.

Further examples of level 3 interventions aimed at women with breast cancer include a nurse-led informational and emotional consultation, evaluated in a controlled study.[34] The intervention comprised a two-hour face-to-face session preoperatively, followed by another session over the telephone three days after surgery. The consultation provided information and support relating to the disease, the treatment and prognosis, and appearance changes following surgery. No significant improvements in body image were reported immediately, but delayed positive effects were seen at two-month follow-up, whereby women felt less self-conscious, more feminine and sexually attractive, and less dissatisfied with their body, appearance, and scarring. Furthermore, a RCT evaluated an eight-week group intervention covering topics including body image, relationships, and sexuality, delivered by a variety of expert health professionals.[35] Positive effects on body image were seen at both postintervention and six-month follow-up. In the UK, the charity Breast Cancer Care currently offers a four-week half-day course as part of its "Moving Forward" program. Delivered by a range of experts, it provides information, support, and guidance on topics including healthy eating, exercise, cancer fatigue, menopausal symptoms, lymphedema, and intimacy and relationships in order to help women adjust to life following completion of active treatment. Body image is explored briefly during the last topic. A noncontrolled two-year evaluation demonstrated improvements across several domains, including confidence and reassurance.[36] Despite these promising findings, a greater focus on body image than what is currently provided in the "Moving Forward" course may be needed.

Patients undergoing cancer treatment often face difficult treatment decisions that can affect their body image. The PEGASUS intervention provides an example of a level 3 intervention to facilitate decision-making about breast reconstruction after mastectomy. This intervention uses a one-to-one goal-focused approach to help trained professionals (coaches) support women in clarifying their expectations and priorities about surgery ahead of a consultation in which the decision about treatment is made as a shared endeavor between the patient and surgical team.[37] This approach has been well received by clinicians and women contemplating breast reconstruction,[37] and the effectiveness of the intervention in terms of patient satisfaction with decision-making and the outcome of surgery, as well as body image, will be determined when ongoing trials are complete.

Amongst the challenges in delivering any face-to-face intervention that involves an element of professional input are the cost and time involved for both the therapist and patient. An additional challenge when providing support for people with cancer who are reporting social anxiety as a result of appearance-related concerns is that traveling to appointments and/or taking part in a group intervention could raise anxieties around being the focus of other people's attention and meeting strangers. Furthermore, some cancer patients find it difficult to seek support and take part in interventions that are provided in settings they associate with their diagnosis and treatment. Researchers have therefore explored the possibility of providing interventions at this level in ways that are more convenient for patients and do not involve face-to-face contact. This work has tended to revolve around the development of online interventions, offering the ability to access interventions at a time and place that suits each individual. However, it is imperative that any new type or mode of delivering an intervention is rigorously tested to ensure it is both acceptable and feasible to deliver support this way.

To date, online interventions have usually been based on a CBT model and are proving to be both acceptable to users and effective in generating and maintaining change. For example, the online Face IT program specifically supports adults with an altered or unusual appearance of any kind.[38] It is based on a CBT model used for face-to-face interventions and comprises eight modules, including sessions on body image anxiety, graded exposure, social skills training, and self-monitoring of outcome. Initially, a health professional was on hand when Face IT was being used in a clinic setting, to help with any technical problems should they arise and clarify any issues raised in the program that were not clear. However, users (including those who were unfamiliar with using computers prior to the study) reported high levels of acceptability. Data of effectiveness was determined by a randomized trial comparing Face IT users with a group receiving normal therapy.[38] The sample included adults with a range of disfigurements, including some with cancer. Both the intervention and control groups showed considerable reduction in anxiety and increased confidence in their own ability to manage their condition. Most importantly, changes in the intervention condition at six months were not only maintained but increased, suggesting that people continued to use and benefit from the skills and approaches they had learned. Notably, Face IT compared favorably with the face-to-face approach delivered by highly trained health professionals, demonstrating that some interventions might be delivered in a more cost-effective yet still appropriate manner. This program has since been further modified for remote use (http://www.faceitonline.org.uk).

The success of Face IT for adults led to interest in its possible use with young people. Health professionals and young people aged 12 to 17 years with a range of visible differences welcomed the prospect of an online intervention specifically to support those whose lives were being negatively affected by anxiety associated with their appearance.[39] However, the program needed to be adapted to meet the specific needs of a younger population and to make it appealing and engaging for them. The subsequent intervention (YP Face IT—www.ypfaceit.co.uk) consists of seven weekly interactive sessions aiming to reduce appearance-related difficulties through advice and by teaching coping skills based on CBT and social skills training. Initial feasibility work has reported very positive feedback from young people, their parents, and health professionals alike,[40] but, at the time of writing, a full randomized trial to evaluate it against treatment as usual is still needed.

EXAMPLE OF A LEVEL 3 INTERVENTION

Tim lost an eye as part of his treatment for cancer as a child. He was settled into a small community where most people knew him, and he experienced few difficulties until he went to a university in a large city. At this stage he felt shy and unused to people staring at him. His fear of negative evaluation increased to the point that he found it easier not to socialize and became isolated. Completing the online Face IT program (discussed earlier) allowed him to consider other explanations for people's responses to him and to challenge his belief that they thought him "odd." Approach strategies based on good social skills were tested gradually and his confidence increased. At the end of the program he reported reduced anxiety and had formed a group of friends that he regularly went out with. Six-month follow-up showed that he had continued to make gains.

LEVEL 4—SUPPORT DELIVERED VIA A SPECIALIST

Support at this level could be provided face-to-face or at a distance via telephone or e-mail and either one to one or in a group setting. Key differences between level 3 and level 4 interventions is that the latter are for patients with a greater level of need and are delivered by specialists with expertise around psychosocial support specifically for people affected by body image-related distress. Level 4 interventions may be warranted, for instance, in patients with high levels of preoccupation about appearance or functional changes who are highly avoidant of viewing themselves in the mirror, frequently engage in social isolation due to body image concerns, or have high levels of relationship distress. Specialists delivering interventions at this level could include a clinical psychologist, psychiatrist, counselor, or social worker with specific training and experience in body image-–related issues, as opposed to a professional with only generalized training in the delivery of mental health interventions.

The benefit of CBT-based support for women who have undergone treatment for breast cancer has already been demonstrated by interventions at lower levels of the CAR framework. Many interventions at level 4 also use CBT, but, importantly, they are delivered by a psychosocial specialist. For example, a controlled evaluation of a 14-week group-based CBT intervention delivered by two psychologists reported significant improvements in body image among women who had undergone surgical treatment.[41] These positive effects were maintained at six-month follow-up. Body image was addressed in five of the sessions that explored concerns relating to altered appearance, presenting oneself to others, changes in sexuality, and facilitating self-acceptance.

Variations of CBT have also been used as a basis for other interventions at this level. For example, a group intervention using rational emotive behavior therapy (a form of CBT) specifically targeted body image among women who had previously undergone a mastectomy. The psychiatrist-led intervention was shown to have large positive effects on body image.[42] Sessions focused on adaptive skills, problem-solving, and muscle relaxation, and participants were required to complete between-session tasks at home. Nonetheless, the absence of a follow-up evaluation impedes understanding of the long-term effects of the intervention, and, although the study was controlled, other aspects of the methodology were less rigorous (e.g., randomization was not conducted and there was no blinding of the participants, facilitator, or outcome assessor), so these findings should be interpreted with caution. In contrast, a more methodologically rigorous study evaluated a group-based mindfulness and yoga program among women with breast cancer.[7] Two-hour sessions based on a mindfulness-based stress reduction program were delivered by two clinical psychologists for eight weeks. Whilst body image was a secondary outcome of the intervention, large postintervention effects were reported on the body image of women in the intervention group, but this improvement was not maintained two months later.

Couple-based interventions at this level have also demonstrated potential for improving body image (see Chapter 15). For example, a RCT evaluated "CanCOPE," a psychologist-delivered intervention for couples within which the woman had been diagnosed with breast or gynecological cancer.[43] Information and counseling aimed to help couples conjointly cope and support one another by teaching communication and partner support, in addition to sexual counseling. It was delivered across five two-hour sessions in the couples' homes and two additional 30-minute telephone calls. However, while the intervention was found to increase women's perceptions of their partners' acceptance of their body, it did not significantly improve their own self-acceptance of it.

An additional example of a level 4 intervention is the program of support offered by the UK charity Changing Faces (see www.changingfaces.org). Managing people remotely via e-mail or telephone calls, highly trained specialists offer informed pragmatic support for people reporting appearance-related anxiety, including those diagnosed and treated for cancer of any kind. Beyond the UK, organizations such as the Sunshine Social Welfare Foundation in Taiwan provide specialist support for people with a range of disfigurements. In 2011, 65% of the charity's clients were oral cancer survivors (https://www.sunshine.org.tw).

EXAMPLE OF A LEVEL 4 INTERVENTION

Martha telephoned a charitable support organization specializing in psychosocial support for people affected by an altered appearance following surgery to remove a basal cell carcinoma on her nose. Unfortunately her treatment resulted in the removal of a significant lesion so that she now described herself as having a large facial disfigurement. She was reluctant to leave the house, feared the comments and questions of others, and could see no way in which she could assume her former lifestyle including job and family responsibilities. Working with Martha, the specialist therapist provided written information outlining common responses to her condition and typical approach strategies that other people with a similar disfigurement had found helpful. Together they agreed on a graded program which she could use to tackle her fears, one step at a time. Details of Martha's progress were recorded and sent back to the therapist by post. Gradually she recovered sufficiently to attend a two-day workshop run by the charity, where a group of patients shared experiences and worked on developing new skills for managing their condition, with a particular focus on dealing with unwanted intrusions or comments from other people. Armed with a set of strategies that she had developed and practiced over time, Martha successfully returned to her previous employment.

LEVEL 5—SYSTEMATIC SPECIALIST-LED THERAPY

Levels 4 and 5 of the framework both refer to interventions delivered by psychosocial specialists trained to support people with body image distress. However, level 5 interventions are delivered face-to-face by fully trained practitioners with additional years of experience who are capable of supporting patients with the highest level of complex needs or comorbidities. Patients in need of interventions at level 5 could include those with suicidal ideation, debilitating levels of anxiety or depression related to body image changes, inability to make treatment decisions that affect body image, or traumatic responses to body image–related treatment changes. These patients are likely to require support from a multidisciplinary team and may also require psychotropic medications.

A psychologist, psychiatrist, or counselor with specialized body image training providing interventions at this level would use an established model of therapy with a good evidence of effectiveness in managing body image and appearance-related concerns. The CBT-based manual developed by Clarke and colleagues[44] was underpinned by the framework developed from a study of 1,265 adults with a range of visible differences,[45] together with examples from clinical practice and relevant components from Clark and Wells' classic model of social phobia (particularly with regard to the management of rumination).[46] The manual describes session-by-session outlines as examples of working with body image problems, which could be adapted to meet the needs of individuals with any type of cancer. First, an assessment of the individual's body image anxiety is made in order to understand the extent to which he or she is affected by appearance-related concerns as a result of cancer and its treatment. This assessment contains three key factors:

- The discrepancy between the individual's current appearance and what he or she considers to be "ideal" or acceptable. Note that it is the discrepancy between *subjective* ratings and ideals of appearance that is important. The *objective* appearance as ranked by observers often bears no relationship to the assessment of appearance made by patients themselves. This fact can be bewildering to health professionals and relatives who tend to offer reassurance that *"it doesn't look too bad"* or *"you look good."* Clinical experience also suggests that psychological adjustment to a change in appearance lags consistently behind the physical process of scar maturation and healing, so that people may still feel very preoccupied with appearance change whilst health professionals and relatives are reassuring them that their wound has healed and they look okay.
- The value the patient places on appearance. Where appearance is generally not regarded as important, the impact of appearance change tends to be less. This is unrelated to age or gender.
- The impact of appearance-related concerns on cognitions, feelings, and behavior on day-to-day life.

After establishing a shared understanding of the rationale for intervention, the therapist then works with the patient to modify the factors identified in the assessment and reduce the impact of the appearance change. Targeting and challenging beliefs about appearance is achieved largely through a focus on recognizing/changing maladaptive behavior, building social skills, using graded exposure in social settings, and using the results of these behavioral experiments to modify prevailing beliefs and underlying assumptions. This approach, laid out in the manual, has been widely used by clinical psychologists but has yet to be evaluated.

Elizabeth was referred to an experienced clinical psychologist with expertise in appearance-related issues following her diagnosis of breast cancer and treatment that included a mastectomy. In a careful, in-depth assessment, the psychologist established that Elizabeth's anxiety centered on the appearance of her breast whilst she awaited reconstructive surgery and the excessive weight that she had put on as a result of chemotherapy. She felt that no one recognized her and that her appearance meant that she was no longer the person she had been before her illness. Thus her body image anxiety led to a challenge of her core beliefs about who she was and whether she could function in the way that she had done previously. Because of this loss of confidence, she no longer felt able to have an intimate relationship with her partner or to return to work, and she was fearful that she would lose her job. The psychologist then worked with her to set out a formulation of her difficulties and to explain how the different emotions, beliefs, and behaviors that she experienced made sense given her history. Over a period of several weeks they challenged her fears that she could no longer function by agreeing on specific tasks that she would complete at home, strategies to support the gradual resumption of intimacy, and tackling her weight management issues through graded exercise and use of food diaries. This was then fed back into the formulation to challenge her beliefs and revise her expectations about herself. At the end of therapy she was less preoccupied with her weight, was able to be more accepting of the appearance of her breast, resumed an intimate relationship with her partner, and had returned to work on a gradual re-entry program, describing herself as much more confident about making a full recovery.

Using the CAR framework has helped demonstrate a range of interventions that could help to meet the needs of cancer patients with varying levels of appearance-related distress. However, evidence-based interventions are not necessarily available or easily accessible to those who may benefit from them. Amongst the possible reasons for this are a number of issues which we believe health professionals and researchers could address. We consider these in the following sections.

CONSIDERATIONS FOR HEALTH PROFESSIONALS

It has been suggested that health professionals may not appreciate the importance of addressing appearance concerns with cancer patients or perhaps are unsure of how to broach the topic with them.[47–49] In addition, the time restrictions on individual consultations during busy clinics can make it extremely difficult for health professionals to assess individuals' needs.[50] This highlights the role for education and training in how to discuss appearance issues appropriately with patients. Yet, whilst raising health professionals' awareness and understanding of the potential impact of appearance and body image issues is key, it is important not to overgeneralize the negative experiences reported by many cancer patients and to assume that all patients with cancer have concerns about their appearance. Knowing when and how to intervene is imperative, since many cancer patients can manage the challenges they face without the need for specialist intervention. This is one of the reasons why a stepped model of care, such as the CAR framework outlined, can be so useful in guiding health professionals toward low-intensity interventions such as clear communication and information provision for *all* their patients, with a gradient of increasingly more intense interventions to meet the individual needs of each patient.

Using a test of implicit (unconscious) attitudes toward appearance, a study of 1,000 nationally representative members of the general public concluded that participants showed a strong bias against people with a visible difference.[51] Relating this finding to the topic at hand, it is important for both health professionals and researchers working within oncology to be conscious and aware of their own attitudes toward appearance, including the importance they place on it and assumptions they make about it, as a first step toward being able to provide appropriate supportive care for their patients with or without appearance-related concerns. Chapter 7 in this volume considers some common "myths" about appearance, particularly those associated with an altered or unusual appearance such as that resulting from cancer treatment.

Health professionals should also carefully consider the language they use in relation to appearance, especially during their interactions with patients. For example, it is common within the medical and surgical professions to use terminology such as "defect," "deformity," "deficit," or "flaw." Whilst issues around the language used in this area has been a topic of considerable discussion and debate for many years, a shift toward language with less negative connotations, for example "changed appearance" or "difference," would be useful. Likewise, phrases such as "looking better" or "improving" when referring to the results of surgery (particularly reconstructive procedures) might inadvertently promote prevailing societal "beauty myths" about the importance of "looking good" and not having visible scars and thereby fuel individual insecurities and influence, albeit unconsciously, a person's evaluation of how he or she looks after surgery and, potentially, decisions about further surgery.

A key issue facing professionals who want to support cancer patients affected by appearance-related and body image concerns is the question of how best to identify those who are likely to benefit from the variety of interventions including those outlined earlier in this chapter. Many professionals (as well as patients' parents/carers) are very aware of physical symptoms, such as pain and nausea, experienced by those for whom they are responsible, and discussing such issues is part and parcel of routine care. In contrast, they may be unaware that appearance concerns are causing their patients distress or fail to realize the extent of such distress and the impact it is having on a person's life. One approach to assessment by psychosocial specialists has been outlined, but it is also important for health professionals who are not experts in this field to be able to gauge the impact of appearance changes on their patients' lives. A useful way of doing this is to proactively explore a patient's body image, even if the patient does not voluntarily bring up any related issues. Fingeret has developed a framework for health professionals to discuss body image difficulties with patients, referred to as "the Three C's."[52] It proposes that at the beginning of the appointment, the patient should be reminded that body image concerns following the diagnosis and treatment of cancer are *common*. Normalizing body image difficulties in this manner is believed to reduce feelings of embarrassment and stigma. Subsequently, through the use of open-ended questions, health professionals are encouraged to ask the patient about the specific nature of the body image *concerns* they are experiencing. These may be associated with appearance- or function-related changes and may also comprise of fears about the effects of impending treatment. Lastly, patients are asked about the *consequences* of their body image concerns. Health professionals should look out for adverse effects upon emotional, social, and occupational functioning.

Screening tools can also be used to identify patients who may benefit from support around appearance-related issues and could indicate the type and level of intervention that they may find helpful. These tools need not be unduly onerous, either for the person with cancer (or the parent/carer) or for health professionals and those potentially providing support. They also need to be rigorously validated so they are underpinned by strong research to support and encourage their use by professionals who want to provide evidence-based practice. One approach that has been shown to help patients identify issues (including body image concerns) that they would like to discuss with health professionals[53,54] is the Patient Concerns Inventory.[55] This was originally developed for use with head and neck cancer patients and has since been used with those with breast cancer and brain tumors. It is a 56-item measure listing an array of possible issues that may be of concern to patients (including one item specifically about appearance) which is completed by patients prior to their consultation, allowing them to indicate their particular concerns which can then be used to promote discussions during the subsequent consultation.

Increasing awareness amongst health professionals of the nature and incidence of appearance issues experienced by their patients is a first step toward improving care, but only if they are confident and able to then put this knowledge into practice. Including this within medical and surgical training and continuing professional development courses could help health professionals to raise these issues with patients. Recently, a range of training materials for health professionals has been developed to raise providers' awareness and understanding of the issues facing their patients (see www.whenlooks.eu). Doing so could be one step toward ensuring patients' appearance-related needs are recognized. Yet, even if these needs are identified, professionals may not address them if they feel unprepared or lack confidence in dealing with them. The phrase "the silencing of disfigurement" was coined to describe health professionals choosing not to discuss appearance issues when working with head and neck cancer patients,[56] in part because they do not feel able to help if patients do report having concerns. This "silencing of appearance" by health professionals, and others, could be a far more widespread issue affecting all cancer patients, and not only those with head and neck cancer. Researchers have also reported general practitioners' difficulty in raising the issue of appearance with young people with visible differences, including those resulting from cancer treatment.[57] The potential consequence is that the issue goes unaddressed, as patients might not raise their concerns about their appearance for fear of being considered vain or ungrateful for the treatment they have received.[58]

Regarding when support about body image issues should be provided, it has been recommended that health professionals consider the stage at which patients are at in their treatment journey. It has been suggested that the needs of women undergoing breast reconstruction would be better met if they were supported according to whether they are awaiting the initial reconstructive surgery, have undergone some surgery, or have completed the whole reconstructive process.[59] This sound advice might also be relevant to patients undergoing other treatments and those with other cancer diagnoses.

Some have suggested that health professionals may overlook, trivialize, or minimize cancer patients' concerns and distress associated with their appearance. A qualitative study with 14 health professionals working in a single pediatric oncology centre and a survey of 48 health professionals from across the UK explored their views on the appearance concerns experienced by young people with cancer and the provision of support and interventions to meet these needs.[58] Most of the interviewees (87%) thought that appearance was a particular concern for their patients throughout every stage of their cancer diagnosis and treatment. Yet it might be assumed that patients with advanced diagnosis, and those with metastatic disease, will not consider appearance-related issues to be important and therefore not candidates for body image interventions. Indeed, some participants in the study admitted to being surprised that appearance concerns were an issue for patients who were terminally ill, and some thought appearance was a low priority for them.[58] However, limited research with this group indicates that it is, for some, a major concern.[60] It is therefore important that interventions are offered to patients even with incurable cancers and that further research is conducted to ensure that interventions are meeting any specific needs this patient group has in terms of their content and delivery.

CONSIDERATIONS FOR RESEARCHERS

A recent systematic review concluded that there is still considerable potential for further development and rigorous evaluation of body image interventions for women treated for breast cancer.[5] We advocate for future intervention research to have an exclusive and explicit focus on body image, rather than including body image as a small component of broader interventions attempting to address the extensive range of psychosocial concerns that can accompany diagnosis, treatment, and recovery. This specific focus has greater potential to validate the concerns of individuals and increase the probability that the interventions will be successful in the long term. Amongst the other recommendations made from this systematic review are that interventions based on physical activity may be attractive, but consideration should be given to whether a psychological approach may be more appropriate for individuals who are physically restricted as a consequence of current treatment. Finally, researchers are encouraged to report the content and delivery format of interventions, so as to enable both replication and assessment of the monetary costs and resources necessary for their implementation. These recommendations can also be directed toward interventions for other cancer groups.

Rigorous methodology is needed to reduce the risk of bias and consequently increase confidence in the validity of positive findings. Accordingly, the use of pretest–posttest designs and control groups is encouraged in order to achieve an acceptable level of internal validity. Further, while the randomization of participants decreases selection bias, ethical issues can arise when individuals with cancer are randomly allocated to conditions (Bottomley provides an overview of considerations regarding the suitablity of randomization in psycho-oncology research).[61] The use of RCTs to evaluate body image interventions can raise particular concerns. Individuals may be in desperate need of support, implying it could be unethical to use a waitlist or passive control group which would delay participants' access to support. These individuals may consequently decide to use other forms of psychosocial or cosmetic support in the meantime, instead of waiting to undergo the evaluated intervention.

Several frameworks are available to direct researchers through the development and evaluation of new health interventions (e.g., the Intervention Mapping protocol;[62] the PRECEDE-PROCEED model;[63]). We recommend the adoption of the Medical Research Council's (MRC) framework for the development and evaluation of complex interventions,[64] which consists of four stages (Development, Feasibility/Piloting, Evaluation, Implementation) that do not need to be pursued in a linear or even cyclical sequence. Following guidelines such as these in the future development of body image interventions for cancer patients will maximize the likelihood that they will be effective and taken up by stakeholders, including funders and policymakers. The MRC framework recognizes the potential usefulness of alternative experimental designs, such as cluster-randomized trials, stepped wedge designs, preference trials, randomized consent designs, and N-of-1 designs, rather than relying on RCTs.[64]

As highlighted in examples throughout this chapter, most studies of the effectiveness of interventions in this field have relied on small sample sizes. A further methodological limitation is the lack of control groups in many studies, making it impossible to know whether any changes in outcomes were due to the intervention alone or could, perhaps, have been due to other factors. To complicate matters further, researchers have, to date, used a wide range of condition-specific and general measures to evaluate the effects of interventions to support cancer patients affected by appearance-related distress and concerns. This variability in the measures used has precluded meta-analysis of results within systematic reviews and thereby prevented definitive conclusions about which are the most effective interventions. Establishing a consensus approach to measurement would alleviate the challenges associated with the comparison of evaluative studies. In the meantime, it is important to continue to employ validated and reliable scales to measure body image. While a single core measure may be preferred, employing a combination of measures may allow the assessment of multiple dimensions of body image, including perceptions, thoughts, feelings, and behavior relating to the body and appearance. Researchers are also encouraged to consider using cancer-specific measures (e.g., the Body Image subscale of the European Organization for Research and Treatment of Cancer Quality of Life Questionnaire Breast Cancer Module[65]), as well as measures developed in the wider body image field (e.g., the Multidimensional Body-Self Relations Questionnaire[66,67]).

Finally, most evaluations of interventions in this field have collected limited follow-up data, thereby restricting our understanding of their longer-term impact including whether interventions that have been shown to be effective in the short-term (posttest) continue to demonstrate sustained improvements on body image or whether those which were noneffective at posttest offer delayed benefits. The Society of Prevention Research recommends follow-up of at least six months in order to establish efficacy,[68] although ideally follow-up will be longer than this since changes to appearance and bodily function, and therefore associated body image, may differ in relation to an individual's stage and regime of treatment. This may consequently influence the timing of the effects of the intervention. Further, researchers are encouraged to include several consistent follow-up points, so as to facilitate comparisons of maintained improvements between studies.

LOOKING AHEAD

Body image and the nature and incidence of appearance-related concerns are dynamic, evolving issues. For example, younger age groups are now reporting anxiety about body image, and growing numbers of men are expressing concern about appearance. Researchers and clinicians need to respond to this shifting landscape, to ensure that the care they provide for their patients is informed by an evidence base and the latest thinking in the fields of both body image and psycho-oncology.

There is still considerable potential for new interventions in this area. It could be fruitful to explore further the use of intervention approaches that have been used in other areas of psycho-oncology but have received less research attention specifically in relation to body image and appearance issues. For example, third-wave CBT approaches such as acceptance and commitment therapy, dialectical behavior therapy, and mindfulness have started to be explored[32] but warrant further studies of their acceptability and feasibility, as well as consideration of which aspects of complex interventions are most effective, for who, and when.

Online interventions outlined (e.g., YP Face IT) are increasing access to interventions and offering the potential for support to be available at any time of day. However, it is important to remember that not all patients will want or be able to use online support and that online provision and further developments should not be at the expense of developments with face-to-face support. Future developments in this area might also include the use of apps and other new and emerging technology.

An exciting development would be to examine whether interventions developed within the broader body image field might be acceptable and effective for use with individuals experiencing body image concerns as a consequence of appearance and bodily changes resulting from cancer and its treatment. For example, a rigorously evaluated and effective group-based CBT program aimed at women in midlife[69] may be appropriate for use with women treated for breast cancer, given that many women with the disease are diagnosed in midlife and are therefore likely to still be vulnerable to similar influences and body image concerns as those without cancer. However, such interventions may require adaption in order to best address any unique body image concerns of specific cancer groups. This is important given the likelihood of condition-specific issues which warrant attention. For example, patients with a stoma often have concerns relating to intimacy, whilst many of those with head and neck cancer may experience anxiety around eating in public.

Finally, since most research in this area has involved women with breast cancer, there is still a need for further studies involving other patient groups and to include greater consideration of interventions to support young people with an altered appearance due to cancer treatment and other groups currently underrepresented in the published research. Further research should also explore the needs and experiences of people close to the person with an altered appearance (e.g., partners, children, siblings, grandparents, teachers, employers) in order to identify if there is a need for intervention or support to help them as well as the patient. Again, a tiered approach might be useful, differing in the type and intensity of support needed.

CONCLUSION

This chapter has introduced a range of interventions, all with the common aim of improving outcomes for cancer patients with appearance-related and body image concerns. By using the framework of a stepped model of care specific to altered appearance, we have shown how patients might be offered access to appropriate interventions to meet their individual, specific needs. The level at which any particular intervention sits on this framework might sometimes be open to debate, but for us the important issue is the translation and implementation of research, so that health professionals and researchers alike all continue to build the evidence base and increase access to resources that patients might benefit from. Clearly, there is still a lot of work to be done, but we remain excited by the possibilities that lie ahead.

REFERENCES

1. Bessell A, Moss, TP. Evaluating the effectiveness of psychosocial interventions for individuals with visible differences: a systematic review of the empirical literature. *Body Image.* 2007;4(3):227–238.

2. Norman A, Moss TP. Psychosocial interventions for adults with visible differences: a systematic review. *Peer J.* 2015;2(3):e870.

3. Muftin Z, Thompson AR. A systematic review of self-help for disfigurement: effectiveness, usability, and acceptability. *Body Image.* 2013;10(4):442–450.

4. Jenkinson E, Williamson H, Byron-Daniel J, Moss TP. Systematic review: psychosocial interventions for children and young people with visible differences resulting from appearance altering conditions, injury, or treatment effects. *J Pediatr Psychol.* 2015;40(10):1017–1033.

5. Lewis-Smith H, Diedrichs PC, Rumsey, N, Harcourt, D. Interventions to improve the body image of women treated for breast cancer: a systematic review. Manuscript submitted for publication.

6. Mehnert A, Veers S, Howaldt D, Braumann KM, Koch U, Schulz KH. Effects of a physical exercise rehabilitation group program on anxiety, depression, body image, and health-related quality of life among breast cancer patients. *Oncol Res Treat.* 2011;34(5):248–253.

7. Rahmani S, Talepasand S. The effect of group mindfulness-based stress reduction program and conscious yoga on the fatigue severity and global and specific life quality in women with breast cancer. *Med J Islam Repub Iran.* 2015;29:175.

8. Speck RM, Gross CR, Hormes JM, et al. Changes in the Body Image and Relationship Scale following a one-year strength training trial for breast cancer survivors with or at risk for lymphedema. *Breast Cancer Res Treat.* 2010;121(2):421–430

9. Campbell A, Mutrie N, White F, McGuire F, Kearney N. A pilot study of a supervised group exercise programme as a rehabilitation treatment for women with breast cancer receiving adjuvant treatment. *Eur J Oncol Nurs.* 2005;9(1):56–63.

10. Courneya KS, Mackey JR, Bell GJ, Jones LW, Field CJ, Fairey AS. Randomized controlled trial of exercise training in postmenopausal breast cancer survivors: cardiopulmonary and quality of life outcomes. *J Clin Oncol.* 2003;21(9):1660–1668.

11. British Psychological Society Division of Clinical Psychology SIGOPAC. *Good Practice Guidance in Demonstrating Quality and Outcomes in Psycho-oncology.* Leicester, UK: British Psychological Society, 2015.

12. Diedrichs PC, Halliwell E. School-based interventions to promote positive body image and the acceptance of diversity in appearance. In: Rumsey N, Harcourt D, eds. *The Oxford Handbook of the Psychology of Appearance*. Oxford: Oxford University Press; 2012:531–550.

13. Appearance Research Collaboration. Factors and processes associated with psychological adjustment to disfiguring conditions. In: Clarke A, Thompson AR, Jenkinson E, Rumsey N, Newell R, eds. *CBT for Appearance Anxiety: Psychosocial Interventions for Anxiety due to Visible Difference*. Oxford: John Wiley; 2013:194–271.

14. Rumsey N, Harcourt D. Where do we go from here? In: Rumsey N, Harcourt D, eds. *The Oxford Handbook of the Psychology of Appearance*. Oxford: Oxford University Press; 2012:679–692.

15. Veale D, Willson R, Clarke A. *Overcoming Body Image Problems Including Body Dysmorphic Disorder*. London: Robinson; 2009.

16. Jarry JL, Ip K. The effectiveness of stand-alone cognitive-behavioural therapy for body image: a meta-analysis. *Body Image*. 2005;2(4):317–331.

17. Robinson E, Rumsey N, Partridge J. An evaluation of the impact of social interaction skills training for facially disfigured people. *J Plast Reconstr Aesthet Surg*. 1996;49:281–289.

18. Partridge J. Persuading the public: new face values for the 21st century. In: Rumsey N, Harcourt D, eds. *The Oxford Handbook of the Psychology of Appearance*. Oxford: Oxford University Press; 2012:468–485.

19. Breast Cancer Care. Body Image Campaign. Breast Cancer Care website, 2014. https://www.breastcancercare.org.uk/get-involved/campaign-us/body-image-breast-cancer. Accessed January 27, 2017.

20. Lewis-Smith H, Diedrichs PC. Exploring attitudes towards individuals with visible differences through the evaluation of the "Changing Faces" poster campaigns. Paper presented at: Appearance Matters 5 Conference; June 2012; Bristol, UK.

21. Sherman KA, Harcourt DM, Lam TC, Shaw LK, Boyages J. BRECONDA: development and acceptability of an interactive decisional support tool for women considering breast reconstruction, *Psychooncology*. 2014;23:835–838.

22. Ziebland S, Wyke S. Health and illness in a connected world: how might sharing experiences on the Internet affect people's health? *Milbank Q*. 2012;90(2):219–249.

23. Katz MR, Irish JC, Devins GM. Development and pilot testing of a psychoeducational intervention for oral cancer patients. *Psychooncology*. 2004;13(9):642–653.

24. Rumsey N, Harcourt D. Visible difference amongst children and adolescents: issues and interventions. *Dev Neurorehabil*. 2007;10(2):113–123.

25. Maddern L, Owen T. The Outlook Summer Group: a social skills workshop for children with a different appearance who are transferring to a secondary school. *Clin Psych*. 2004;33:25–29.

26. Jenkinson E. Therapeutic interventions: evidence of effectiveness. In: Rumsey N, Harcourt D, eds. *The Oxford Handbook of the Psychology of Appearance*. Oxford: Oxford University Press; 2012:551–567.

27. Cash TF. *The Body Image Workbook: An 8-Step Program for Learning to Like Your Looks*, 2nd ed. Oakland, CA: New Harbinger; 2008.

28. Ucok O. The meaning of appearance in surviving breast cancer. *Hum Stud*. 2005;28(3):291–316.

29. Taggart LR, Ozolins L, Hardie H, Nyhof-Young J. Look good feel better workshops: a "big lift" for women with cancer. *J Cancer Educ*. 2009;24(2) 94–99.

30. Huang S, Liu HE. Effectiveness of cosmetic rehabilitation on the body image of oral cancer patients in Taiwan. *Support Care Cancer*. 2008;16(9):981–986.

31. Pilkington M, Harcourt D, Rumsey N, O'Connor D, Brennan J. "Your hair's your crowning glory": breast cancer patients' experiences of treatment-related hair loss and a camouflage based support service. *Psychooncology*. 2014;23:181–182.

32. Przezdziecki A, Sherman KA. Modifying affective and cognitive responses regarding body image difficulties in breast cancer survivors using a self-compassion-based writing intervention. *Mindfulness.* 2016;7(5):1142–1155.

33. Clarke A. *Social rehabilitation in head and neck cancer* (DPsych thesis). London: City University, 2001.

34. Hsu SC, Wang HH, Chu SY, Yen HF. Effectiveness of informational and emotional consultation on the psychological impact on women with breast cancer who underwent modified radical mastectomy. *J Nurs Res.* 2010;18(3):215–226.

35. Helgeson VS, Cohen S, Schulz R, Yasko J. Education and peer discussion group interventions and adjustment to breast cancer. *Arch Gen Psychiatry.* 1999;56(4):340–347.

36. Scanlon K, McCoy M, Jupp D. A nationwide survivorship intervention for women with breast cancer: results from a 2 year evaluation of Breast Cancer Care's "Moving Forward courses." *Psychooncology.* 2013;22:6.

37. Harcourt D, Griffiths C, Baker E, Hansen E, White P, Clarke A. The acceptability of PEGASUS: an intervention to facilitate patient-centred consultations and shared decision-making with women contemplating breast reconstruction. *Psychol Health Med.* 2016;21(2):248–253.

38. Bessell A, Clarke A, Harcourt D, Moss TP, Rumsey N. Incorporating user perspectives in the design of an online intervention tool for people with visible differences: Face IT. *Behav Cogn Psychother.* 2010;38:577–596.

39. Williamson H, Griffiths C, Harcourt D. Developing young person's Face IT: online psychosocial support for adolescents struggling with conditions or injuries affecting their appearance. *Health Psychol Open.* 2015;2(2). doi:10.1177/2055102915619092

40. Williamson H, Hamlet C, White P, et al. Supporting adolescents struggling with appearance-altering conditions: the feasibility of using an online psychosocial intervention (YP Face IT) in primary care. Manuscript submitted for publication.

41. Sebastián J, Manos D, Bueno M, Mateos N. Body image and self esteem in women with breast cancer participating in psychosocial intervention program. *Psychol Spain.* 2008;12(1):13–28.

42. Fadaei S, Janighorban M, Mehrabi T, Ahmadi SA, Mokaryan F, Gukizade A. Effects of cognitive behavioral counseling on body image following mastectomy. *J Res Med Sci.* 2011;16(8):1047–1054.

43. Scott JL, Halford WK, Ward BG. United we stand? The effects of a couple-coping intervention on adjustment to early stage breast or gynecological cancer. *J Consult Clin Psychol.* 2004;72(6):1122–1135.

44. Clarke A, Thompson AR, Jenkinson E, Rumsey N, Newell R. *CBT for Appearance Anxiety: Psychosocial Interventions for Anxiety due to Visible Difference.* Oxford: John Wiley; 2014.

45. Appearance Research Collaboration. Factors and processes associated with psychological adjustment to disfiguring conditions. In: Clarke A, Thompson AR, Jenkinson E, Rumsey N, Newell R, eds. *CBT for Appearance Anxiety: Psychosocial Interventions for Anxiety due to Visible Difference.* Oxford: John Wiley; 2014:194–271.

46. Clark DM, Wells A. A cognitive model of social phobia. In: Liebowitz M, Heimberg RG, eds. *Social Phobia: Diagnosis, Assessment, and Treatment.* New York: Guilford Press; 1995:69–93.

47. Cadogan J. Changing provision of healthcare settings in the United Kingdom. In: Rumsey N, Harcourt D, eds. *The Oxford Handbook of the Psychology of Appearance.* Oxford: Oxford University Press; 2012:486–501.

48. Clarke A, Cooper C. Psychosocial rehabilitation after disfiguring injury or disease: investigating the training needs of specialist nurses. *J Adv Nurs.* 2001;34(1):18–26.

49. Randall J, Ream E. Hair loss with chemotherapy: at a loss over its management? *Eur J Cancer Care.* 2005;14(3):223–231.

50. Fingeret MC, Teo I, Epner DE. Managing body image difficulties of adult cancer patients: lessons from available research. *Cancer.* 2014;120:633–641.

51. Goode A, Ellis R, Coutinho W, Partridge J. The face equality campaign—the evidence. Public attitudes survey, 2008. http://www.changingfaces.org.uk/downloads/FE%20Campaign,%20Public%20Attitudes%20survey.pdf. Accessed January 28, 2017.

52. Fingeret MC. Body image and disfigurement. In: Duffy J, Valentine A, eds. *MD Anderson Manual of Psychosocial Oncology*. Columbus, OH: McGraw-Hill; 2010:271–288.

53. Flexen J, Ghazali N, Lowe D, Rogers SN. Identifying appearance-related concerns in routine follow-up clinics following treatment for oral and oropharyngeal cancer. *Br J Oral Maxillofac Surg.* 2012;50(4):314–320.

54. Kanatas A, Lowe D, Velikova G, et al. Issues patients would like to discuss at their review consultation in breast cancer clinics—a cross-sectional survey. *Tumori.* 2014;100(5):568–579.

55. Rogers SN, El-Sheikha J, Lowe D. The development of a Patients Concerns Inventory (PCI) to help reveal patients concerns in the head and neck clinic. *Oral Oncol.* 2009;45(7):555–561.

56. Konradsen H, Kirkevold M, Zoffmann V. Surgical facial cancer treatment: the silencing of disfigurement in nurse–patient interactions. *J Adv Nurs.* 2009;65(11):2409–2418.

57. Hamlet C, Williamson H, Harcourt D. Recruiting young people with a visible difference to the YP Face IT feasibility trial: a qualitative exploration of primary care staff experiences. *Prim Health Care Res Dev.* 2017;18(6):541–548.

58. Williamson H, Rumsey N. The perspectives of health professionals on the psychosocial impact of an altered appearance among adolescents treated for cancer and how to improve appearance-related care. *J Psychosoc Oncol.* 2016;35(1):47–60.

59. Teo I, Reece GP, Christie IC, et al. Body image and quality of life of breast cancer patients: influence of timing and stage of breast reconstruction. *Psychooncology.* 2015;25:1106–1112.

60. McClelland SI, Holland KJ, Griggs JJ. Quality of life and metastatic breast cancer: the role of body image, disease site, and time since diagnosis. *Qual Life Res.* 2015;24(12):2939–2943.

61. Bottomley A. To randomise or not to randomise: methodological pitfalls of the RCT design in psychosocial intervention studies. *Eur J Cancer Care.* 1997;6(3):222–230.

62. Eldredge LKB, Parcel, GS, Kok, G, Gottlieb, NH. *Planning Health Promotion Programs: An Intervention Mapping Approach*. 3rd ed. San Francisco, CA: John Wiley; 2011.

63. Green LW, Kreuter MW. *Health Program Planning: An Educational and Ecological Approach*, 4th ed. New York: McGraw-Hill; 2005.

64. Craig P, Dieppe P, Macintyre S, Michie S, Nazareth I, Petticrew M. Developing and evaluating complex interventions: the new Medical Research Council guidance. *BMJ.* 2008;337:979–983.

65. Sprangers MA, Groenvold M, Arraras JI, et al. The European Organization for Research and Treatment of Cancer breast cancer-specific quality-of-life questionnaire module: first results from a three-country field study. *J Clin Oncol.* 1996;14(10):2756–2768.

66. Brown TA, Cash TF, Mikulka PJ. Attitudinal body-image assessment: factor analysis of the Body-Self Relations Questionnaire. *J Pers Assess.* 1990;55(1–2):135–144.

67. Cash TF. *Users' Manual for the Multidimensional Body-Self Relations Questionnaire*. Norfolk, VA: Author; 2000.

68. Flay BR, Biglan A, Boruch RF, et al. Standards of evidence: Criteria for efficacy, effectiveness and dissemination. *Prev Sci.* 2005;6(3):151–175.

69. McLean SA, Paxton SJ, Wertheim EH. A body image and disordered eating intervention for women in midlife: a randomized controlled trial. *J Consult Clin Psychol.* 2011;79(6):751–758.

CHAPTER 5

BODY IMAGE ISSUES ACROSS CANCER TYPES

Vicky Lehmann and Marrit A. Tuinman

Medical advances in cancer treatment have led to improved survival and a growing population of currently more than 15 million cancer survivors in the United States alone.[1] However, in many cases survival comes at the cost of various medical and psychological late effects. This has encouraged psychosocial oncology research focusing on various aspects surrounding the diagnosis of cancer and potential consequences for long-term survivorship. Body image is one such concept that is related to domains such as sexual functioning and health-related quality of life. However, how do we characterize and interpret body image changes among various types of cancer, and how do we determine whether body image may have changed as a consequence of cancer?

The general body image literature[2] has raised an important question: *Does a change to the body inherently change a person's body image?* Cancer and its treatment constitute a disruptive and life-threatening event that can alter the body in various ways. However, these effects can be very diverse, as some cancer survivors live relatively symptom free and/or cope well with body image changes, while others struggle with various medical late-effect or chronic conditions. For many survivors, there can be physical remainders of their cancer experience, such as permanent scarring, disfigurement, or alterations to functioning (e.g., speech and swallowing) that fuel ongoing distress and difficulty coping. Accordingly, survivors can feel uncomfortable and ashamed in social situations, while many also fear that, even after having overcome cancer, the physical remainders of cancer may be interpreted by others as ongoing sickness.[3] Throughout this chapter, we use the terms "patient" and "survivor" somewhat interchangeably, as the National Cancer Institute considers every cancer patient a survivor from the day of diagnosis onward.[4]

Physical remainders may indeed display that cancer survivors are different from healthy peers. A recent review encompassing 25 studies on body image in cancer survivors relative to controls without an illness history[5] indicated that cancer survivors may have a somewhat more negative body image than controls. However, numerous methodological problems were identified among the included studies. The main concerns were missing conceptualizations of body image, usage of unstandardized questionnaires with poor psychometric properties, comparisons to (sociodemographically) different control groups, varying sample sizes, and others (see review[5]). Therefore, firm conclusions were not warranted.

VISIBILITY-STABILITY CONTINUUM

When considering disease-specific effects of cancer on body image, we conceptualize cancer and its treatment as altering the body on two primary dimensions: (a) visibility of physical changes (i.e., where and which body part(s) is affected) and (b) temporal stability (i.e., whether the physical change is permanent, temporary, or delayed). Figure 5.1 presents the visibility-stability continuum of body image changes resulting from cancer and its treatment. Within this continuum a focus is given to appearance, but for a comprehensive consideration of the potential impact of cancer and its treatment on body image, one must also consider whether and which *body functions* are altered. Functional body changes include the degree to which these changes hinder (a) daily functioning (e.g., self-care, household tasks), (b) social functioning (e.g., going out in public, meeting friends,

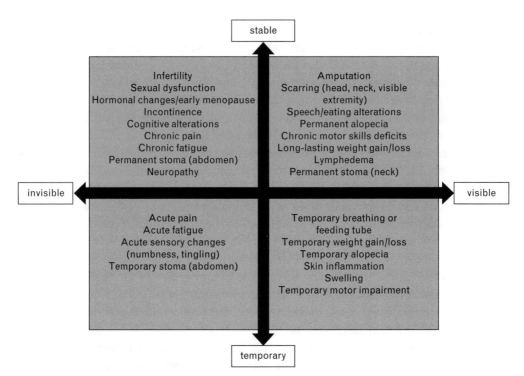

FIGURE 5.1: Visibility-stability continuum of body image changes resulting from cancer and its treatment.

spending time with family), (c) physical functioning (e.g., participation in sports, exercise, other fitness activities/hobbies), (d) occupational functioning (e.g., returning to work, specific work tasks), and (e) functioning in intimate relationships (e.g., finding a partner, sexual functioning).

Case Example: High Visibility/High Stability

Lisa is a 62-year-old female with a history of orbital cancer, who underwent total removal of her left eye and the contents of the eye socket (orbital exenteration) followed by immediate reconstruction using a full-thickness skin graft. Her body changes are highly visible and in a socially significant part of her body (i.e., the face). She now wears an eye patch whenever leaving her home. She has permanent functional changes to her vision (i.e., monocular instead of binocular), making her, for example, too afraid to drive. She has engaged in long-term body image counseling to help her with adjusting to these significant changes to her appearance and lifestyle.

Case Example: Low Visibility/High Stability

Jose is a 35-year-old man with rectal cancer who has undergone chemotherapy and radiation treatment and is expected to have a permanent colostomy following abdominoperitoneal surgical resection. The patient presents for a body image consultation to discuss his concerns about the upcoming surgery and ways of coping with permanent body changes. Even though the colostomy bag can be readily concealed under clothing and is not visible to others, he is extremely distressed about how these changes will affect his active lifestyle (e.g., he regularly competes in bike races) and the relationship with his romantic partner. He is specifically concerned about odors and leakage from the colostomy bag. He is considering declining surgery due to his body image concerns and potential limitations.

Case Example: High Visibility/Low Stability

Juanita is a 45-year-old woman with left breast cancer. She has just completed neoadjuvant chemotherapy and is expected to undergo mastectomy and radiation treatment. She presents for body image counseling at this time because she is having significant difficulties coping with hair loss from chemotherapy. Prior to cancer treatment, Juanita had long hair and indicated it was an extremely important part of her identity and something she was known for by friends and family. She works as a beautician and is refusing to return to work because she believes her clients will be extremely uncomfortable about her changed appearance. She understands her hair will most likely grow back once she has completed treatment, but this issue remains a very significant source of distress for her and is affecting her daily functioning.

Case Example: Low Visibility/Low Stability

Chris is a 68-year old man with thyroid cancer who is undergoing radiation treatment. He is concerned that there may be indications for him to receive a feeding tube in the future, which is why he is highly resistant to agreeing to treatment if this becomes necessary. He enjoys eating and works in the food service industry. He is extremely fearful that a feeding tube could become permanent. His treatment team has assured him that in most cases, if a feeding tube is required during treatment, it is removed shortly after treatment. Chris indicated he is not bothered by any appearance changes resulting from treatment but rather the impact of stigma and functional changes that a feeding tube represent to him.

The manner in which an individual evaluates his or her own appearance and functional changes is extremely variable and inherently subjective. Consequently, individuals with similar types of physical changes may experience very different levels of body image adjustment. As such, one can conceptualize body image after cancer as being a function of a survivor's subjective evaluation of the physical changes caused by cancer and its treatment (Box 5.1).

Thus, even the same type of cancer with identical treatments could lead to different levels of body image adaptation among survivors (and will further depend on the individual's body image before cancer diagnosis). Nevertheless, certain types of cancers share commonalities in how they affect the body. Accordingly, the majority of research on body image issues in the oncology setting is conducted with patients that have the same cancer type. Fewer studies compare body image between groups of patients with different cancer types, as it does not seem to have as much theoretical or clinical relevance.

In this chapter, we first describe several patient characteristics and treatment factors that can affect body image outcomes, then we discuss relevant findings on body image clustered by disease site (i.e., tumor location). For each cluster, we describe the potential *physical changes* due to cancer and its treatment alongside *emotional reactions* that can be relevant for body image and that are typically shared by survivors of the same type of cancer.

PATIENT CHARACTERISTICS AND TREATMENT FACTORS THAT AFFECT BODY IMAGE

AGE

Findings that cancer may affect body image differently depending on a patient's age are mixed. First, it is important to note that studies among healthy individuals show that body dissatisfaction is rather stable across all age groups.[6] Nevertheless, younger people are more likely to place greater importance on body shape, weight, and appearance.[6] Several studies in cancer populations show no associations between age and body image,[7-10] while others report worse body image among younger survivors.[11-14] However, the use of different measures in these studies potentially emphasizing different aspects of body image may be relevant to consider. It is noteworthy that age has been reported to moderate the relationship between body image and emotional distress, such that negative body image and increased emotional distress were associated in younger but not older breast cancer patients.[7] See Chapters 12 and 13 in this book, which are specifically dedicated to body image in younger and older cancer populations.

SEX

Historically, research on body image issues largely focused on women and girls in the general population, although increasing focus is being given to evaluating male body image outcomes. When considering cancer and its treatment side effects, one might assume that issues such as losing one's hair or extensive weight changes might be more relevant to women. While this reasoning was supported in some studies reporting more negative body image in women than men,[15,16] others have found no sex differences.[16-18] It may be speculated that both sexes can experience negative body image following cancer but due to different reasons/mechanisms. While it has typically been assumed that appearance changes may be related to body image issues in women, more attention is warranted to studying treatment side effects that could also affect the male gender identity (e.g., muscular atrophy, erectile dysfunction) and resulting body image outcomes. Overall, sex differences are not frequently the focus of studies in cancer populations, perhaps due to preselections based on cancer type that at times include one sex only. Furthermore, a recent review indicated that female cancer survivors do not report particularly worse body image than female controls.[5] For example, half of the six higher quality studies indicated no differences between female survivors and female controls, while the rest reported mixed findings or subscale differences only. Only two studies focused on male survivors and controls and provided insufficient evidence to draw any conclusion.[5]

WEIGHT CHANGE

Weight gain is often observed as an unwanted, highly visible side effect of cancer treatment, especially among patients receiving chemotherapies or hormone replacement therapies.[19] Treatments with corticosteroids (e.g., prednisone) also cause swelling especially in the facial area and torso, which is often experienced as distressing. However, the extent to which cancer patients may gain weight also depends on age, menopausal stage, or the duration of treatment. Along with that, other consequences of cancer treatment such as a different diet, reduced physical activity, and general (emotional) distress may also be related to weight gain. Given a thin body ideal in most Western cultures, weight gain can be experienced as a negative side effect of cancer, contributing to higher levels of body image distress/dissatisfaction.

Contrarily, some patients experience distress due to weight loss which can occur for various reasons (e.g., recurrent vomiting, loss of appetite, negative mood). Weight loss has anecdotally been reported as positive, especially in women who initially welcome being thinner. However, prolonged weight loss can result in cancer anorexia-cachexia syndrome (cachexia), which is observed among 60% to 80% of advanced cancer patients.[20] Cachexia is characterized by a loss of appetite and status of malnutrition (i.e., loss of muscle and fat tissue). Supplemental nutrition can typically not counteract cachexia, which indicates complex metabolic changes in cancer patients that are not entirely understood.[21–23] Other side effects such as pain, nausea, fatigue, and psychological factors (e.g., shame) can potentially play a role as well and may further discourage appetite. This may develop into a downward spiral, and cachexia may also cause social challenges, as others may not understand why the patient would not "just" eat or interpret a restricted food intake as a sign of giving up. As a consequence, social isolation initiated by the patient has been commonly observed.[24,25]

FATIGUE

Fatigue is recognized as one of the most prevalent and distressing symptoms reported by individuals with cancer, and it has significant deteriorating effects on overall quality of life.[26,27] Fatigue among cancer patients is different from that experienced by the general population, as cancer-related fatigue (CRF) is disproportionate to the exertion level and cannot be reduced by rest or sleep.[28] The National Comprehensive Cancer Network describes CRF as "an unusual, persistent, subjective sense of tiredness related to cancer or cancer treatment that interferes with usual functioning."[29] CRF may persist for months or years even after treatment has been completed.

Fatigue represents an invisible physical change that has significant impact on daily functioning. Moreover, fatigue can be considered as an important mechanism contributing to physical changes and thus body image changes accordingly. For example, if patients are fatigued, they may not have sufficient energy to exercise, participate in leisure activities, or perform routine household tasks. Such significant reductions in physical activity can be further associated with weight gain and pain. Concurrently, fatigued cancer patients also reduce their daily activity in an attempt to recover from their fatigue.[26,30] As a result patients may become more socially isolated and spend fewer hours in occupational and self-care activities.

ALOPECIA

Alopecia is a common visible side effect of chemotherapy and related to poor body image.[31] It is often experienced as distressing as it is associated with social stigma and immediately reveals to the (social) environment that the patient/survivor is "not healthy." At the same time, baldness is reported as especially distressing among female patients, since one's natural hair is associated with beauty/femininity. However, alopecia is typically temporary, and many patients can hope for the regrowth of their hair. Yet, many survivors describe their regrown hair as altered in structure (i.e., often termed "chemo hair") and mourn the loss of their original hair. Accordingly, a prospective study found that body image scores worsened and did not return to baseline even when patients experienced regrowth of their hair.[32] Some survivors experience persistent, stable alopecia (i.e., they remain bald permanently). This treatment side effect can result in long-lasting negative implications for body image.

TIME AND TREATMENT PHASE

Time since treatment is an important factor, as many studies have found body image of cancer survivors to improve over time,[17,33,34] which may especially be true for longer follow-up periods.[35] For example, some studies have found that long-term cancer survivors (i.e., >5 years postdiagnosis) report similar body image scores to controls, which suggests that body image problems, if present during treatment, may subside over time. This was supported by longitudinal studies where women with breast and genital cancers reported greatest body image concerns shortly after diagnosis.[31,36] These findings seem intuitive and further suggest that body image experiences will differ as a result of a patient's treatment phase and time since treatment. Patients recently diagnosed and on active treatment are likely to experience the greatest impact on body image due to the acute nature of physical changes from the illness and its treatment. In contrast, long-term survivors will have found temporary body image changes to be resolved and will have had time to develop coping strategies for managing more stable/lasting physical changes. Nevertheless, this pattern may not hold true for all cancers. For instance, it has been reported that oral cancer patients became significantly more concerned about body image over time,[37] perhaps due to increasing exposure and difficulties in social contexts and environments. Even in the palliative treatment phase, body image seems an important issue for cancer patients, as body image dissatisfaction has also been reported to occur frequently in advanced cancer patients.[38] See Chapter 6 in this book, which is specifically dedicated to body image in treatment phases.

OVERVIEW OF DISEASE-SPECIFIC BODY IMAGE ISSUES

We present an overview of research on body image issues resulting from the following clusters of cancer types: sexual organ-related (including breast), gastrointestinal, head and neck, skin, brain sarcomas, ocular, and systemic cancers. Within each cluster we present specific types of physical changes in relation to the visibility-stability continuum (see Figure 5.1) and identify when a change affects visibility, stability, and/or functioning before describing common evaluations/emotional reactions to these physical changes that are relevant to body image.

SEXUAL ORGAN-RELATED CANCERS

PHYSICAL CHANGES

Sexual organ-related cancers include diagnoses that affect the primary sexual organs, such as testicular, penile, prostate, vaginal, endometrial, cervical, or ovarian cancers. Many of these cancers are treated with minimal surgical incisions or laparoscopic surgeries and thus leave small scars, which are only visible if survivors are fully naked and can otherwise be hidden under clothes (*visibility, stability*). However, some of the "interior alterations" can be quite extensive, such as hysterectomies. In addition, physical alterations for example in testicular cancer are more visible as it often includes the removal of one/both testicles (*visibility*), although implants are often offered to minimize changes in appearance (*visibility*). Similarly, surgeries for vaginal cancers can be more extensive and alter the appearance of the labia (*visibility*). All sexual organ-related cancers can impair sexual functioning or also cause the permanent loss of fertility (*functioning, stability*). The impact on other daily functioning, such as work, is usually minimal, but hormone imbalances could cause some difficulties in this area, if survivors experience menopausal symptoms for example.

BODY IMAGE ADJUSTMENT

Overall, and although appearance alterations are often minimal, self-consciousness about scarring could negatively affect leisure time activities (e.g., sports, swimming) or more intimate activities such as sex. Particularly, testicular cancer survivors have been reported to feel self-conscious about a removed testicle (i.e., orchiectomy),[39,40] while side effects of other sexual organ-related cancers are less visible. However, many patients treated with hysterectomy, orchiectomy, oophorectomy, and so on are potentially left infertile and with tremendous hormonal changes. In these cases, negative feelings about the body are more likely a reflection of experiencing a loss of wholeness (e.g., loss of testicle[39] or uterus[41–43]), loss of functioning (i.e., infertility[44]), and/or a loss of masculinity[45] or femininity[46] rather than feelings about the body's appearance. Survivors of gynecological cancers in particular describe the removal of inner organs as leaving some "emptiness."[41] Some gynecological cancers are also treated with extensive surgeries and removal of gastrointestinal/urinal systems leaving survivors with extensive changes in bodily functioning and more negative body image.[47] Other side effects among patients of sexual organ–related cancers might be pain during sex, vaginal dryness, sexual dysfunction, or erectile dysfunction.[36,44,48] Such symptoms can be related to feelings of shame,[39] regret, or concerns about sexual attractiveness[36] that are closely related to overall negative body image. Studies among prostate cancer patients seem to indicate that body image is not particularly negative among survivors overall but among those that receive hormone therapies.[49,50]

Interestingly, some patients anecdotally describe a separation/dissociation from their bodies from constantly showing their intimate parts to medical health personnel. As such, the body is experienced as a medical object that is being treated. This might be adaptive for patients during the medical procedures, but the process of reconnecting with the body once treatment is completed has not been a focus of study.

BREAST CANCER

The majority of research on cancer and body image has focused on breast cancer, a type of cancer that is closely related to sexual organ–related cancers in terms of physical and emotional impact. Breasts, as secondary sexual organs, do not limit the physical act of sex itself or interfere with fertility but are considered essential to femininity and sexuality. Partial or complete removal of the breast, scarring, or other alterations of the breast due to radiation (e.g., skin discoloration) affect a part of the body that is visible to the patient only when naked as well as in the context of intimate or sexual encounters (*visibility, stability*). Accordingly, extensive effects on intimacy and sexuality are reported among breast cancer survivors.[31] Many female survivors report feelings of self-consciousness and discomfort during sexual encounters,[51] shame,[52,53] or worries about reactions from sexual partners to their scars (*visibility*). The type of treatment has also been found to be important in body image outcomes among breast cancer survivors.[11] Breast cancer treatments often include surgery but vary from breast-conserving surgery to radical mastectomy (*visibility*). Chemotherapy, radiation, and/or hormone replacement therapies often accompany surgical treatment.

Studies have reported that women with mastectomies experience more negative body image or more body image concerns than those receiving breast-conserving therapies,[54–58] but the severity of surgical side effects may also play a vital role.[54] Even more fine-grained aspects of the mastectomy, such as undergoing a nipple-sparing procedure, appears to enhance body image outcomes.[59] However, although the effects of mastectomy are experienced as very negative, subsequent reconstruction offers an opportunity for recovery,[60] and more positive body image is typically found in women with immediate reconstruction.[61]

Given diverse findings of body image outcomes among breast cancer patients, considerations must be given to factors beyond treatment variables that can account for differences,[62] such as age, prognosis, or disease stage.[5,11,63,64] For example, younger women with breast cancer tend to report more negative body image,[11] and women with less severe forms of breast cancer (i.e., ductal carcinoma in situ) were found to report similar body image to healthy controls.[63] Personal characteristics such as body investment may also play an important role in body image dissatisfaction, such that women treated with mastectomy reported comparable body image to women treated with breast-conserving surgery if they had low levels of body investment.[65]

Other treatment side effects, such as lymphedema, are important to examine to better understand associations with body image outcomes. Although literature in this area is relatively sparse,[66] qualitative studies indicate that survivors' body image can be burdened by the presence of lymphedema. Other studies found no differences in overall body image between breast cancer survivors with and without lymphedema, but it was indicated that groups differed on some aspects of body dissatisfaction,[67] and that body image could be improved by physical exercise training.[68] See Chapter 10 for information on lymphedema and body image. Women with greater internalization of traditional gender roles have reported greater body image disturbance due to breast cancer treatment.[52,69] Additionally, patients of childbearing age who undergo mastectomy might experience the consequences as more detrimental if they desire children in the future (e.g., inability to breastfeed, higher risk for second malignancies). Finally, breast cancer, although seldom, can also occur in men and is associated with greater self-consciousness, shame, and distress[70] in part due to breast cancer being considered a "female" type of cancer.

GASTROINTESTINAL TUMORS

PHYSICAL CHANGES

Gastrointestinal tumors subsume malignant diseases of the digestive tract, including the stomach, gall bladder, liver, pancreas, intestine, colon, rectum, or anus. Treatments can be very extensive and diverse. Depending on the location of the tumor, side effects commonly interfere with either nutrition/diet (i.e., upper digestive tract) or digestion/fecal matters (i.e., lower digestive tract), causing various problems in physiological functioning such as eating, digesting, and/or defecating (*functioning, stability*). Most treatment side effects, such as removal of parts of the stomach/bowel are typically internal and therefore invisible, but they are marked by scars that can typically be hidden under clothes (*visibility*). Moreover, these physical alterations are irreversible and cause extensive alterations in the digestive process (*stability*). Many patients receive a stoma (e.g., colostomy), which can be either temporary or permanent (*stability*). More importantly, this procedure means that parts of the bowel and its secretions are placed in a bag outside of the body, although the bag can be hidden under clothes (*visibility*). Stomas require much attention as they need to be replaced/cleaned daily. Common side effects from radiation are irritated skin and bowels, which are often reported in relation to nausea and diarrhea but are in many cases only temporary (*stability*).

BODY IMAGE ADJUSTMENT

Many treatment effects of gastrointestinal tumors are related to disturbances in the digestive process and are associated with great discomfort, shame, and an experienced loss of dignity.[71] Diarrhea, fecal incontinence/leakage, inflamed bowels, self-consciousness about stomas, loud bowel movements, and associated body image concerns are common[12] and impair functioning across various domains. Generally, colorectal cancer patients with any postoperative complications (e.g., wound complications, infections) report worse body image compared to those without postoperative complications.[72] Patients treated with laparoscopic (vs. open) techniques report more positive body image,[73] but larger studies are needed. Research efforts have also focused on comparing cancer patients with and without stomas, consistently showing that those with stomas report more negative body image,[74-77] which does not improve[78] or even declines over time.[74] In contrast, rectal cancer patients with stomas also report fewer gastrointestinal problems and a higher health status than those without stomas.[79] The vast majority of rectal/anal as well as colorectal cancer patients report body image problems that are strongly related to problems with sexual functioning.[12,13] Given the extensive impact of gastrointestinal tumors on both romantic functioning as well as nutrition/digestion, they can also cause significant social distress and avoidance.

UROLOGICAL CANCERS

PHYSICAL CHANGES

Urological cancers include bladder and kidney/renal cancer.[a] Treatment for bladder and kidney cancers can be diverse but typically include surgery (i.e., cystectomy or partial/complete nephrectomy, respectively) potentially followed by adjuvant treatments. If cystectomy is performed in patients with bladder cancers, these are followed by any type of permanent urine diversion (e.g., construction of a neobladder, conduit, or pouch [*stability, functioning*]). Incision from surgeries are typically minimal to moderate (*visibility, stability*), but depending on the type of urine diversion, body alterations might be more visible: stoma bags outside the body (i.e., conduits), reservoirs under the skin and occasional catheterization to empty the reservoir (i.e., pouches), or neobladders that closely resemble the function of a bladder but are often related to incontinence (*stability, visibility, functioning*).

BODY IMAGE ADJUSTMENT

Research on body image of bladder cancer survivors is limited and samples are often small. Studies among bladder cancer patients typically focus on comparing the body image of patients with conduits versus neobladders. It is often assumed that survivors with neobladders have more positive body image, because the urination process closely resembles the natural process (vs. pouches/reservoirs that have to be emptied). Although evidence is scarce, more recent studies seem to support this notion.[80] While significant differences in body image between patients with neobladders versus conduits have been found within the first year postdiagnosis, both groups did not differ beyond this one-year follow-up.[81] Another long-term follow-up study (i.e., eight years) showed that both survivors with neobladder or conduits reported worse body image scores directly after cystectomy, which improved over time, but the neobladder group never returned to baseline.[17] These findings might be explained by the fact that many neobladder patients experience incontinence especially shortly after receiving the neobladder, which, in some cases, never subsides. This distressing side effect is known to induce shame and feelings of a loss of dignity. Accordingly, qualitative research has indicated the most challenging domains for bladder cancer survivors are changes in body functioning, body image, sexuality, and intimacy.[82] In addition, survivors with conduits versus those with different types of pouches do not differ on body image,[83] possibly because both techniques require emptying a reservoir. Interestingly, the type of surgery for radical cystectomy (i.e., open vs. robot-assisted) does not seem to be related to different levels of body image.[84]

Studies focusing on body image among kidney/renal cancer patients could not be found. Apart from immediate surgical side effects (e.g., bleeding), long-term physical alterations due to removal of a partial/whole kidney are minimal (*stability*). Typically the other kidney

[a]Please note that sometimes the term genitourinary cancer is used to subsume bladder and kidney, together with prostate and penile cancer. Given the direct involvement of the latter two on the physical sexual act and therefore its direct and indirect associations with body image, we believe their inclusion in sexual organ-related cancers is more meaningful here (see previous discussion).

takes over full functioning and effects on body image are probably minimal, apart from potential self-consciousness about scars.

HEAD AND NECK CANCERS

PHYSICAL CHANGES

Head and neck cancers subsume different types of malignant tumors around the throat, nose, and mouth/jaw (e.g., including laryngeal, oral cavity, or oesophageal cancers). These tumors often require radical surgical resection that can alter the appearance of the facial area and/or neck, which is highly visible to others (*visibility*). The extent of disfigurement from scarring can range from minimal to severe depending on the location and size of the tumor. Along with cosmetic alterations, these cancers and their treatment can also impair speech and/or swallowing depending on the tumor location (*functioning*). Speech and swallowing impairment can be considered a visible change because it is obvious to others when these functions are compromised. A patient's daily functioning can be extensively impaired (*functioning*) particularly in social arenas. Many of the physical changes due to head and neck cancers are intense and permanent (*stability*). Although reconstructive surgery can be used to minimize appearance alterations or functional defects, some degree of disfigurement or functional loss can persist (*stability*). Treatment of head and neck cancer can also include radiation therapy and/or chemotherapy, and in many cases patients may need multimodal treatment. Additional oral complications of head and neck treatments include mucositis (painful inflammation and ulceration of mucous membranes lining the digestive track), xerostomia (dry mouth associated with change in the composition of saliva or reduced salivary flow), osteoradionecrosis (which usually occurs in the mandible, where bone does not heal from irradiation), lymphedema, and trismus (lock-jaw, or tonic contraction of the muscles of mastication). These oral complications can range from being temporary and mild through more lasting and severe in nature (*stability*).

BODY IMAGE ADJUSTMENT

An individual's inherent uniqueness, and thus identity, is very much tied to his or her facial appearance. The physical alterations due to head and neck cancer and its treatment can come with great psychological burden. Increased research attention is being given to evaluating body image outcomes of patients with head and neck cancer, and qualitative methods are being used to investigate the process of psychological adjustment to head and neck cancer.[85–88] Observational and descriptive studies have confirmed the importance of considering body image outcomes for patients with head and neck cancer and demonstrate that head and neck cancer disfigurement is significantly associated with worsened relationships with partners, impaired sexuality, and clinical levels of depression and anxiety.[89–92] Body image difficulties are highly prevalent, as for example 75% of patients with head and neck cancer undergoing surgical treatment were concerned or embarrassed by one or more types of bodily changes they experienced following diagnosis.[93,94] Many patients have reported feeling discounted or stigmatized, are preoccupied with appearance changes, or avoid social situations due to changes in appearance and functioning.[94] Recently, two types of body image concerns experienced by head and neck cancer patients have been identified, suggesting that appearance distress and functional difficulties are fundamental areas of concerns for patients as they prepare for head and neck reconstruction.[95]

SKIN CANCERS

PHYSICAL CHANGES

Skin cancers (i.e., melanomas and basal-/squamous-cell carcinomas) can be found anywhere on the body and, depending on the location, may or may not be visible to others (*visibility*). Treatment includes surgery that could leave survivors with minimal or extensive scarring depending on the size of the lesion (*visibility*). For larger excisions, a skin transplant from another body part (typically, the leg) can be necessary for wound closure. Having larger scars (with or without skin transplants) may be especially visible in the summer time (*visibility*). If scarring can be hidden under clothes, it may only be visible to intimate partners or during leisure activities/sports. Yet the scarring is permanent (*stability*). Surgical excision might also have functional consequences, for example when skin has been removed from body areas that are frequently moved/stretched such as shoulders or ankles (*functioning*). When a skin cancer is located in the facial region, psychosocial effects might be similar to head and neck cancers. Finally, if lymph nodes are affected, these may need to be resected too, potentially causing other side effects such as lymphedema (*visibility*).

BODY IMAGE ADJUSTMENT

The impact of skin cancers on body image depends not only on tumor location and size but more importantly on the patient's subjective perception of resulting disfigurement. As described earlier, alterations due to skin cancers can significantly affect physical appearance and are related to dissatisfaction, distress, and/or appearance concerns.[96,97] The negative psychosocial impact might be more extensive if scars are larger than anticipated.[98] In addition, skin cancer survivors described worries about being in the sun,[99] which may also affect their social functioning. However, studies about body image in skin cancer populations are scarce.

BRAIN TUMORS

PHYSICAL CHANGES

Brain or central nervous system (CNS) tumors are commonly diagnosed in children, but many adults are affected as well. Depending on the age at diagnosis and type of treatment, effects of CNS tumors and their treatment can be very diverse. CNS tumors can be treated with the whole array of surgery, chemotherapy, and/or radiation, which can alter the physical appearance of the head (e.g., scars, alopecia) and may differ in their temporal stability (*visibility, stability*). Other treatment effects on the body can be hearing loss, loss of speech, seizures, chronic headaches, or endocrine impairments (*stability, functioning*). If patients are very young at the time of treatment, there is an increased risk for impairments in cognitive functioning and development (*stability, functioning*).

BODY IMAGE ADJUSTMENT

Studies about body image in CNS tumor survivors are scarce, perhaps due to late effects being typically related to (cognitive) functioning rather than appearance alterations. Available studies are often conducted among survivors of childhood cancer. For example, adult survivors of childhood CNS tumors reported more negative body image than the general population,[100] while problems with body image were reported by only 3 (out of 54) survivors in another study.[101] Interestingly, in adults with brain tumors, body image was reported among the top five concerns/needs for additional support.[102]

SYSTEMIC CANCERS

PHYSICAL CHANGES

This cluster subsumes malignancies of the blood or lymphoid tissues, such as leukemia and lymphoma. These malignancies are commonly diagnosed in children, but many adults are affected too. Survivors of hematological and lymphoid cancers may have difficulties similar to those survivors of CNS tumors, if they are treated with similarly extensive chemotherapy and radiation (directed to the head/whole body). Scarring is usually minimal as many survivors only have scars from a port which can be hidden under clothes (*visibility*). However, bone marrow or homeostatic stem cell transplants can immensely alter appearance in some patients but also the general relationship with one's body (see later discussion).

BODY IMAGE ADJUSTMENT

Overall, limited research is available focusing on body image in patients with systemic cancer, perhaps due to functional/endocrine rather than appearance alterations. In addition, studies including childhood or adolescent and young adult (AYA) cancer populations usually combine different groups of diagnoses and do not reports findings specific to systemic cancers. Nevertheless, it was found that adolescent survivors of childhood leukemia reported better body image than matched controls,[103] while poorer body image in survivors of AYA leukemia compared to norms has been reported as well.[104] Interestingly, one study showed that female leukemia survivors were not different from matched controls on quantitative measures of body image, but interviews revealed impaired body image in about 70% of the sample.[105] Additionally, the type of treatment might be important for potential effects on body image as leukemia survivors who had been treated with radiation in addition to toxic chemotherapies reported worse body image than those receiving chemotherapy only.[106] It was further reported that body image of young adult survivors of childhood lymphoma did not differ from leukemia survivors,[107] which seems logical given that treatments are rather comparable.

Bone marrow transplants (BMT) or *hematopoietic stem cell transplants* (HSCT) require extensive immunosuppressing treatments that precede the actual transplant. These treatments can drastically alter quality of life and have been described by survivors as a "violation to one's body" or like "being dead."[108] Some common immediate side effects include puffiness (due to corticosteroid use) or muscle weakness which can affect patients' feelings toward their body. Depending on the age of the patient, long-term effects on the body may differ. Particularly among survivors treated at a young age, many impairments have been observed in their physical development caused by endocrine and metabolic changes (often expressed in a short stature, delayed puberty, hypothyroidism, infertility, etc.). Yet, studies closely examining how survivors feel about their bodies are scarce. It was reported that BMT survivors had similar body image to other cancer patients, while both groups reported worse body image than healthy subjects.[104,109] In addition, survivors of adult lymphoma noted many appearance changes shortly after bone marrow transplant, which they felt had subsided over time.[110] In contrast, one longitudinal study found that body image scores remained the same from one-month pre-transplant to one-year post-transplant in adult patients with hematological malignancies.[111]

One particular side effect of transplants are acute or chronic graft-versus-host disease (GvHD), which are found in about one-third of patients treated with BMTs or HSCTs. Chronic GvHD was identified as the strongest predictor of adverse medical late effects and poor health[112] and can develop in the skin, liver, eyes, or gastrointestinal tract. Acute GvHD (typically rashes) and chronic GvHD of the skin (typically visible as irregular pigmentation) are often visible to others, which might be experienced as stressful, especially if present in the facial area, head and neck, or arms (*visibility*). However, studies are scarce and often include small samples. Yet it was indicated that survivors with chronic GvHD reported somewhat more negative body image than those who never or previously had GvHD.[113]

SARCOMAS

Sarcomas (including bone and soft-tissue sarcomas) are very rare in adults and more common in children. Many times they require lower (or sometimes upper) limb amputations and several studies have investigated body image among amputated survivors versus those with limb salvage surgeries. Findings reveal that survivors who received limb salvage surgery reported more positive body image than those with an amputation, while those with a "late amputation" (i.e., salvage surgeries were revisited and the limb was amputated after all) reported the worst body image scores.[114] However, another study reported similar body image among survivors with limb salvage surgery versus amputation, while both groups still reported scores below population norms.[115] In addition, 30% to 50% of all sarcoma survivors with a rotationplasty (i.e., a large margin amputation of the knee, where the remaining lower limb is reattached backward so the foot can function as a knee) reported negative effects of their surgeries on body image and sexuality.[116] Overall, survivors are likely to express concerns about extensive and visible alterations (*visibility, stability*) and feel the need to hide body changes in order to appear normal, attractive, and healthy.[117] In contrast, qualitative studies highlighted that survivors who had received limb salvage surgeries reported "excellent" perceptions of body image and physical attractiveness[118] and that overall body image scores improved over one year.[119]

OCULAR/EYE CANCERS

Eye/ocular cancers are specific cases of skin cancers (i.e., uveal melanomas) where survivors not only have to cope with disfigurement (e.g., loss of an eye [*visibility*]), but also impaired physical functioning (i.e., loss of binocular vision [*functioning*]). Studies on body image among these patients are scarce, but these survivors have been found to have difficulties adjusting to and accepting their altered body and appearance.[120,121] In general, the impact of uveal melanomas on body image may be comparable to that reported among patients of head and neck cancers (instead of skin cancers) due to the visible nature of body alterations in a socially significant part of the body (i.e., the face). However, there are other effects specific to uveal melanomas (e.g., visual hallucinations after enucleation)[120] that may also affect how survivors feel about their bodies.

CONCLUSION

Throughout this chapter, we have proposed and utilized a visibility-stability framework to explain a wide range of body image changes that result from various types of cancer and their treatment. We also demonstrated the central importance of considering functional changes and survivors' subjective evaluations as key aspects of body image. We provided an overview of the body image literature across the clusters of certain cancers, including sexual organ–related (including breast), gastrointestinal, urological, head and neck, skin, brain, systemic, sarcomas, and ocular cancers. While many of these cancer types have been underrepresented in the literature on body image and cancer, we can nonetheless conclude that survivors across these cancer types are at risk for experiencing difficulties adjusting to body changes.

At the outset of this chapter we raised a question as to whether a change to the body inherently changes a person's body image. This will clearly depend on the patient's subjective evaluation of the physical changes caused by the illness and its treatment. To the extent that these changes are distressing or a source of concern for the patient, they are likely to significantly alter the patient's body image. The patient's subjective experience of body image can help explain some of the diverse and at times contradictory findings regarding body image outcomes within a specific cancer population.

Although there are numerous studies concerning body image, few generic conclusions can be drawn. Many types of cancer are underrepresented in the literature, while the majority focus on patients and survivors of breast cancer. Nevertheless, numerous cancer survivors have difficulties adjusting to body changes due to cancer and its treatment, and this may be particularly true for the time shortly after diagnosis and treatment. Adjustment may improve over time, and, with that, body image can improve too, as long-term survivors (on a group level) report similar body image to their peers. Other generic aspects such as age at diagnosis or common side effects (e.g., alopecia, weight changes, etc.) may also play vital roles for survivors' body image. In addition to considering changes to body image as a consequence of cancer and treatment, a patient's body image may also be vital in treatment-related decisions (e.g., choosing between treatment options) or even refusing treatment.

Importantly, even if patients receive the same diagnosis and treatment, the impact on their body image can be vastly different. Considering the impact of cancer on body image as a function of survivors' subjective evaluation of the physical impact of cancer and its treatment could be useful for researchers to disentangle cancer-specific factors related to body image, as well as for healthcare professionals who can anticipate certain treatment effects and outcomes that may indicate which patients are at risk for body image problems.

Case Example: LaToya

LaToya is a 35-year-old woman with acute myeloblastic leukemia. She has previously undergone an allogenic stem cell transplant and has achieved remission. She is having difficulty coping with significant weight loss and "the new physical me." She spends a great deal of time worrying about her weight and has become consumed by dissatisfaction with the way her body now looks. In addition to the challenges she is encountering in coping with visible changes to her body shape and size, she is also highly distressed by less visible body changes related to chronic fatigue and low energy levels. These body changes have persisted for over a year, and she reports they are negatively affecting her functioning at work and her social life and have led to fights with her partner and problems with intimacy. Before LaToya was diagnosed, she and her partner had been talking about having a baby. Due to having to rush into treatment, LaToya did not opt for fertility preservation and has not been told she will most likely be infertile after treatment. Given all of her physical symptoms and body changes, she also does not feel able, either physically or emotionally, to have a child in the near future; adding additional burden to her relationship.

Case Example: Justin

Justin is a 70-year-old man with a history of squamous cell carcinoma of the left oral tongue. His treatment history includes left partial glossectomy and left neck dissection followed by postoperative radiation therapy. He presents for body image treatment because of concerns about changes to the quality of his speech and significant distress related to physical appearance changes to his neck as a side effect of lymphedema. He reports that his speech and appearance changes are significantly interfering with his social functioning. For example, he avoids family gatherings and feels very ashamed in front of wife but also does not want to share any of these feelings with her. He is needing to further manage his expectations at this point, as he anticipated these changes would be temporary but now recognizes that they are likely to be long-lasting.

Case Example: Ling

Ling is a 40-year-old woman with breast cancer who has undergone neoadjuvant chemotherapy, unilateral mastectomy (without reconstruction), and radiation treatment. She is scheduled for delayed reconstruction in a few months' time. Ling has experienced a large number of physical changes to her body from breast cancer treatment, which include temporary hair loss and peripheral neuropathy from chemotherapy, loss of a breast and visible scarring from mastectomy, and skin discoloration from radiation. In addition, she has developed symptoms of lymphedema. She has been engaged in body image counseling since the outset of her treatment, providing her with a supportive environment to discuss the manner in which these physical changes are affecting her daily functioning and emotional well-being.

REFERENCES

1. American Cancer Society. Cancer treatment & survivorship facts & figures 2016–2017. Atlanta: American Cancer Society; 2016.

2. Cash TF, Smolak L. *Body Image: A Handbook of Science, Practice, and Prevention*. New York: Guilford Press; 2011.

3. Rasmussen DM, Hansen HP, Elverdam B. How cancer survivors experience their changed body encountering others. *Eur J Oncol Nurs*. 2010;14(2):154–159.

4. National Cancer Institute. Survivorship definitions. https://cancercontrol.cancer.gov/ocs/statistics/definitions.html. Updated 2014. Accessed 2017.

5. Lehmann V, Hagedoorn M, Tuinman MA. Body image in cancer survivors: a systematic review of case-control studies. *J Cancer Surviv*. 2015;9(2):339–348.

6. Tiggemann M. Body image across the adult life span: stability and change. *Body Image*. 2004;1(1):29–41.

7. Miller SJ, Schnur JB, Weinberger-Litman SL, Montgomery GH. The relationship between body image, age, and distress in women facing breast cancer surgery. *Palliat Support Care*. 2014;12(5):363–367.

8. Pendley JS, Dahlquist LM, Dreyer Z. Body image and psychosocial adjustment in adolescent cancer survivors. *J Pediatr Psychol*. 1997;22(1):29–43.

9. DeFrank JT, Mehta CC, Stein KD, Baker F. Body image dissatisfaction in cancer survivors. *Oncol Nurs Forum*. 2007;34(3):E36–E41.

10. Myers VS, Manne SL, Ozga M, et al. Cancer-related concerns among women with a new diagnosis of gynecological cancer: an exploration of age group differences. *Int J Gynecol Cancer*. 2014;24(1):165–171.

11. Paterson CL, Lengacher CA, Donovan KA, Kip KE, Tofthagen CS. Body image in younger breast cancer survivors: a systematic review. *Cancer Nurs*. 2016;39(1):E39–E58.

12. Bailey CE, Tran Cao HS, Hu CY, et al. Functional deficits and symptoms of long-term survivors of colorectal cancer treated by multimodality therapy differ by age at diagnosis. *J Gastrointest Surg*. 2015;19(1):180–188.

13. Benedict C, Philip EJ, Baser RE, et al. Body image and sexual function in women after treatment for anal and rectal cancer. *Psychooncology*. 2016;25(3):316–323.

14. Champion VL, Wagner LI, Monahan PO, et al. Comparison of younger and older breast cancer survivors and age-matched controls on specific and overall quality of life domains. *Cancer*. 2014;120(15):2237–2246.

15. Clarke SA, Newell R, Thompson A, Harcourt D, Lindenmeyer A. Appearance concerns and psychosocial adjustment following head and neck cancer: a cross-sectional study and nine-month follow-up. *Psychol Health Med*. 2014;19(5):505–518.

16. Fan SY, Eiser C. Body image of children and adolescents with cancer: a systematic review. *Body Image*. 2009;6(4):247–256.

17. Hedgepeth RC, Gilbert SM, He C, Lee CT, Wood DP Jr. Body image and bladder cancer specific quality of life in patients with ileal conduit and neobladder urinary diversions. *Urology*. 2010;76(3):671–675.

18. Barrera M, Teall T, Barr R, Silva M, Greenberg M. Gender differences in sexual function in adolescent and young adult survivors of pediatric bone cancer. *Psychooncology*. 2009;18:S155.

19. Goodwin PJ, Ennis M, Pritchard KI, et al. Adjuvant treatment and onset of menopause predict weight gain after breast cancer diagnosis. *J Clin Oncol*. 1999;17(1):120–129.

20. Argilés JM, López-Soriano FJ. The role of cytokines in cancer cachexia. *Med Res Rev*. 1999;19(3):223–248.

21. Argilés JM, Busquets S, Moore-Carrasco R, López-Soriano FJ. The role of cytokines in cancer cachexia. In: *Cachexia and Wasting: A Modern Approach*. New York: Springer; 2006:467–475.

22. Ramos EJ, Suzuki S, Marks D, Inui A, Asakawa A, Meguid MM. Cancer anorexia-cachexia syndrome: cytokines and neuropeptides. *Curr Opin Clin Nutr Metab Care*. 2004;7(4):427–434.

23. Bennani-Baiti N, Davis M. Cytokines and cancer anorexia cachexia syndromes. *Am J Hospice Pall Med*. 2008;25:407–411.

24. Hinsley R, Hughes R. "The reflections you get": an exploration of body image and cachexia. *Int J Palliat Nurs*. 2007;13(2):84–89.

25. McClement S. Cancer anorexia-cachexia syndrome: psychological effect on the patient and family. *J Wound Ostomy Cont*. 2005;32(4):264–268.

26. Goedendorp M, Gielissen M, Verhagen S, Bleijenberg G. Development of fatigue in cancer survivors: a prospective follow-up study from diagnosis into the year after successful cancer treatment. *J Pain Symptom Manage*. 2011;45(2):213–222.

27. Kangas M, Bovbjerg DH, Montgomery GH. Cancer-related fatigue: a systematic and meta-analytic review of non-pharmacological therapies for cancer patients. *Psychol Bull*. 2008;134(5):700.

28. Servaes P, Gielissen M, Verhagen S, Bleijenberg G. The course of severe fatigue in disease-free breast cancer patients: a longitudinal study. *Psychooncology*. 2007;16(9):787–795.

29. National Comprehensive Cancer Network, https://Www.nccn.org/patients/resources/life_with_cancer/managing_symptoms/fatigue.aspx. Updated 2017. Accessed 2017.

30. Meeske K, Smith AW, Alfano CM, et al. Fatigue in breast cancer survivors two to five years post diagnosis: a HEAL study report. *Qual Life Res*. 2007;16(6):947–960.

31. Fobair P, Stewart SL, Chang S, D'Onofrio C, Banks PJ, Bloom JR. Body image and sexual problems in young women with breast cancer. *Psychooncology*. 2006;15(7):579–594.

32. Munstedt K, Manthey N, Sachsse S, Vahrson H. Changes in self-concept and body image during alopecia induced cancer chemotherapy. *Support Care Cancer*. 1997;5(2):139–143.

33. Da Silva GM, Hull T, Roberts PL, et al. The effect of colorectal surgery in female sexual function, body image, self-esteem and general health: a prospective study. *Ann Surg*. 2008;248(2):266–272.

34. Gopie JP, ter Kuile MM, Timman R, Mureau MA, Tibben A. Impact of delayed implant and DIEP flap breast reconstruction on body image and sexual satisfaction: a prospective follow-up study. *Psychooncology*. 2014;23(1):100–107.

35. Den Oudsten BL, Pullens MJJ, Van DS, Roukema JA, De Vries J. Personality and not type of surgery affects body image in women with breast problems. *Eur J Cancer Suppl*. 2010;8(3):82–83.

36. Hawighorst-Knapstein S, Fusshoeller C, Franz C, et al. The impact of treatment for genital cancer on quality of life and body image—results of a prospective longitudinal 10-year study. *Gynecol Oncol*. 2004;94(2):398–403.

37. Fingeret M, Reece G, Gillenwater A, Li Y, Palla S, Gritz E. A prospective examination of body image outcomes for patients with oral cancer. *Psychooncology*. 2009;18:S64.

38. Rhondali W, Chisholm GB, Filbet M, et al. Screening for body image dissatisfaction in patients with advanced cancer: a pilot study. *J Palliat Med*. 2015;18(2):151–156.

39. Skoogh J, Steineck G, Cavallin-Ståhl E, et al. Feelings of loss and uneasiness or shame after removal of a testicle by orchidectomy: a population-based long-term follow-up of testicular cancer survivors. *Int J Androl*. 2011;34(2):183–192.

40. Carpentier MY, Fortenberry JD. Romantic and sexual relationships, body image, and fertility in adolescent and young adult testicular cancer survivors: a review of the literature. *J Adolesc Health.* 2010;47(2):115–125.

41. Sekse RJT, Gjengedal E, Raheim MÇ. Living in a changed female body after gynecological cancer. *Health Care Women Int.* 2013;34(1):14–33.

42. Pinar G, Okdem S, Dogan N, Buyukgonenc L, Ayhan A. The effects of hysterectomy on body image, self-esteem, and marital adjustment in Turkish women with gynecologic cancer. *Clin J Oncol Nurs.* 2012;16(3):E99–E104.

43. Aydin Avci I, Altinel B, Gunestas I. Women's body perceptions and self-esteem before and after hysterectomy due to gynecological cancer. *Eur J Cancer.* 2011;47:S310.

44. Wortel RC, Ghidey AW, Incrocci L. Orchiectomy and radiotherapy for stage I-II testicular seminoma: a prospective evaluation of short-term effects on body image and sexual function. *J Sex Med.* 2015;12(1):210–218.

45. Gurevich M, Bishop S, Bower J, Malka M, Nyhof-Young J. (Dis)embodying gender and sexuality in testicular cancer. *Social Sci Med.* 2004;58(9):1597–1607.

46. Gilbert E, Ussher JM, Perz J. Sexuality after gynaecological cancer: a review of the material, intrapsychic, and discursive aspects of treatment on women's sexual-wellbeing. *Maturitas.* 2011;70(1):42–57.

47. Dessole M, Petrillo M, Lucidi A, et al. Quality of life in women after pelvic exenteration for gynecological malignancies: a multicentric study. *Int J Gynecol Cancer.* 2016;28(2):267–273.

48. Rossen P, Pedersen AF, Zachariae RH. Sexuality and body image in long-term survivors of testicular cancer. *Eur J Cancer.* 2012;48(4):571–578.

49. Taylor-Ford M, Meyerowitz BE, D'Orazio LM, Christie KM, Gross ME, Agus DB. Body image predicts quality of life in men with prostate cancer. *Psychooncology.* 2013;22(4):756–761.

50. Ervik B, Asplund K. Dealing with a troublesome body: a qualitative interview study of men's experiences living with prostate cancer treated with endocrine therapy. *Eur J Oncol Nurs.* 2012;16(2):103–108.

51. Fallbjork U, Rasmussen BH, Karlsson S, Salander P. Aspects of body image after mastectomy due to breast cancer—a two-year follow-up study. *Eur J Oncol Nurs.* 2012;17(3):340–345.

52. Esplen MJ, Toner B, Wong J, Warner E, Boquiren V. A group approach to address the influence of gender-role socialization and body consciousness on body image in breast cancer survivors: experiences from a randomized controlled trial. *Asia-Pac J Clin Oncol.* 2012;8:195.

53. Moreira H, Canavarro MC. A longitudinal study about the body image and psychosocial adjustment of breast cancer patients during the course of the disease. *Eur J Oncol Nurs.* 2010;14(4):263–270.

54. Collins KK, Liu Y, Schootman M, et al. Effects of breast cancer surgery and surgical side effects on body image over time. *Breast Cancer Res Treat.* 2011;126(1):167–176.

55. Reaby LL, Hort LK, Vandervord J. Body image, self-concept, and self-esteem in women who had a mastectomy and either wore an external breast prosthesis or had breast reconstruction and women who had not experienced mastectomy. *Health Care Women Int.* 1994;15(5):361–375.

56. Fang SY, Shu BC, Chang YJ. The effect of breast reconstruction surgery on body image among women after mastectomy: a meta-analysis. *Breast Cancer Res Treat.* 2013;137(1):13–21.

57. Rosenberg SM, Tamimi RM, Gelber S, et al. Body image in recently diagnosed young women with early breast cancer. *Psychooncology.* 2013;22(8):1849–1855.

58. Ganz PA, Schag AC, Lee JJ, Polinsky ML, Tan SJ. Breast conservation versus mastectomy: Is there a difference in psychological adjustment or quality of life in the year after surgery? *Cancer.* 1992;69(7):1729–1738.

59. Didier F, Radice D, Gandini S, et al. Does nipple preservation in mastectomy improve satisfaction with cosmetic results, psychological adjustment, body image and sexuality? *Breast Cancer Res Treat.* 2009;118(3):623–633.

60. Piot-Ziegler C, Sassi ML, Raffoul W, Delaloye JF. Mastectomy, body deconstruction, and impact on identity: a qualitative study. *Br J Health Psychol*. 2010;15:479–510.

61. Teo I, Reece GP, Christie IC, et al. Body image and quality of life of breast cancer patients: influence of timing and stage of breast reconstruction. *Psychooncology*. 2015;25:1106–1112.

62. Helms RL, O'Hea EL, Corso M. Body image issues in women with breast cancer. *Psychol Health Med*. 2008;13(3):313–325.

63. Bober SL, Giobbie-Hurder A, Emmons KM, Winer E, Partridge A. Psychosexual functioning and body image following a diagnosis of ductal carcinoma in situ. *J Sex Med*. 2013;10(2):370–377.

64. Male DA, Fergus KD, Cullen K. Sexual identity after breast cancer: sexuality, body image, and relationship repercussions. *Curr Opin Support Palliat Care*. 2016;10(1):66–74.

65. Kraus PL. Body image, decision making, and breast cancer treatment. *Cancer Nurs*. 1999;22(6): 421–427.

66. Fu MR, Ridner SH, Hu SH, Stewart BR, Cormier JN, Armer JM. Psychosocial impact of lymphedema: a systematic review of literature from 2004 to 2011. *Psychooncology*. 2013;22(7):1466–1484.

67. Martin SM, Hanson C. The differences in body image between patients with and without lymphedema following breast cancer treatment. *Occup Ther Ment Health*. 2000;15(2):49–69.

68. Speck RM, Gross CR, Hormes JM, et al. Changes in the body image and relationship scale following a one-year strength training trial for breast cancer survivors with or at risk for lymphedema. *Breast Cancer Res Treat*. 2010;121(2):421–430.

69. Boquiren VM, Esplen MJ, Wong J, Toner B, Warner E. Exploring the influence of gender-role socialization and objectified body consciousness on body image disturbance in breast cancer survivors. *Psychooncology*. 2013;22(10):2177–2185.

70. Iredale R, Brain K, Williams B, France E, Gray J. The experiences of men with breast cancer in the United Kingdom. *Eur J Cancer*. 2006;42(3):334–341.

71. Rozmovits L, Ziebland S. Expressions of loss of adulthood in the narratives of people with colorectal cancer. *Qual Health Res*. 2004;14(2):187–203.

72. Mathew R, Keding A, Brown S, Thorpe H, Brown J, Jayne DG. Quality of life following postoperative complications of colorectal cancer surgery. *Colorectal Dis*. 2011;13:11.

73. Polle SW, Dunker MS, Slors JFM, et al. Body image, cosmesis, quality of life, and functional outcome of hand-assisted laparoscopic versus open restorative proctocolectomy: long-term results of a randomized trial. *Surg Endosc*. 2007;21(8):1301–1307.

74. Sharpe L, Patel D, Clarke S. The relationship between body image disturbance and distress in colorectal cancer patients with and without stomas. *J Psychosom Res*. 2011;70(5):395–402.

75. Whistance RN, Gilbert R, Fayers P, et al. Assessment of body image in patients undergoing surgery for colorectal cancer. *Int J Colorectal Dis*. 2010;25(3):369–374.

76. Cotrim H, Pereira G. Impact of colorectal cancer on patient and family: implications for care. *Eur J Oncol Nurs*. 2008;12(3):217–226.

77. Bullen TL, Sharpe L, Lawsin C, Patel DC, Clarke S, Bokey L. Body image as a predictor of psychopathology in surgical patients with colorectal disease. *J Psychosom Res*. 2012;73(6):459–463.

78. Gervaz P, Bucher P, Konrad B, et al. A prospective longitudinal evaluation of quality of life after abdominoperineal resection. *J Surg Oncol*. 2008;97(1):14–19.

79. Bloemen JG, Visschers RGJ, Truin W, Beets GL, Konsten JLM. Long-term quality of life in patients with rectal cancer: association with severe postoperative complications and presence of a stoma. *Dis Colon Rectum*. 2009;52(7):1251–1258.

80. Gosh A, Somani BK. Recent trends in postcystectomy health-related quality of life (QoL) favors neobladder diversion: systematic review of the literature. *Urology*. 2016;93:22–26.

81. Huang Y, Pan X, Zhou Q, et al. Quality-of-life outcomes and unmet needs between ileal conduit and orthotopic ileal neobladder after radical cystectomy in a Chinese population: a 2-to-1 matched-pair analysis. *BMC Urol.* 2015;15:117.

82. Fitch MI, Miller D, Sharir S, McAndrew A. Radical cystectomy for bladder cancer: a qualitative study of patient experiences and implications for practice. *Can Oncol Nurs J.* 2010;20(4):177–181.

83. Hart S, Skinner EC, Meyerowitz BE, Boyd S, Lieskovsky G, Skinner DG. Quality of life after radical cystectomy for bladder cancer in patients with an ileal conduit, cutaneous or urethral kock pouch. *J Urol.* 1999;162(1):77–81.

84. Aboumohamed AA, Raza SJ, Al-Daghmin A, et al. Health-related quality of life outcomes after robot-assisted and open radical cystectomy using a validated bladder-specific instrument: a multi-institutional study. *Urology.* 2014;83(6):1300–1308.

85. Lang H, France E, Williams B, Humphris G, Wells M. The psychological experience of living with head and neck cancer: a systematic review and meta-synthesis. *Psychooncology.* 2013;22(12):2648–2663.

86. Henry M, Ho A, Lambert SD, et al. Looking beyond disfigurement: the experience of patients with head and neck cancer. *J Palliat Care.* 2014;30(1):5–15.

87. Costa EF, Nogueira TE, de Souza Lima, Nathália Caroline, Mendonça EF, Leles CR. A qualitative study of the dimensions of patients' perceptions of facial disfigurement after head and neck cancer surgery. *Spec Care Dentistry.* 2014;34(3):114–121.

88. McGarvey A, Osmotherly P, Hoffman G, Chiarelli P. Lymphoedema following treatment for head and neck cancer: impact on patients, and beliefs of health professionals. *Eur J Cancer Care.* 2014;23(3):317–327.

89. Gamba A, Romano M, Grosso IM, et al. Psychosocial adjustment of patients surgically treated for head and neck cancer. *Head Neck.* 1992;14(3):218–223.

90. Hagedoorn M, Molleman E. Facial disfigurement in patients with head and neck cancer: the role of social self-efficacy. *Health Psychol.* 2006;25(5):643–647.

91. Katz MR, Irish JC, Devins GM, Rodin GM, Gullane PJ. Psychosocial adjustment in head and neck cancer: the impact of disfigurement, gender and social support. *Head Neck.* 2003;25(2):103–112.

92. Rumsey N, Harcourt D. Body image and disfigurement: issues and interventions. *Body Image.* 2004;1(1):83–97.

93. Fingeret MC, Vidrine DJ, Reece GP, Gillenwater AM, Gritz ER. Multidimensional analysis of body image concerns among newly diagnosed patients with oral cavity cancer. *Head Neck.* 2010;32(3):301–309.

94. Fingeret MC, Yuan Y, Urbauer D, Weston J, Nipomnick S, Weber R. The nature and extent of body image concerns among surgically treated patients with head and neck cancer. *Psychooncology.* 2012;21(8):836–844.

95. Teo I, Fronczyk KM, Guindani M, et al. Salient body image concerns of patients with cancer undergoing head and neck reconstruction. *Head Neck.* 2016;38(7):1035–1042.

96. Atkinson TM, Noce NS, Hay J, Rafferty BT, Brady MS. Illness-related distress in women with clinically localized cutaneous melanoma. *Ann Surg Oncol.* 2013;20(2):675–679.

97. Noce NS, Atkinson TM, Hay J, Rafferty B, Brady MS. Illness-related distress in women with clinically localized cutaneous melanoma. *Pigm Cell Melanoma Res.* 2010;23(6):966–967.

98. Cassileth BR, Lusk EJ, Tenaglia AN. Patients' perceptions of the cosmetic impact of melanoma resection. *Plast Reconstr Surg.* 1983;71(1):73–75.

99. Stamataki Z, Brunton L, Lorigan P, Green AC, Newton-Bishop J, Molassiotis A. Assessing the impact of diagnosis and the related supportive care needs in patients with cutaneous melanoma. *Support Care Cancer.* 2015;23(3):779–789.

100. Hornquist L, Rickardsson J, Lannering B, Gustafsson G, Boman KK. Altered self-perception in adult survivors treated for a CNS tumor in childhood or adolescence: population-based outcomes compared with the general population. *Neuro Oncol.* 2015;17(5):733–740.

101. Dreyer ZE, Yan J, Carroll M, et al. Psychosocial well being in pediatric brain tumor survivors. *Neuro Oncol.* 2010;12(6):ii110.

102. Bunston T, Mings D, Laperriere N, Malcolm J, Williams D. The impact of psychosocial need and needs resolution on quality of life in patients with brain tumors. *Neurosurg Focus.* 1998;4(6):e7.

103. Maggiolini A, Grassi R, Adamoli L, et al. Self-image of adolescent survivors of long-term childhood leukemia. *J Pediatr Hematol Oncol.* 2000;22(5):417–421.

104. Mumma GH, Mashberg D, Lesko LM. Long-term psychosexual adjustment of acute leukemia survivors: impact of marrow transplantation versus conventional chemotherapy. *Gen Hosp Psychiatry.* 1992;14(1):43–55.

105. Puukko LR, Sammallahti PR, Siimes MA, Aalberg VA. Childhood leukemia and body image: interview reveals impairment not found with a questionnaire. *J Clin Psychol.* 1997;53(2):133–137.

106. Hill JM, Kornblith AB, Jones D, et al. A comparative study of the long term psychosocial functioning of childhood acute lymphoblastic leukemia survivors treated by intrathecal methotrexate with or without cranial radiation. *Cancer.* 1998;82(1):208–218.

107. Lehmann V, Hagedoorn M, Gerhardt CA, et al. Body issues, sexual satisfaction, and relationship status satisfaction in long-term childhood cancer survivors and healthy controls. *Psychooncology.* 2016;25(2):210–216.

108. Potrata B, Cavet J, Blair S, Howe T, Molassiotis A. Understanding distress and distressing experiences in patients living with multiple myeloma: an exploratory study. *Psychooncology.* 2011;20(2):127–134.

109. Molassiotis A, van den Akker, O.B., Milligan DW, Boughton BJ. Gonadal function and psychosexual adjustment in male long-term survivors of bone marrow transplantation. *Bone Marrow Transplant.* 1995;16(2):253–259.

110. Vose JM, Kennedy BC, Bierman PJ, Kessinger A, Armitage JO. Long-term sequelae of autologous bone marrow or peripheral stem cell transplantation for lymphoid malignancies. *Cancer.* 1992;69(3):784–789.

111. Caocci G, Pisano V, Vacca A, et al. Health-related quality of life assessment during high-dose chemotherapy and stem cell transplantation in patients with haematologic malignancies. *Bone Marrow Transplant.* 2011;46:S172–S173.

112. Baker KS, Gurney JG, Ness KK, et al. Late effects in survivors of chronic myeloid leukemia treated with hematopoietic cell transplantation: results from the bone marrow transplant survivor study. *Blood.* 2004;104(6):1898–1906.

113. Pallua S, Giesinger J, Oberguggenberger A, et al. Impact of GvHD on quality of life in long-term survivors of haematopoietic transplantation. *Bone Marrow Transplant.* 2010;45(10):1534–1539.

114. Robert RS, Ottaviani G, Huh WW, Palla S, Jaffe N. Psychosocial and functional outcomes in long-term survivors of osteosarcoma: a comparison of limb-salvage surgery and amputation. *Pediatr Blood Cancer.* 2010;54(7):990–999.

115. Eiser C, Darlington AE, Stride CB, Grimer R. Quality of life implications as a consequence of surgery: Limb salvage, primary and secondary amputation. *Sarcoma.* 2001;5(4):189–195.

116. Veenstra KM, Sprangers MA, van der Eyken, J.W., Taminiau AH. Quality of life in survivors with a Van Ness-Borggreve rotationplasty after bone tumour resection. *J Surg Oncol.* 2000;73(4):192–197.

117. Fauske L, Lorem G, Grov EK, Bondevik H. Changes in the body image of bone sarcoma survivors following surgical treatment—a qualitative study. *J Surg Oncol.* 2016;113(2):229–234.

118. Henderson ER, Pepper AM, Marulanda GA, Millard JD, Letson GD. What is the emotional acceptance after limb salvage with an expandable prosthesis? *Clin Orthop Relat Res.* 2010;468(11):2933–2938.

119. Sasidharan SM, Srinivasan V, Narayanaswamy K, Veeraiah S. Quality of life and functional status of patients treated with limb salvage surgery for lower limb bone tumors. *Asia-Pac J Clin Oncol.* 2012;8:126.

120. Rasmussen MLR. The eye amputated–consequences of eye amputation with emphasis on clinical aspects, phantom eye syndrome and quality of life. *Acta Ophthalmol.* 2010;88(2):1–26.

121. Brandberg Y, Kock E, Oskar K, Af Trampe E, Seregard S. Psychological reactions and quality of life in patients with posterior uveal melanoma treated with ruthenium plaque therapy or enucleation: a one year follow-up study. *Eye.* 2000;14:839–846.

CHAPTER 6

BODY IMAGE AND THE CANCER TREATMENT TRAJECTORY

Kerry A. Sherman and Laura-Kate E. Shaw

INTRODUCTION

An individual's cancer journey can be conceptualized as occurring in a number of stages, each of which present unique physical and psychological challenges. Detection and diagnosis of cancer may entail a combination of approaches from self- (e.g., skin cancer checks) and physician (e.g., for prostate cancer) examination, to routine screening (e.g., mammogram for breast cancer, Pap smear for cervical cancer), and other diagnostic tests (e.g., endoscopy for gastrointestinal cancer). Following diagnosis, active treatment is usually initiated, with the treatment approach and duration depending on the type, location, and staging of the cancer; previous treatment received; and the individual's medical characteristics and overall personal preferences. Importantly, not everyone's cancer journey is the same, as treatment modalities and dosage depend on cancer characteristics. Some patients are unable to receive cancer treatment due to extensive disease, and others experience cancer recurrence following treatment. Moreover, some patients have a strong family history of cancer and thus are at increased risk of developing a particular cancer type due to genetic risk—these patients may be offered a range of options for managing their risk such as risk-reducing surgery (e.g., mastectomy for breast cancer risk) and chemoprevention, if available, to reduce their likelihood of developing cancer in the future. Irrespective of the underlying cancer story, there are commonly experienced psychological and social challenges that reflect the changes that occur to an individual's body, in terms of appearance, function, and sensation. These challenges wax and wane across the cancer trajectory, reflecting both real and anticipated body image changes.

Body image disturbance arises when there is a perceived discrepancy between an individual's perception of an idealized body shape, size, and function and his or her actual body, leading to body dissatisfaction and the experience of distress.[1] This discrepancy can be exacerbated following surgery and treatment for cancer that frequently leads to disfigurement and changes in the appearance (e.g., loss of a breast following breast cancer), function (e.g., incontinence following bladder cancer), and sensation (e.g., pain) of one's body. Fear, shame, and embarrassment regarding one's altered body are commonly experienced, particularly when treatment leads to unfamiliar bodily changes and sensations and the feeling that one's body is "alien."[2] Bodily changes that are highly visible (e.g., loss of a limb from bone cancer; tracheotomy tube for head and neck cancers) are likely to further challenge the individual due to the inherent difficulties of managing social interactions with strangers so as to minimize feelings of shame and embarrassment.[3] There is extensive evidence linking cancer-related body image disturbance with psychological distress, both in the short and long term.[4,5] Aside from needing to adjust to a new post-cancer body, these bodily changes can serve as a constant reminder of the cancer experience and may heighten feelings of anxiety about a possible future cancer recurrence.[3] Accommodating and accepting the post-cancer bodily changes to one's self-concept is a key feature of survivorship;[2] yet this process is often difficult, frequently necessitating specific support and assistance in adjusting and accepting these changes.[6]

Over time, body image disturbance and associated psychological distress can impact other aspects of the individual's life, including sexuality and intimate relations[7–9] and personal relationships.[10,11] Similarly, early-onset menopause, decreased physical fitness, increased pain, or limited mobility can interfere with a variety of life areas including job productivity, leisure activities, house duties, sleep quality, independence levels, and general life satisfaction.[12] Even work-related activities may be negatively impacted by body image following cancer treatment. For example, individuals with head and neck cancer have difficulties and reluctance to resume paid employment following treatment due to concerns regarding visible scarring and eating difficulties,[13] and for urology patients' concerns about bowel functioning predict longer delays in return to work following the completion of cancer treatment.[14] This chapter provides an overview of body image–related concerns and challenges that can arise across the cancer trajectory.

CANCER DETECTION/DIAGNOSIS

The cancer journey typically starts with detection and diagnosis, which may entail a number of different procedures, many of which can be embarrassing, anxiety-provoking, uncomfortable, and at times painful.[15] For example, breast cancer screening mammograms entail a radiographer firmly pressing each breast between two plates on the mammography machine,[16] and endoscopy (used to detect irregularities in the bile ducts, stomach, and duodenum) involves inserting a thin, flexible tube down the throat and into the digestive system.[17] Although cancer screening and detection itself does not necessarily lead to body image disturbance, there is a growing body of research suggesting that poor body image negatively impacts on screening intentions.[18] In particular, body image disturbance has been associated with lower rates of skin and breast self-examination and reluctance to participate in screening for breast, colorectal, and cervical cancers.[19] Moreover, women who fall outside the generally accepted healthy weight range (i.e., BMI <18.5 or >24.9) are more likely to delay Pap smear testing, mammography, and clinical breast examination,[20] suggesting that appearance-related concerns may underlie this reluctance to be screened. However, body image concerns do not appear to influence men's testicular self-examination behaviors,[19] suggesting that there may be gender differences in the extent to which these concerns impact cancer detection behaviors. In light of these findings, women with specific manifestations of body image disturbances relating to body shame and body avoidance may be less likely to engage in regular cancer screening behaviors.[21] These findings have important clinical implications, and specific interventions to encourage screening attendance and overcome appearance-related barriers to screening of these individuals are warranted. Interventions that focus on diminishing body image concerns through cognitive and behavioral treatment strategies as outlined in Chapter 4 may assist in improving screening attendance in this context.

ACTIVE CANCER TREATMENT

Following diagnosis, surgery is often the first line of treatment for many patients. Surgery by its very nature is an invasive approach leading to acute and potentially extensive changes to bodily appearance and/or function (e.g., mastectomy for breast cancer; partial removal of the jaw or tongue for head and neck cancer; resection of the bowel and colostomy for bowel cancer). Typically, surgery may be followed by any number of active treatment approaches entailing radiation therapy (using high-energy rays to destroy or damage cancer cells), chemotherapy (using drugs to destroy cancer cells), and hormone therapy (using drugs to either suppress the body's hormone production on which cancers rely or block the effect of hormones on tumor cells). Increasingly, neoadjuvant therapy (including radiation therapy and chemotherapy) is being used as a first step to shrink tumors prior to surgery. For some cancers (e.g., breast, prostate), hormone treatments are prescribed for many years after surgery is completed.[22]

PRESURGERY

Not surprisingly, cancer treatment has implications for how an individual perceives his or her body, and concerns about body image may develop before surgery and active cancer treatment take place.[23] Unfortunately, these anticipatory pretreatment body image concerns can adversely impact the cancer treatment process; for example, female cancer patients' expectations and anticipatory concerns about treatment-related bodily changes and anticipated hair loss (alopecia) have led to chemotherapy treatment refusal.[24]

Anticipatory concerns about changed body image have also been shown to increase psychological distress prior to surgery taking place. In one study of head and neck cancer patients, 77% reported experiencing current and/or future appearance-related concerns related to impending surgery and consequent scarring, loss of teeth and hair, and speech concerns.[23] These anticipatory body image concerns negatively impact presurgical psychological functioning and are associated with increased psychological distress and low levels of postoperative coping effectiveness.[23,25] Presurgical body image–related distress is concerning, as there is extensive evidence that patients who experience heightened presurgical distress tend to have longer and slower recovery times and more postsurgical complications.[26] Clearly, experiencing anticipatory body image concerns not only jeopardizes the individual's self-concept but may have implications for physical well-being postsurgery.

Although anticipatory body image concerns have the potential to increase psychological distress, on the flipside, this anticipation may provide an opportunity for affected individuals to initiate anticipatory coping, preparing psychologically for these changes. A qualitative study exploring perceptions of hair loss in women about to undergo chemotherapy for breast cancer found that as the women were anticipating hair loss they were simultaneously engaging in anticipatory or proactive coping processes.[27] In particular, these women were enhancing their sense of control over the anticipated hair loss situation by pre-emptively engaging in emotional and behavioral rehearsal of the situation. Therefore, by encouraging the anticipation of body image concerns as a means of bolstering future coping approaches, it may serve to enhance, rather than detract from, the recovery from surgery and treatment.[28]

SURGERY

Given the invasive nature of surgery as a treatment approach, it is not surprising that individuals affected with cancer typically experience some of the greatest body image difficulties in the period immediately following surgery. These can be described as acute body image changes in response to the immediate changes that have occurred and may either resolve over time or develop into a more chronic concern.[29] Many surgical interventions can be disfiguring. Mastectomy, entailing the removal of a breast (or breasts) for treating breast cancer, is typically associated with greater body image concerns than for women undergoing breast-conserving surgery.[30] Following mastectomy, women have reported feeling less attractive and less sexually desirable, compared with women receiving breast-conserving surgery.[31] Gynecological cancer, which includes cancers of the cervix, ovaries, uterus, fallopian tubes, vagina, and vulva, can have a profound impact on a woman's body image and sexual functioning,[32] particularly for cervical cancer patients.[33] Body image concerns in these gynecological cancer populations are also associated with questioning of self-identity and distancing in intimate relationships.[34] Men undergoing surgical removal of their testes also report negative changes in body image and associated decreased erectile rigidity, sexual interest, activity, and pleasure.[35] Surgery for prostate cancer can have adverse impacts on body image, particularly due to penile shortening following radical prostatectomy.[36]

To a great extent body image concerns also reflect anxieties about being seen in public with post-surgical bodily changes. For example, bowel cancer patients who have a stoma (i.e., the end of their bowel brought out into an opening on the abdomen) experience poor body image, depression, and anxiety, particularly related to social situations and concerns about stoma leakage.[37] Similarly, survivors of bone sarcoma who undergo surgical treatment[38] report feeling the need to hide their appearance alterations (e.g., scars, hernias, skinnier legs, skin discoloration), as they no longer feel attractive and are unable to accept these changes.[38] Individuals who undergo surgery for head and neck cancers experience similar concerns of being seen in public.[39] Surgical treatment for head and neck cancer can entail removal of parts of the jaw, tongue, nose, or skin and have potential impact on the ability to chew, swallow, or talk.[39,40] As these physical changes occur in a highly visible and socially significant part of the body (i.e., the face), it is unsurprising that such changes profoundly affect a patient's body image. One study found that 75% of head and neck cancer patients reported concerns or embarrassment with bodily changes[41] regarding speaking, scarring/disfigurement, social eating, loss of teeth, and swelling and that as a consequence they avoided social activities.[29] Individuals with speech and eating concerns reported the highest levels of body image/appearance dissatisfaction. Moreover, head and neck cancer–related disfigurement is associated with feelings of shame, prejudice, and stigma.[42]

Brief Clinical Vignette

Jeff (54 years) is diagnosed with Stage III laryngeal (throat) cancer after he notices his voice often sounds hoarse and that he is losing weight without trying. Jeff visits his local cancer center and undergoes a total laryngectomy to remove his larynx. He has a permanent surgically made tracheostomy (stoma) in his neck and requires a speech aid to communicate. After Jeff is released from hospital, he has considerable difficulties adjusting to his previous routine. He avoids being around friends and family since his voice no longer sounds normal, and he worries people will not understand him. He is particularly fearful of returning to work as a part-time retail manager. Jeff's oncologist refers him to a psychologist to begin weekly counseling sessions to address his body image concerns. Jeff finds these sessions to be helpful for managing his anxiety about what others may think about him now that he has an electronic voice and facilitating his adjustment to his "new normal" following cancer treatment. Although he still feels worried and self-conscious of his stoma when he is around others, he is able to resume working and enjoys occasional social outings with close friends.

The extent of cancer surgery will moderate the extent to which an individual's body image is disturbed, with less invasive surgery typically minimizing body image changes. For example, there are more favorable body image outcomes for breast cancer patients who undergo breast-conservation surgery as opposed to mastectomy[29,43] and who have minimal removal of lymph nodes, compared with extensive node removal.[44] Similarly, women with vulval cancer who are treated with partial lymph node removal experience less body image disturbance then those who have complete lymph node dissection.[45] Better body image and fewer sexual functioning concerns have also been documented for invasive bladder cancer survivors who undergo bladder-sparing surgery and treatment, compared with those having surgical removal of the entire bladder[46] and with rectal cancer patients who undergo endoscopic microsurgery compared with total mesorectal excision, whose more positive body image is associated with less bowel dysfunction.[47]

To some extent, the negative effects of cancer surgery on body image may be minimized through reconstructive surgery, if appropriate.[48] For breast cancer, women undergoing reconstructive surgery after mastectomy typically have better body image postsurgery than those opting for no reconstruction.[48] Similarly, men who undergo surgical prosthetic implantation following removal of the testes for testicular cancer report greater body esteem.[49] However, reconstructive surgery does not guarantee better body image outcomes. Within the context of head and neck cancer treatment, reconstructive surgery tends to be required when patients have an extensive tumor requiring radical surgical ablation that affects critical facial structures. As such it is unsurprising that one study of head and neck cancer patients found that those who received reconstructive surgery were more likely to report negative body image two years postdiagnosis.[50] However, similar results have been reported with breast cancer patients where reconstruction is an elective procedure, such that women who had undergone breast reconstruction, or intended to have reconstruction, reported poorer body image.[51] Some consideration can be given as to whether individuals who opt for reconstructive surgery (when it can be elected and is not required for restoring form and function) may be more concerned about their physical appearance from the outset and possibly hold higher expectations for the surgical outcome, which fuels postreconstruction dissatisfaction. In support of this view, one study of women who had nipple-sparing mastectomy and immediate breast reconstruction found that higher levels of body image–related distress were evident in women with a high level of investment in their physical appearance.[52] Another factor that likely impacts body image satisfaction from reconstructive surgery is the aspect of time, as it generally entails more extensive surgery that may require a long period of appearance altering procedures.[53] Hence, reconstruction should not be regarded as a "universal panacea" for emotional and psychological recovery after cancer surgery[54] or as the only means of improving one's body image.[55]

ADJUVANT TREATMENT

For many individuals diagnosed with cancer, treatment entails not only surgery but a combination of other treatments including chemotherapy, radiation therapy, and hormonal therapy for hormone-sensitive cancers (including breast, prostate, ovarian, uterine, and kidney). The side effects of these adjuvant treatments also frequently involve direct changes to an individual's appearance and the way in which his or her body functions.

CHEMOTHERAPY

In general, quality of life of cancer patients treated with chemotherapy tends to initially diminish but then gradually returns to prediagnosis levels within the first year.[56] Regarding body image, although for many cancer patients initial acute chemotherapy-induced body image disturbances may resolve over time, this is not the case for all patients some of whom may develop long-lasting, chronic body image concerns, or for all treatment-related bodily changes.[57]

Hair is a key component of our physical appearance, being simultaneously public and personal and reflecting cultural norms and personal preferences.[58] The extent of hair loss varies between patients and by specific chemotherapy used, ranging from complete hair loss to thinning hair or patches of baldness. Many patients experience loss of eyelashes and eyebrows, which can be exceptionally distressing and more difficult to disguise than hair located on the torso or legs. Despite the usual impermanence of alopecia during chemotherapy, its impact is far-reaching; it is considered one of the most burdensome, traumatizing, and distressing aspects of treatment,[59] irrespective of the extent of hair loss.[60] Even when chemotherapy treatment leads to uncomfortable physical side effects, such as vomiting, hair loss remains one of the most impactful side effects.[61] Alopecia can impact body image significantly, with studies of breast cancer patients reporting that it often signifies changes in feelings of femininity, sexuality, and attractiveness; in turn, this leads to body dissatisfaction and poor adjustment posttreatment.[59] Breast cancer patients report feeling "unattractive" and "alien" upon losing their hair,[62] and male patients with testicular cancer similarly report that hair loss can denote a loss of attractiveness and sexuality.[63] Hair loss following chemotherapy has been associated with loss of self-esteem and a threat to self-identity[64] and a consequent curtailing of, and reluctance to engage in, social activities and employment.[65] Alopecia appears to be a particular concern for women,[24] perhaps reflecting the greater emphasis that women place on their hair as reflecting physical appearance and social identity[58] and, therefore, possible losses in aspects of womanhood and sexual attractiveness.[66]

In contrast, for some individuals, hair loss is regarded positively and as a sign that the chemotherapy is working.[61] Chemotherapy-induced hair loss is generally unavoidable, although there is some evidence that interventions such as scalp cooling (cryotherapy) may minimize hair loss and subsequent psychological distress.[67] One caveat regarding research on alopecia, however, is that the majority of this research has assessed the impact of hair loss as a secondary outcome, and not specifically on body image–related concerns; clearly, more investigations are needed that focus on the impact of hair loss on body image as a primary outcome.[61]

Another, less known, negative side effect of certain types of chemotherapy (e.g., anthracyclines, taxanes) and targeted cancer therapies is hand-foot syndrome. This condition is characterized by tingling or burning, redness, swelling, pain, and blistering primarily on the palms and soles of the feet, although it can more broadly affect parts of the body where tight-fitting clothing is worn, such as in the groin.[68] It ranges in extent from mild skin symptoms to severe and debilitating symptoms characterized by ulceration, bleeding, swelling, and pain.[69] Individuals severely affected will typically experience difficulties carrying out usual daily activities and diminished quality of life,[70] although no studies to date have specifically investigated the impact of hand-foot syndrome on body image. Since this chemotherapy side effect involves the hands, a highly visible part of the body, and is similar in appearance to atopic eczema and psoriasis for which body image disturbance is common,[71] it is likely that hand-foot syndrome will lead to significant body image concerns in affected individuals, although specific investigations focused on these body image concerns are clearly warranted.

Brief Clinical Vignette

Lori, a single mother of two young children, is diagnosed with bowel cancer at age 37. She had experienced rectal bleeding for three months prior to her diagnosis, and a subsequent colonoscopy reveals a large tumor. Lori undergoes chemotherapy for several months and experiences several side effects including hand-foot syndrome and hair thinning. Lori feels unprepared for the emotional difficulties she has upon seeing herself in the mirror and the debilitating nature of pain and discomfort on the palms and soles of her feet. She allows herself to be supported by friends and family, particularly when it comes to help with getting her children to and from school. Throughout active treatment Lori feels highly fatigued and is also fearful of how other parents will react to her changed appearance. Lori is particularly scared that her life will be changed forever and she will never feel or look like herself again. She finds her oncology nurses to be a wonderful source of support and encouragement as she goes in for her treatments, as they directly address and talk with her about her body image concerns. Five months later, Lori is pleasantly surprised that she is feeling more confident about her body image—her hair is growing back and her skin is starting to heal.

RADIATION THERAPY

Patients undergoing radiation therapy will also often experience many negative side effects that contribute to body image concerns, including skin changes such as discoloration, blistering, peeling, dryness, and itching at the targeted site.[72] As with chemotherapy, for many cancer patients the greatest impact of radiotherapy is felt at the time of treatment and immediately following completion.[73] Along with increased psychological distress, particularly anxiety, during radiotherapy, cancer patients frequently report decreased body image satisfaction at the conclusion of this treatment.[74] When used to treat cancers in the mouth, throat, neck, and upper chest region, radiation treatment can affect the oral cavity and teeth, causing difficulties with eating and swallowing.[75] Radiation treatment–related decayed and discolored teeth, tooth removal in the targeted area, and loss of oral function are likely to worsen disturbances in body image in individuals with head and neck cancer and are of particular concern for the increasing number of young patients who experience oral health complications from HPV-associated cancer. Moreover, facial appearance changes occur in a highly visible part of the body that is critical for one's identity and social interactions, yet it is an area that is difficult to hide from view.[75]

Radiation therapy to treat cancers in the stomach, lower abdomen, or pelvic area may lead to urinary/bladder symptoms, such as incontinence and/or diarrhea, which have implications for body image. For example, bowel cancer patients report a range of long-term treatment side effects including incontinence (39%), pad wearing (41%), and inability to defer defecation (78%).[8] Despite overall improvements in quality of life of rectal cancer patients, one-year postradiation or chemoradiation treatment, body image concerns persist and are associated with sexual dysfunction, particularly for male patients.[76] Women with gynecological cancer who are treated with radiotherapy also report poorer long-term body image than women treated with surgery alone.[77] Concerns about bodily functioning, particularly urinary and bowel incontinence, are strongly associated with poor body image,[78,79] which is exacerbated by the stigma associated with unpredictable bowel movements, particularly in social situations.[80]

Radiotherapy for a diversity of cancers (e.g., bladder, breast, lung, liver, prostate) frequently entails the individual receiving dark ink tattoos to guide the placement of the radiation beam for each treatment.[81,82] Unfortunately, as with any tattoos, these are permanent marks which serve as a constant reminder of the cancer experience, as well as impacting on physical appearance. One approach to overcoming these visible tattoo concerns is to use tattoo markers that are invisible to the naked eye using fluorescent ink that is visible only under ultraviolet light. One trial of women with breast cancer receiving radiotherapy[83] found that, compared with women receiving the dark ink tattoos, those with the "invisible" tattoos reported more positive changes in their body image up to six months following treatment completion.

Other concerns have been raised about the possible deleterious effects on surgical outcomes when radiotherapy is given postsurgery, particularly for women following breast surgery. Women receiving breast irradiation report faster deterioration and more prolonged body image disturbance and dissatisfaction with breast surgery[57] compared with women not receiving radiotherapy.[84] There is also a greater risk of delayed wound healing and postsurgery infection, which impact body image.[85] The adverse impact of radiotherapy is particularly relevant given that for the popular implant-based type of reconstruction there is an increased risk of capsular contracture, a complication whereby scar tissue forming around the implant distorts the shape of the breast. This complication has a direct and adverse impact on the cosmetic appearance of the breast reconstruction and is a key reason for breast reconstruction failure.[84] Capsular contracture has been associated with diminished satisfaction with breast surgery outcomes and body image. It is important to note that not every woman will experience these side effects and that many women are prepared to risk the possibility of these radiation-related complications in light of the potential gains in enhanced body image provided by immediate breast reconstruction.[86] Moreover, the use of partial, as opposed to whole, breast irradiation may lessen the negative impact on the surgical cosmetic result and the woman's body image.[87]

HORMONE THERAPY

Another type of cancer treatment known to impact body image is hormone therapy, entailing the use of certain drugs to block the effects of hormones for cancers that are hormone sensitive or hormone dependent, such as breast, endometrial, kidney, ovarian, and prostate cancers.[88] Hormone therapy has a range of appearance-related and general side effects that can impact both men and women including tiredness, hot flushes, weight gain, memory problems, breast tenderness and testicular shrinkage (men), labile mood, and hair thinning (women).[89] Women with breast cancer express concern and worry about the body image-related side effects of hot flushes and loss of libido.[90,91] Younger women are particularly at risk of experiencing adverse side effects of hormone therapy, physically and psychologically, as they are effectively experiencing premature menopause and need to manage the symptoms of hot flushes, loss of fertility, vaginal dryness, and weight gain.[92] This can present many challenges, given younger women are often at a stage in their life characterized by the cementing of personal relationships and starting a family,[93,94] and such bodily changes have been associated with diminished sexual activity and quality of intimate relationships.[90] Unfortunately, there is a paucity of research addressing ways to alleviate these hormone therapy–related side effects for younger women,[95] although one trial reported benefits in terms of fewer menopause-related symptoms, and an increase in sexual activity, for women receiving a cognitive-behavioral therapy and/or physical exercise.[96] However, this intervention was not found to provide benefits in terms of improving the body image of these women. The extent and type of hormone therapy–related side effects varies from individual to individual, as does the impact on body image,[97] but nonadherence to hormone therapy for breast cancer has been strongly associated with the extent of side effects experienced.[98]

Body image is also an important aspect of prostate cancer with men receiving androgen deprivation therapy (ADT) experiencing greater body image dissatisfaction compared to those without ADT.[99] Negative changes in body image occurring within the first month of receiving hormone treatment for prostate cancer have been shown to predict poorer quality of life up to two years later.[97] From a qualitative perspective, the impact of hormone therapy for men with prostate can has been described as having a troublesome body, and coping with the alterations may lead to feelings of loss of identity.[100]

POSTTREATMENT CANCER SURVIVORSHIP

Posttreatment cancer survivorship is defined here as the timepoint when a patient has completed cancer treatment with no evidence of active disease. During this stage, most patients will witness a cessation of temporary side effects that occur exclusively during treatment but may be faced with a number of delayed or long-term treatment side effects.[101] With regard to cessation of temporary side effects, skin irritations such as blistering, peeling, and dryness will typically resolve within weeks of treatment completion.[102] Chemotherapy-induced alopecia also tends to be short-lived, with hair regrowth rates typically returning to prechemotherapy levels within months following the cessation of treatment,[103] although some concerns may remain regarding changes in hair texture, form (e.g., curly, straight), or color (e.g., grey) compared with pretreatment.[104]

However, other treatment-related difficulties and side effects can persist long into cancer survivorship, becoming chronic concerns and hindering an individuals' ability to resume their precancer lifestyle and profoundly impacting their body image and self-perception. Many individuals who undergo cancer surgery are left with long-term, permanent disfigurements, for example scarring, loss of a breast(s), or a stoma. The degree to which body image is affected in the long term depends upon the type of cancer and surgery undertaken. Breast cancer patients tend to experience greater body image concerns in the immediate posttreatment period. For most individuals, these concerns subside and remain stable after about two years,[29] although approximately one in three women experience ongoing body image concerns post–breast cancer.[51] These findings are relatively consistent across most breast cancer surgery types (mastectomy with reconstruction, mastectomy without reconstruction, breast conservation therapy), with the exception of radical mastectomy which is associated with greater body image disturbance in the long term.[105] Similarly, in female anal and rectal cancer survivors, most women report at least one problem related to body image up to four years after treatment, with younger age and poorer sexual functioning significantly associated with body image disturbance.[106] Colorectal cancer patients with a permanent stoma are also significantly more likely to report negative feelings about body appearance compared to non-stoma survivors (25% vs. 12%) four years posttreatment.[107]

In addition to permanent physical disfigurement, many cancer survivors must learn to cope with long-term treatment side effects that impact body perception and overall quality of life. For example, some colorectal cancer patients permanently lose control of defecation functions as a result of surgical treatment,[108] with up to half of these individuals suffering from chronic diarrhea.[8,107] Rectal cancer patients undergoing an anterior resection (a sphincter-saving operation performed on the rectum as an alternative to a stoma) also report long-term difficulties with increased bowel movements, changes to frequency and urgency of evacuation, and inability to differentiate between stool and gas; such difficulties are associated with poor body image and low self-confidence.[8,9] Adjuvant postoperative radiation therapy, combined with chemotherapy, is being increasingly used for rectal cancer patients and can also significantly impact bowel functioning for a number of years after surgery.[8] Importantly, difficulties with bowel functioning can greatly affect an individual's ability to go about his or her daily activities, thus hindering efforts to resume a pre-cancer lifestyle. A qualitative study of patients who underwent surgical resection of their rectal cancer 12 months earlier found that individuals often felt stigmatized and avoided social situations due to embarrassment around the unpredictable nature of their bowel difficulties.[108] Head and neck cancer patients who undergo radiation therapy may also experience long-term treatment-related difficulties impacting on body image, such as permanent glandular changes causing an inability to secrete saliva, leading to dry mouth syndrome, oral infections, and tooth decay.[109]

Unlike chemotherapy and radiation therapy, hormone therapy is typically continued for a number of years after initial cancer treatment; as such, the side effects of this treatment can endure for many years. In breast cancer patients, this can involve a sudden onset of menopausal symptoms, including sexual difficulties (loss of libido and vaginal dryness), significant weight changes, night sweats, and vasomotor hot flashes.[22] These menopausal symptoms tend to be more severe among women who become menopausal from treatment, compared to those women experiencing a normal menopausal transition, due to the sudden onset.[95] In prostate cancer patients, hormone therapy can elicit similar sexual difficulties, including low interest in sexual intercourse, erectile dysfunction, and hot flashes whose spontaneous presentation can be debilitating, making the individual feel self-conscious and socially avoidant.[110]

Given that body image is an integral component of sexuality, it is unsurprising that body image disturbances following cancer treatment are associated with sexual dysfunction (see also Chapter 9). Total mesorectal excision surgery in colorectal cancer patients has been linked with long-term sexual dysfunction, difficulties in erectile and ejaculatory function in men, and dyspareunia (difficult or painful intercourse) and vaginal dryness in women.[8,9] Similarly, among testicular cancer survivors three years posttreatment, high levels of sexual dysfunction were evident in terms of reduced sexual activity (43%) and enjoyment (14%), erectile dysfunction (18%), ejaculatory problems (7%), and sexual discomfort (3%); each of these concerns were associated with body image disturbance.[111] In the long term, one in three head and neck cancer patients report substantial problems with sexual interest and enjoyment and one in four with intimacy.[112] Treatment for breast cancer typically affects parts of the body that are universally linked to female sexuality and womanhood (i.e., a woman's breasts and reproductive system), which may offer some explanation as to why body image difficulties are associated with sexual problems in this population. Women who are less satisfied with their body image are up to two and a half times more likely to experience sexual problems after breast cancer,[113] with approximately 83% of survivors reporting sexual difficulties three to four years after diagnosis.[114] Here, body stigma is significantly associated with sexual arousal, orgasm, satisfaction, and overall sexual functioning.[114]

Brief Clinical Vignette

Anne is 36 when she is diagnosed with breast cancer. She lives with her husband, Adam, and works as a personal trainer at her local gym. She is very invested in her body and takes pride in being fit and physically active. Anne opts to undergo a single mastectomy with immediate breast reconstruction using an implant. Following surgery, she undergoes six cycles of chemotherapy. After completing treatment, Anne has considerable difficulty adjusting to her new body. She is dissatisfied with the look and feel of her reconstructed breast. She has difficulty viewing her breasts and showing them to her husband. She is distressed that her breasts are no longer symmetrical; one nipple is completely gone and she has lost sensation in her operated breast. Two years following treatment, Anne continues to experience difficulties being intimate with Adam. Not only does she feel self-conscious about the way her breasts look, she is also experiencing significant problems with lack of desire for sex. Anne knows she needs help dealing with these problems but does not know who to turn to for assistance. She wishes a member of her healthcare team would ask her about these sensitive issues because she is too uncomfortable to bring them up on her own.

Another potentially long-term adverse impact of cancer on body image is due to treatment-related weight fluctuations, both weight loss and weight gain. For example, in oesophageal cancer patients, continuous weight *loss* has been shown to occur for up to three years postsurgery, with overweight patients being particularly at risk for malnutrition.[117] Importantly, across all cancer patients, weight loss of 10% of usual weight has been linked with body image dissatisfaction.[118] Conversely, weight *gain* is a common side effect of chemotherapy, especially in women who enter early menopause, and may persist for many years after surgery is completed.[119] Breast cancer survivors who receive chemotherapy are 65% more likely to gain weight compared to patients who do not undergo this treatment type, and the more weight a woman gains, the less likely she is to return to her prediagnosis weight.[120] Results from a review and meta-analysis suggest difficulty for breast cancer patients in returning to their pre-cancer weight, even when participating in moderate aerobic exercise and/or resistance training.[121,122] Postdiagnosis weight gain is associated with embarrassment about appearance and body image disturbance in this cancer population.[123] Patients with high levels of cortisol (due to either corticosteroid prescription or an adrenal tumor) also tend to gain weight in the face (Cushing syndrome), impacting significantly on body image.[115,116] In prostate cancer patients, BMI and waist circumference has been found to impact body image disturbance two years after treatment.[124]

Lymphedema, another long-term cancer treatment side effect, is characterized by chronic swelling caused by damage or blockage to the lymphatic system, rendering it unable to transport lymph fluid out of the interstitial tissues[125] (see Chapter 10). It is one of the few treatment-related side effects that occurs outside of the active treatment period and may manifest months or even years following treatment completion. Cancer patients who have undergone extensive surgical or radiation treatment to lymph nodes are at increased lifetime risk for developing lymphedema,[125] with lymphoma and cancers of the breast (occurring in 17%–21% of patients), gynecologic (20%), genitourinary (10%), melanoma (16%), and head and neck (up to 75%) at most risk.[126] As yet there is no cure for lymphedema, and affected individuals must learn to manage their symptoms on a daily basis. Physically, lymphedema can be debilitating, causing poor mobility and leading to significant pain and heaviness/ numbness in the affected area.[127] In severe cases, lymphedema causes extensive and visibly noticeable swelling. Finding clothing to fit the enlarged area can be particularly challenging and a great source of distress for many cancer patients. Head and neck lymphedema can involve external (skin, soft tissue of the face or neck) and/or internal (laryngeal, pharyngeal, oral cavity) sites; the former can cause reduced range of motion in the neck and shoulders, while the latter can lead to airway obstruction and consequent swallowing difficulties. Aside from the obvious physical difficulties associated with lymphedema, its highly visible and disfiguring nature means that it often has a profound impact on a patient's body perception and sense of self, being consistently associated with poor body image, reduced self-esteem and body confidence, and sexual difficulties across various cancer contexts.[128–130] As is the case for individuals with disfigurement arising from cancer surgery and treatment, those with lymphedema may become socially isolated and avoidant.[131,132] Younger women and those whose weight is outside of the normal (either over- or underweight) have been found to experience higher levels of body image concerns[133] and poorer social well-being.[132] Qualitative studies of individuals affected also point to significant stigma around lymphedema, which further exacerbates feelings of self-consciousness.[134] Women affected with breast cancer–related lymphedema have described their changed body shape as "ugly," "horrible," and "damaged" and noted that their altered appearance placed a significant strain on their personal relationships.[135] Poor body image in patients with breast cancer–related lymphedema has been linked with increased depression, anxiety, and stress[4] and has been shown to mediate the relationships between pain and body integrity beliefs and pain and depression.[136] While there is no cure for lymphedema, there are a number of strategies available to help manage its progression including manual lymphatic drainage, daily bandaging, skin care, exercise, and compression,[137] which has been shown to improve overall quality of life.[138] However, to date there is no evidence as to the impact of this type of therapy on body image of affected individuals.[139]

Brief Clinical Vignette

Mary is 58 when she undergoes breast cancer treatment. One year after her treatment, Mary hopes she is well on her way to resuming her pre-cancer life—she starts going out with friends more often, joins her local gym, and returns to her job as a receptionist in a medical practice. She is beginning to feel generally optimistic about her future. One afternoon, Mary notices her shirt cuff feels tight around her arm. Her arm feels heavy and somewhat achy. Mary makes an appointment to see her doctor who diagnoses her with Stage II lymphedema. She feels distraught and keeps thinking how unfair this is, given her traumatic breast cancer journey only a year earlier. Things progress to where Mary must now perform regular massage (manual lymphatic drainage) on her affected arm and use a compression garment daily. She feels frustrated as she is unable to carry shopping bags with her affected arm and cannot complete simple tasks such as hanging out the wash on her clothes line. Mary feels self-conscious at work and when socializing. She spends lots of time searching for and purchasing long-sleeved shirts that fit her arm to try and cover the swelling. She feels anxious and "trapped," unsure if her lymphedema will continue to worsen over time. Mary has just been referred to a rehabilitation therapist for lymphedema treatment. She felt comforted during the consultation session because this healthcare provider appeared understanding and sensitive to her body image concerns.

Managing the long-term difficulties of cancer survivorship and resuming a pre-cancer lifestyle can be particularly challenging and can take a significant toll on an individual's emotions and overall psychosocial well-being. Individuals may continue to feel uncomfortable in social situations and struggle with survivorship milestones such as returning to work. For example, breast cancer patients in paid employment report poorer body image and greater appearance distress compared with unemployed survivors; this likely reflects the increased exposure to social and public situations for women who are employed, who are unable to hide their changed bodies as easily as unemployed women who may be able to avoid such contact more readily by staying at home, out of the public eye.[140] An inability to adjust to bodily changes and prolonged body image concerns can also be detrimental to an individual's psychological well-being. Research indicates that approximately one fifth of cancer patients report clinically relevant depressive symptomology 6 to 10 years' posttreatment,[141] and long-term body image concerns in breast cancer survivors are associated with depressed mood,[142] anxiety, fatigue, fear of cancer recurrence, and impairment in social functioning and relationships.[51] Qualitative studies also suggest that women experience relationship difficulties during breast cancer survivorship, and unpartnered women in particular report that body image concerns are a significant barrier in forming future romantic relationships.[5,10,11]

BODY IMAGE AND RISK-REDUCING SURGERY FOR INDIVIDUALS AT HEREDITARY RISK FOR CANCER

In consideration of the short and longer term impact of cancer treatment on body image, it is important to consider the experience of individuals found to be at hereditary risk of cancer and who opt for specific risk reduction procedures. Genetic testing aims to identify whether an individual with a family history of cancer carries specific gene faults known to increase his or her cancer risk[143] and is increasingly available for many cancers including breast, ovarian, melanoma, bowel, and prostate. For individuals found to have a specific gene mutation(s), several cancer risk-reducing options may be available ranging from regular surveillance and screening to surgery and chemoprevention. For example, risk-reducing mastectomy and oophorectomy (ovary removal) may be offered to women with increased risk for breast and/or ovarian cancer and surgical removal of the large bowel for individuals at high risk of bowel cancer. As with surgical curative treatment for cancer, risk-reducing surgery will likely have implications for the body image of the affected individual.

Risk-reducing mastectomy usually entails the removal of both breasts (bilateral prophylactic mastectomy) and in many instances the nipple, areola, and surrounding skin. Women may opt for breast reconstruction following mastectomy, as well as surgical reconstruction of the nipple. The findings from research examining the impact of risk-reducing mastectomy typically reports that this surgery does not adversely impact physical and psychological functioning, including depression and anxiety, particularly beyond 12 months' postsurgery.[144] However, body image concerns are prevalent in the longer term, particularly regarding overall perceptions of attractiveness, embarrassment, and satisfaction with one's body and feeling sexually attractive.[145] Moreover, the average age of women opting for risk-reducing surgery is younger than for those diagnosed with cancer; hence, these women may face additional challenges in terms of bodily changes in the context of personal relationships.

Surgical removal of the ovaries (i.e., risk-reducing salpingo-oophorectomy) is another procedure that can adversely impact body image. As this surgery impacts directly on the female reproductive system, it is not surprising that sexual dysfunction is particularly prevalent in this population with more than 70% of women experiencing these concerns.[144,146] In particular, women who are premenopausal at the time of the surgery experience higher rates of sexual distress and psychological and emotional distress than postmenopausal women,[147] presumably due to the sudden onset of menopause due to surgical removal of the ovaries. Women experiencing sexual dysfunction following risk-reducing salpingo-oophorectomy are also more likely to report compromised and diminished body image and gender identity.[146,148] Persistent negative impacts on body image have also been reported by men and women who undergo surgical removal of the stomach (gastrectomy) to reduce hereditary risk of gastric cancer.[149]

As is the case with curative surgery for breast cancer, women who experience greater body image disturbance following risk-reducing mastectomy and salpingo-oophorectomy are more likely to experience regret about their decision to undergo this surgery.[144] Given the apparent lack of information about the possible adverse impacts on body image and sexual functioning following risk-reducing surgery, this finding is not surprising. Clearly, there is a need to provide patients with comprehensive information and psychosocial support regarding the likely outcomes of their risk-reducing surgery, not just in terms of cancer risk reduction and physical outcomes but importantly to raise awareness of potential long-term decrements in both body image and sexual functioning of these individuals.

SUMMARY

This chapter has highlighted the myriad of ways in which cancer and its treatment can impact body image. These effects have been seen to occur across cancer sites as a consequence of curative and preventive treatment approaches and vary in both their duration and type, impacting on the aesthetic, sensory, and functional aspects of body image. Of particular consequence is that cancer-related body image changes can have pervasive and long-lasting adverse impact on other aspects of individuals' functioning, including their social and occupational lives and personal and intimate relationships. There is a direct relationship between body image concerns in cancer patients and poor psychological adjustment and distress. As cancer patients come to terms with and cope with their changed body image, there is a need for psychosocial support to assist these individuals with bodily acceptance strategies.[6] Unfortunately, body image and sexuality concerns are rarely discussed in typical oncology and postsurgical consultations, possibly deriving from a reluctance amongst oncology health professionals who may feel inadequately trained or prepared to broach these issues with patients.[7,55,116] Furthermore, relevant support and interventions may not be routinely available within healthcare systems, and existing psychosocial care may be reactive rather than preventive.[150] There is clearly a need in the oncology context to increase aware-ness of these concerns amongst health professionals and to provide easy-to-implement screening processes to identify body image concerns held by patients early on in their treatment cycle. Referral pathways to health professionals who are trained to manage these treatment-related body image concerns, such as psychologists, social workers, psychiatrists, mental health counselors, and other allied health professionals, need to be developed and implemented as part of the standard oncology care pathway. Moreover, consideration of how cancer-related body image disturbance can be prevented is an important step in better managing this life-impacting side effect of cancer and its treatment. In sum, a greater under-standing of the body image–related difficulties that individuals with cancer face throughout the cancer treatment trajectory, and a focus on enhancement of their new relationship with their changed bodies in a cost-effective manner, could dramatically improve quality of life and facilitate psychosocial adjustment to body image.

REFERENCES

1. Higgins ET. Self-discrepancy: a theory relating self and affect. *Psychol Rev.* 1987;94(3):319–340.

2. Hefferon K, Grealy M, Mutrie N. Transforming from cocoon to butterfly: the potential role of the body in the process of posttraumatic growth. *J Human Psychol.* 2010;50(2):224–247.

3. Bolton MA, Lobben I, Stern TA. The impact of body image on patient care. *Prim Care Compan J Clin Psychiatry.* 2010;12(2):PCC.10r00947.

4. Alcorso J, Sherman KA. Factors associated with psychological distress in women with breast cancer-related lymphoedema. *Psychooncology.* 2016;25(7):865–872.

5. Przezdziecki A, Sherman KA, Baillie A, Taylor A, Foley E, Stalgis-Bilinski K. My changed body: breast cancer, body image, distress and self-compassion. *Psychooncology.* 2013;22(8):1872–1879.

6. Grogan S, Mechan J. Body image after mastectomy: a thematic analysis of younger women's written accounts. *J Health Psychol.* 2016;22(11):1480–1490.

7. Bartula I, Sherman KA. Screening for sexual dysfunction in women diagnosed with breast cancer: system-atic review and recommendations. *Breast Cancer Res Treat.* 2013;141(2):173–185.

8. Denlinger CS, Barsevick AM. The challenges of colorectal cancer survivorship. *J Natl Comp Cancer Netw.* 2009;7(8):883–894.

9. Guren MG, Eriksen MT, Wiig JN, et al. Quality of life and functional outcome following anterior or abdominoperineal resection for rectal cancer. *Eur J Surg Oncol.* 2005;31(7):735–742.

10. Shaw L-K, Sherman K, Fitness J. Dating concerns among women with breast cancer or with genetic breast cancer susceptibility: a review and meta-synthesis. *Health Psychol Rev.* 2015;9(4):491–505.

11. Shaw L-K, Sherman KA, Fitness J, Breast Cancer Network Australia. Women's experiences of dating after breast cancer. *J Psychosoc Oncol.* 2016;34(4):318–335.

12. Fobair P, Spiegel D. Concerns about sexuality after breast cancer. *Cancer J.* 2009;15(1):19–26.

13. Isaksson J, Salander P, Lilliehorn S, Laurell G. Living an everyday life with head and neck cancer 2–2.5 years post-diagnosis—a qualitative prospective study of 56 patients. *Social Sci Med.* 2016;154:54–61.

14. Cooper AF, Hankins M, Rixon L, Eaton E, Grunfeld EA. Distinct work-related, clinical and psycho-logical factors predict return to work following treatment in four different cancer types. *Psychooncology.* 2013;22(3):659–667.

15. Zavotsky KE, Banavage A, James P, Easter K, Pontieri-Lewis V, Lutwin L. The effects of music on pain and anxiety during screening mammography. *Clin J Oncol Nurs*. 2014;18(3):E45–E49.

16. Keemers-Gels ME, Groenendijk RP, van den Heuvel JH, Boetes C, Peer PG, Wobbes TH. Pain experienced by women attending breast cancer screening. *Breast Cancer Res Treat*. 2000;60(3):235–240.

17. Vitale GC, Davis BR, Tran TC. The advancing art and science of endoscopy. *Am J Surg*. 2005;190(2):228–233.

18. Clark MA, Rogers ML, Armstrong GF, et al. Comprehensive cancer screening among unmarried women aged 40–75 years: results from the cancer screening project for women. *J Womens Health*. 2009;18(4):451–459.

19. Brewer G, Dewhurst AM. Body esteem and self–examination in British men and women. *Int J Prevent Med*. 2013;4(6):684–689.

20. Fontaine KR, Heo M, Allison DB. Body weight and cancer screening among women. *J Womens Health Gender-Based Med*. 2001;10(5):463–470.

21. Ridolfi DR, Crowther JH. The link between women's body image disturbances and body-focused cancer screening behaviors: a critical review of the literature and a new integrated model for women. *Body Image*. 2013;10(2):149–162.

22. Ward JH. Duration of adjuvant endocrine therapy of breast cancer: how much is enough? *Curr Opin Obstetr Gynecol*. 2010;22(1):51–55.

23. Fingeret MC, Vidrine DJ, Reece GP, Gillenwater AM, Gritz ER. A multidimensional analysis of body image concerns among newly diagnosed patients with oral cavity cancer. *Head Neck*. 2010;32(3):301–309.

24. Trueb RM. Chemotherapy-induced hair loss. *Skin Ther Letter*. 2010;15(7):5–7.

25. Dropkin MJ. Body image and quality of life after head and neck cancer surgery. *Cancer Pract*. 1999;7(6):309–313.

26. Sherman KA, Winch CJ, Koukoulis A, Koelmeyer L. The effect of monitoring "processing style" on post-surgical neuropathic pain in women with breast cancer. *Eur J Pain*. 2015;19(4):585–592.

27. Frith H, Harcourt D, Fussell A. Anticipating an altered appearance: women undergoing chemotherapy treatment for breast cancer. *Eur J Oncol Nurs*. 2007;11(5):385–391.

28. Ouwehand C, de Ridder DT, Bensing JM. A review of successful aging models: proposing proactive coping as an important additional strategy. *Clin Psychol Rev*. 2007;27(8):873–884.

29. Fingeret MC, Teo I, Epner DE. Managing body image difficulties of adult cancer patients: lessons from available research. *Cancer*. 2014;120(5):633–641.

30. Arndt V, Stegmaier C, Ziegler H, Brenner H. Quality of life over 5 years in women with breast cancer after breast-conserving therapy versus mastectomy: a population-based study. *J Cancer Res Clin Oncol*. 2008;134(12):1311–1318.

31. Margolis G, Goodman RL, Rubin A. Psychological effects of breast-conserving cancer treatment and mastectomy. *Psychosomatics*. 1990;31(1):33–39.

32. Juraskova I, Butow P, Robertson R, Sharpe L, McLeod C, Hacker N. Post-treatment sexual adjustment following cervical and endometrial cancer: a qualitative insight. *Psychooncology*. 2003;12(3):267–279.

33. Mirabeau-Beale KL, Viswanathan AN. Quality of life (QOL) in women treated for gynecologic malignancies with radiation therapy: a literature review of patient-reported outcomes. *Gynecolog Oncol*. 2014;134(2):403–409.

34. Sacerdoti RC, Lagana' L, Koopman C. Altered sexuality and body image after gynecological cancer treatment: how can psychologists help? *Prof Psychol Res Pract*. 2010;41(6):533–540.

35. Wortel RC, Ghidey Alemayehu W, Incrocci L. Orchiectomy and radiotherapy for stage I-II testicular seminoma: a prospective evaluation of short-term effects on body image and sexual function. *J Sex Med*. 2015;12(1):210–218.

36. Savoie M, Kim SS, Soloway MS. A prospective study measuring penile length in men treated with radical prostatectomy for prostate cancer. *J Urology*. 2003;169(4):1462–1464.

37. Sharpe L, Patel D, Clarke S. The relationship between body image disturbance and distress in colorectal cancer patients with and without stomas. *J Psychosom Res*. 2011;70(5):395–402.

38. Fauske L, Lorem G, Grov EK, Bondevik H. Changes in the body image of bone sarcoma survivors following surgical treatment—a qualitative study. *J Surg Oncol*. 2016;113(2):229–234.

39. Fingeret MC, Teo I, Goettsch K. Body image: A critical psychosocial issue for patients with head and neck cancer. *Curr Oncol Rep*. 2015;17(1):422.

40. Teo I, Fronczyk KM, Guindani M, et al. Salient body image concerns of patients with cancer undergoing head and neck reconstruction. *Head Neck*. 2016;38(7):1035–1042.

41. Fingeret MC, Yuan Y, Urbauer D, Weston J, Nipomnick S, Weber R. The nature and extent of body image concerns among surgically treated patients with head and neck cancer. *Psychooncology*. 2012;21(8):836–844.

42. Costa EF, Nogueira TE, de Souza Lima NC, Mendonca EF, Leles CR. A qualitative study of the dimensions of patients' perceptions of facial disfigurement after head and neck cancer surgery. *Spec Care Dentistry*. 2014;34(3):114–121.

43. Fingeret MC, Nipomnick SW, Crosby MA, Reece GP. Developing a theoretical framework to illustrate associations among patient satisfaction, body image and quality of life for women undergoing breast reconstruction. *Cancer Treat Rev*. 2013;39(6):673–681.

44. Arraras JI, Manterola A, Asin G, et al. Quality of life in elderly patients with localized breast cancer treated with radiotherapy. A prospective study. *Breast*. 2016;26:46–53.

45. Novackova M, Halaska MJ, Robova H, et al. A prospective study in the evaluation of quality of life after vulvar cancer surgery. *Int J Gynecolog Cancer*. 2015;25(1):166–173.

46. Mak KS, Smith AB, Eidelman A, et al. Quality of life in long-term survivors of muscle-invasive bladder cancer. *Int J Radiat Oncol Biol Phys*. 2016;96(5):1028–1036.

47. D'Ambrosio G, Paganini AM, Balla A, et al. Quality of life in non-early rectal cancer treated by neoadjuvant radio-chemotherapy and endoluminal loco-regional resection (ELRR) by transanal endoscopic microsurgery (TEM) versus laparoscopic total mesorectal excision. *Surg Endoscopy*. 2016;30(2):504–511.

48. Fang SY, Shu BC, Chang YJ. The effect of breast reconstruction surgery on body image among women after mastectomy: a meta-analysis. *Breast Cancer Res Treat*. 2013;137(1):13–21.

49. Turek PJ, Master VA. Safety and effectiveness of a new saline filled testicular prosthesis. *J Urology*. 2004;172(4 Pt. 1):1427–1430.

50. Chen SC, Yu PJ, Hong MY, et al. Communication dysfunction, body image, and symptom severity in postoperative head and neck cancer patients: factors associated with the amount of speaking after treatment. *Support Care Cancer*. 2015;23(8):2375–2382.

51. Falk Dahl CA, Reinertsen KV, Nesvold IL, Fossa SD, Dahl AA. A study of body image in long-term breast cancer survivors. *Cancer*. 2010;116(15):3549–3557.

52. Sherman KA, Woon S, French J, Elder E. Body image and psychological distress in nipple-sparing mastectomy: the roles of self-compassion and appearance investment. *Psychooncology*. 2017;26(3):337–345.

53. Chua A, DeSantis S, Teo I, Fingeret M. Body image investment in breast cancer patients undergoing reconstruction: taking a closer look at the Appearance Schemas Inventory Revised. *Body Image*. 2015;13:33–37.

54. Sheehan J, Sherman K, Lam T, Boyages J. Regret associated with the decision for breast reconstruction: the association of negative body image, distress and surgery characteristics with decision regret. *Psychology Health*. 2008;23(2):207–219.

55. Jorgensen L, Garne J, Sogaard M, Laursen B. The experience of distress in relation to surgical treatment and care for breast cancer: an interview study. *Eur J Oncol Nurs*. 2015;19:612–618.

56. Lam WW, Soong I, Yau TK, et al. The evolution of psychological distress trajectories in women diagnosed with advanced breast cancer: a longitudinal study. *Psychooncology*. 2013;22(12):2831–2839.

57. Hamidou Z, Dabakuyo-Yonli TS, Guillemin F, et al. Impact of response shift on time to deterioration in quality of life scores in breast cancer patients. *PLoS One*. 2014;9(5):e96848.

58. Weitz T, Estes CL. Adding aging and gender to the women's health agenda. *J Women Aging*. 2001;13(2):3–20.

59. Choi EK, Kim IR, Chang O, et al. Impact of chemotherapy-induced alopecia distress on body image, psychosocial well-being, and depression in breast cancer patients. *Psychooncology*. 2014;23(10):1103–1110.

60. Lindley C, McCune JS, Thomason TE, et al. Perception of chemotherapy side effects cancer versus noncancer patients. *Cancer Practice*. 1999;7(2):59–65.

61. Lemieux J, Maunsell E, Provencher L. Chemotherapy-induced alopecia and effects on quality of life among women with breast cancer: a literature review. *Psychooncology*. 2008;17(4):317–328.

62. Frith H, Harcourt D, Fussell A. Anticipating an altered appearance: women undergoing chemotherapy treatment for breast cancer. *Eur J Oncol Nurs*. 2007;11(5):385–391.

63. Kuzbit, P. The importance of hair. *Cancer Nurs Pract*. 2004;3(8):10–13.

64. Williams J, Wood C, Cunningham-Warburton P. A narrative study of chemotherapy-induced alopecia. *Oncol Nurs Forum*. 1999;26(9):1463–1468.

65. Luoma ML, Hakamies-Blomqvist L. The meaning of quality of life in patients being treated for advanced breast cancer: a qualitative study. *Psychooncology*. 2004;13(10):729–739.

66. Helms RL, O'Hea EL, Corso M. Body image issues in women with breast cancer. *Psychol Health Med*. 2008;13(3):313–325.

67. Protière C, Evans K, Camerlo J, et al. Efficacy and tolerance of a scalp-cooling system for prevention of hair loss and the experience of breast cancer patients treated by adjuvant chemotherapy. *Support Care Cancer*. 2002;10(7):529–537.

68. Degen A, Alter M, Schenck F, et al. The hand-foot-syndrome associated with medical tumor therapy—classification and management. *J Deutschen Dermatologischen Gesellschaft = J German Society Dermatol*. 2010;8(9):652–661.

69. Miller KK, Gorcey L, McLellan BN. Chemotherapy-induced hand-foot syndrome and nail changes: a review of clinical presentation, etiology, pathogenesis, and management. *J Am Acad Dermatol*. 71(4):787–794.

70. Sibaud V, Dalenc F, Chevreau C, et al. HFS-14, a specific quality of life scale developed for patients suffering from hand–foot syndrome. *Oncologist*. 2011;16(10):1469–1478.

71. Khoury LR, Danielsen PL, Skiveren J. Body image altered by psoriasis. a study based on individual interviews and a model for body image. *J Dermatolog Treat*. 2014;25(1):2–7.

72. Collen EB, Mayer MN. Acute effects of radiation treatment: skin reactions. *Can Vet J*. 2006;47(9):931–935.

73. Marijnen CA, Kapiteijn E, van de Velde CJ, et al. Acute side effects and complications after short-term preoperative radiotherapy combined with total mesorectal excision in primary rectal cancer: report of a multicenter randomized trial. *J Clin Oncol*. 2002;20(3):817–825.

74. Versmessen H, Vinh-Hung V, Van Parijs H, et al. Health-related quality of life in survivors of stage I-II breast cancer: randomized trial of post-operative conventional radiotherapy and hypofractionated tomotherapy. *BMC Cancer*. 2012;12:495.

75. Deng J, Jackson L, Epstein JB, Migliorati CA, Murphy BA. Dental demineralization and caries in patients with head and neck cancer. *Oral Oncol*. 2015;51(9):824–831.

76. McLachlan S-A, Fisher RJ, Zalcberg J, et al. The impact on health-related quality of life in the first 12 months: a randomised comparison of preoperative short-course radiation versus long-course chemoradiation for T3 rectal cancer (Trans-Tasman Radiation Oncology Group Trial 01.04). *Eur J Cancer*. 2016;55:15–26.

77. Korfage IJ, Essink-Bot ML, Mols F, van de Poll-Franse L, Kruitwagen R, van Ballegooijen M. Health-related quality of life in cervical cancer survivors: a population-based survey. *Int J Radiat Oncol Biol Phys.* 2009;73(5):1501–1509.

78. Lezoche E, Paganini AM, Fabiani B, et al. Quality-of-life impairment after endoluminal locoregional resection and laparoscopic total mesorectal excision. *Surg Endoscopy.* 2014;28(1):227–234.

79. Sclafani F, Peckitt C, Cunningham D, et al. Short- and long-term quality of life and bowel function in patients with MRI-defined, high-risk, locally advanced rectal cancer treated with an intensified neoadjuvant strategy in the randomized phase 2 EXPERT-C trial. *Int J Radiat Oncol Biol Phys.* 2015;93(2):303–312.

80. Dancey CP, Hutton-Young SA, Moye S, Devins GM. Perceived stigma, illness intrusiveness and quality of life in men and women with irritable bowel syndrome. *Psychology Health Med.* 2002;7(4):381–395.

81. Elsner K, Francis K, Hruby G, Roderick S. Quality improvement process to assess tattoo alignment, set-up accuracy and isocentre reproducibility in pelvic radiotherapy patients. *J Med Radiation Sci.* 2014;61(4):246–252.

82. Foster R, Meyer J, Iyengar P, et al. Localization accuracy and immobilization effectiveness of a stereotactic body frame for a variety of treatment sites. *Int J Radiat Oncol Biol Phys.* 2013;87(5):911–916.

83. Landeg SJ, Kirby AM, Lee SF, et al. A randomized control trial evaluating fluorescent ink versus dark ink tattoos for breast radiotherapy. *Br J Radiology.* 2016;89(1068):20160288.

84. Cordeiro PG, Albornoz CR, McCormick B, Hu Q, Van Zee K. The impact of postmastectomy radiotherapy on two-stage implant breast reconstruction: an analysis of long-term surgical outcomes, aesthetic results, and satisfaction over 13 years. *Plastic Reconstruct Surg.* 2014;134(4):588–595.

85. Haubner F, Ohmann E, Pohl F, et al. Wound healing after radiation therapy: review of the literature. *Radiation Oncol.* 2012;7(1):162

86. Brennan ME, Flitcroft K, Warrier S, Snook K, Spillane AJ. Immediate expander/implant breast reconstruction followed by post-mastectomy radiotherapy for breast cancer: aesthetic, surgical, satisfaction and quality of life outcomes in women with high-risk breast cancer. *Breast.* 2016;30:59–65.

87. Perrucci E, Lancellotta V, Bini V, et al. Quality of life and cosmesis after breast cancer: whole breast radiotherapy vs partial breast high-dose-rate brachytherapy. *Tumori.* 2015;101(2):161–167.

88. Li, Pan Z, Gao KUN, et al. Impact of post-operative hormone replacement therapy on life quality and prognosis in patients with ovarian malignancy. *Oncol Lett.* 2012;3(1):244–249.

89. Cancer Research UK. General side effects of hormone therapy 2014; http://www.cancerresearchuk.org/about-cancer/cancers-in-general/treatment/hormone/general-side-effects-of-hormone-therapy -5HmgGYLsWOKEXHI0.99eneral side effects hormone therapy - women.

90. Biglia N, Moggio G, Peano E, et al. Effects of surgical and adjuvant therapies for breast cancer on sexuality, cognitive functions, and body weight. *J Sex Med.* 2010;7(5):1891–1900.

91. Hunter MS, Grunfeld EA, Mittal S, et al. Menopausal symptoms in women with breast cancer: prevalence and treatment preferences. *Psychooncology.* 2004;13(11):769–778.

92. Rosenberg SM, Tamimi RM, Gelber S, et al. Body image in recently diagnosed young women with early breast cancer. *Psychooncology.* 2013;22(8):1849–1855.

93. Hopwood P, Haviland J, Mills J, Sumo G, J MB. The impact of age and clinical factors on quality of life in early breast cancer: an analysis of 2208 women recruited to the UK START Trial (Standardisation of Breast Radiotherapy Trial). *Breast.* 2007;16(3):241–251.

94. Paterson CL, Lengacher CA, Donovan KA, Kip KE, Tofthagen CS. Body image in younger breast cancer survivors: a systematic review. *Cancer Nurs.* 2016;39(1):E39–E58.

95. Rosenberg SM, Partridge AH. Premature menopause in young breast cancer: Effects on quality of life and treatment interventions. *J Thorac Dis.* 2013;5(Suppl. 1):S55–S61.

96. Duijts SF, Stolk-Vos AC, Oldenburg HS, van Beurden M, Aaronson NK. Characteristics of breast cancer patients who experience menopausal transition due to treatment. *Climacteric.* 2011;14(3):362–368.

97. Taylor-Ford M, Meyerowitz BE, D'Orazio LM, Christie KM, Gross ME, Agus DB. Body image predicts quality of life in men with prostate cancer. *Psychooncology*. 2013;22(4):756–761.

98. Wouters H, Stiggelbout AM, Bouvy ML, et al. Endocrine therapy for breast cancer: assessing an array of women's treatment experiences and perceptions, their perceived self-efficacy and nonadherence. *Clin Breast Cancer*. 2014;14(6):460–467.e462.

99. Harrington JM, Jones EG, Badger T. Body image perceptions in men with prostate cancer. *Oncol Nurs Forum*. 2009;36(2):167–172.

100. Ervik B, Asplund K. Dealing with a troublesome body: a qualitative interview study of men's experiences living with prostate cancer treated with endocrine therapy. *Eur J Oncol Nurs*. 2012;16(2):103–108.

101. Dirven L, van de Poll-Franse LV, Aaronson NK, Reijneveld JC. Controversies in defining cancer survivorship. *Lancet Oncol*. 16(6):610–612.

102. Qiao J, Fang H. Hand-foot syndrome related to chemotherapy. *CMAJ*. 2012;184(15):E818–E818.

103. Kanti V, Nuwayhid R, Lindner J, et al. Analysis of quantitative changes in hair growth during treatment with chemotherapy or tamoxifen in patients with breast cancer: a cohort study. *Br J Dermatol*. 2014;170(3):643–650.

104. Roe H. Chemotherapy-induced alopecia: advice and support for hair loss. *Br J Nurs*. 2011;20(10):S4–S11.

105. Parker PA, Youssef A, Walker S, et al. Short-term and long-term psychosocial adjustment and quality of life in women undergoing different surgical procedures for breast cancer. *Ann Surg Oncol*. 2007;14(11):3078–3089.

106. Benedict C, Philip EJ, Baser RE, et al. Body image and sexual function in women after treatment for anal and rectal cancer. *Psychooncology*. 2016;25(3):316–323.

107. Schneider EC, Malin JL, Kahn KL, Ko CY, Adams J, Epstein AM. Surviving colorectal cancer: patient-reported symptoms 4 years after diagnosis. *Cancer*. 2007;110(9):2075–2082.

108. DeSnoo L, Faithfull S. A qualitative study of anterior resection syndrome: the experiences of cancer survivors who have undergone resection surgery. *Eur J Cancer Care*. 2006;15(3):244–251.

109. Tolentino E, Centurion BS, Ferreira LHC, de Souza AP, Damante JH, Rubira-Bullen IRF. Oral adverse effects of head and neck radiotherapy: literature review and suggestion of a clinical oral care guideline for irradiated patients. *J Applied Oral Sci*. 2011;19(5):448–454.

110. Kumar RJ, Barqawi A, Crawford ED. Adverse events associated with hormonal therapy for prostate cancer. *Rev Urology*. 2005;7(Suppl. 5):S37–S43.

111. Rossen P, Pedersen AF, Zachariae R, von der Maase H. Sexuality and body image in long-term survivors of testicular cancer. *Eur J Cancer*. 2012;48(4):571–578.

112. Low C, Fullarton M, Parkinson E, et al. Issues of intimacy and sexual dysfunction following major head and neck cancer treatment. *Oral Oncology*. 2009;45(10):898–903.

113. Panjari M, Bell RJ, Davis SR. Sexual function after breast cancer. *J Sex Med*. 2011;8(1):294–302.

114. Boquiren VM, Esplen MJ, Wong J, Toner B, Warner E, Malik N. Sexual functioning in breast cancer survivors experiencing body image disturbance. *Psychooncology*. 2016;25(1):66–76.

115. Alcalar N, Ozkan S, Kadioglu P, et al. Evaluation of depression, quality of life and body image in patients with Cushing's disease. *Pituitary*. 2013;16(3):333–340.

116. Bartula I, Sherman KA. Development and validation of the Female Sexual Function Index adaptation for breast cancer patients (FSFI-BC). *Breast Cancer Res Treat*. 2015;152(3):477–488.

117. Stratakis C. Cushing syndrome caused by adrenocortical tumors and hyperplasias (corticotrophin-independent Cushing syndrome). *Endocrine Develop*. 2008;13:117–132.

118. Rhondali W, Chisholm GB, Daneshmand M, et al. Association between body image dissatisfaction and weight loss among patients with advanced cancer and their caregivers: a preliminary report. *J Pain Symptom Manage*. 2013;45(6):1039–1049.

119. Makari-Judson G, Judson CH, Mertens WC. Longitudinal patterns of weight gain after breast cancer diagnosis: observations beyond the first year. *Breast J*. 2007;13(3):258–265.

120. Saquib N, Flatt SW, Natarajan L, et al. Weight gain and recovery of pre-cancer weight after breast cancer treatments: evidence from the Women's Healthy Eating and Living (WHEL) study. *Breast Cancer Res Treat*. 2007;105(2):177–186.

121. Kim CJ, Kang DH, Park JW. A meta-analysis of aerobic exercise interventions for women with breast cancer. *West J Nurs Res*. 2009;31(4):437–461.

122. De Backer IC, Schep G, Backx FJ, Vreugdenhil G, Kuipers H. Resistance training in cancer survivors: a systematic review. *Int J Sports Med*. 2009;30(10):703–712.

123. Mikkelsen TB, Sorensen B, Dieperink KB. Prediction of rehabilitation needs after treatment of cervical cancer: What do late adverse effects tell us? *Support Care Cancer*. 2017;25(3): 823–831

124. van den Driessche H, Mattelaer P, van Oyen P, et al. Changes in body image in patients with prostate cancer over 2 years of treatment with a gonadotropin-releasing hormone analogue (triptorelin): results from a Belgian non-interventional study. *Drugs Real World Outcomes*. 2016;3(2):183–190.

125. Taghian NR, Miller CL, Jammallo LS, O'Toole J, Skolny MN. Lymphedema following breast cancer treatment and impact on quality of life: a review. *Crit Rev Oncol Hematol*. 2014;92(3):227–234.

126. Cormier JN, Askew RL, Mungovan KS, Xing Y, Ross MI, Armer JM. Lymphedema beyond breast cancer: a systematic review and meta-analysis of cancer-related secondary lymphedema. *Cancer*. 2010;116(22):5138–5149.

127. O'Toole J, Jammallo LS, Skolny MN, et al. Lymphedema following treatment for breast cancer: a new approach to an old problem. *Crit Rev Oncol Hematol*. 2013;88(2):437–446.

128. Deng J, Murphy BA, Dietrich MS, et al. The impact of secondary lymphedema after head and neck cancer treatment on symptoms, functional status, and quality of life. *Head Neck*. 2013;35(7):1026–1035.

129. Speck RM, Gross CR, Hormes JM, et al. Changes in the Body Image and Relationship Scale following a one-year strength training trial for breast cancer survivors with or at risk for lymphedema. *Breast Cancer Res Treat*. 2010;121(2):421–430.

130. Chachaj A, Malyszczak K, Pyszel K, et al. Physical and psychological impairments of women with upper limb lymphedema following breast cancer treatment. *Psychooncology*. 2010;19(3):299–305.

131. Deng J, Murphy BA, Dietrich MS, et al. Impact of secondary lymphedema after head and neck cancer treatment on symptoms, functional status, and quality of life. *Head Neck*. 2013;35(7):1026–1035.

132. Pusic AL, Cemal Y, Albornoz C, et al. Quality of life among breast cancer patients with lymphedema: a systematic review of patient-reported outcome instruments and outcomes. *J Cancer Survivor*. 2013;7(1):83–92.

133. McGarvey AC, Osmotherly PG, Hoffman GR, Chiarelli PE. Lymphoedema following treatment for head and neck cancer: impact on patients, and beliefs of health professionals. *Eur J Cancer Care*. 2014;23(3):317–327.

134. Winch CJ, Sherman KA, Koelmeyer LA, Smith KM, Mackie H, Boyages J. Sexual concerns of women diagnosed with breast cancer-related lymphedema. *Support Care Cancer*. 2015;23(12):3481–3491.

135. Burckhardt M, Belzner M, Berg A, Fleischer S. Living with breast cancer-related lymphedema: a synthesis of qualitative research. *Oncol Nurs Forum*. 2014;41(4):E220–E237.

136. Teo I, Novy DM, Chang DW, Cox MG, Fingeret MC. Examining pain, body image, and depressive symptoms in patients with lymphedema secondary to breast cancer. *Psychooncology*. 2015;24(11):1377–1383.

137. Shaitelman SF, Cromwell KD, Rasmussen JC, et al. Recent progress in cancer-related lymphedema treatment and prevention. *CA Cancer J Clin*. 2015;65(1):55–81.

138. Lasinski BB, McKillip Thrift K, Squire D, et al. A systematic review of the evidence for complete decongestive therapy in the treatment of lymphedema from 2004 to 2011. *PM R*. 2012;4(8):580–601.

139. Brown JC, John GM, Segal S, Chu CS, Schmitz KH. Physical activity and lower limb lymphedema among uterine cancer survivors. *Med Sci Sports Exer*. 2013;45(11):2091–2097.

140. Chang O, Choi EK, Kim IR, et al. Association between socioeconomic status and altered appearance distress, body image, and quality of life among breast cancer patients. *Asian Pacific J Cancer Prevent*. 2014;15(20):8607–8612.

141. Philip EJ, Merluzzi TV, Zhang Z, Heitzmann CA. Depression and cancer survivorship: importance of coping self-efficacy in post-treatment survivors. *Psychooncology*. 2013;22(5):987–994.

142. Begovic-Juhant A, Chmielewski A, Iwuagwu S, Chapman LA. Impact of body image on depression and quality of life among women with breast cancer. *J Psychosoc Oncol*. 2012;30(4):446–460.

143. Bancroft EK. Genetic testing for cancer predisposition and implications for nursing practice: narrative review. *J Adv Nurs*. 2010;66(4):710–737.

144. Heiniger L, Butow PN, Coll J, et al. Long-term outcomes of risk-reducing surgery in unaffected women at increased familial risk of breast and/or ovarian cancer. *Familial Cancer*. 2015;14(1):105–115.

145. Unukovych D, Johansson H, Johansson E, Arver B, Liljegren A, Brandberg Y. Physical therapy after prophylactic mastectomy with breast reconstruction: a prospective randomized study. *Breast*. 2014;23(4):357–363.

146. Johansen N, Liavaag AH, Tanbo TG, Dahl AA, Pripp AH, Michelsen TM. Sexual activity and functioning after risk-reducing salpingo-oophorectomy: impact of hormone replacement therapy. *Gynecolog Oncol*. 2016;140(1):101–106.

147. Tucker PE, Bulsara MK, Salfinger SG, Tan JJ, Green H, Cohen PA. The effects of pre-operative menopausal status and hormone replacement therapy (HRT) on sexuality and quality of life after risk-reducing salpingo-oophorectomy. *Maturitas*. 2016;85:42–48.

148. Hallowell N, Mackay J, Richards M, Gore M, Jacobs I. High-risk premenopausal women's experiences of undergoing prophylactic oophorectomy: a descriptive study. *Genet Test*. 2004;8(2):148–156.

149. Worster E, Liu X, Richardson S, et al. The impact of prophylactic total gastrectomy on health-related quality of life: a prospective cohort study. *Ann Surg*. 2014;260(1):87–93.

150. Mouradian WE. The face of a child: children's oral health and dental education. *J Dental Educ*. 2001;65(9):821–831.

SECTION II

CANCER-SPECIFIC SEQUELAE ASSOCIATED WITH BODY IMAGE DISTURBANCE

CHAPTER 7

ALTERED APPEARANCE FROM CANCER

Nicole Paraskeva, Alex Clarke, and Diana Harcourt

THE PSYCHOLOGICAL IMPACT OF AN ALTERED APPEARANCE

Poor body image and appearance-related concerns are highly prevalent among people with cancer. For example, Nozawa and colleagues[1] reported that 80.3% of patients were concerned about changes in appearance as a result of treatment. In recent years, the body of research into the experiences of people living with visible differences of any sort has grown considerably by focusing on the experiences of adults and young people with congenital conditions (e.g., cleft lip and/or palate and neurofibromatosis type 1), skin conditions (such as acne, atopic eczema, vitiligo, and psoriasis), and the consequences of disease (such as cancer) or trauma (such as burns). One of the striking features of this literature is the consistency of the challenges reported by people whose appearance is somewhat different to most other people, irrespective of the cause or type of the disfigurement.[2] These include concerns about social interactions and having to deal with the reactions of other people (including unsolicited comments, questions, and staring). Many people manage these challenges very well. Indeed, a study of 1,265 adults with a range of visible differences concluded that around one-third of participants reported levels of social anxiety and avoidance considered to be in the "normal" range.[3] However, approximately two-thirds reported levels of distress that indicate a potential need for intervention and support. Those who are struggling with the challenges they face can respond with negative emotions (e.g., social anxiety, particularly about intimate relationships), maladaptive thought processes (e.g., fear of negative evaluation by others), unfavorable self-perceptions (e.g., lowered self-esteem, feeling unattractive), and negative behavior patterns (e.g., social avoidance, hostility).[2]

Cancer-related changes to appearance can be varied and extensive, including scarring, weight changes, hair loss, ridges in nail beds, discoloration of nails and skin, menopausal symptoms, and changes to physical development. These changes have been associated with increased levels of distress, anxiety, and depression across cancer types, negatively impacting on how individuals interact and behave.[4–7] Furthermore, the impact can be long lasting and sustained beyond the point of treatment.[8] The following section outlines how cancer, its treatment, and side effects can result in a range of permanent (e.g., scarring) or temporary (e.g., hair loss) changes to the body and how these impact an individual's body image.

The purpose of this chapter is to delineate a broad array of appearance alterations that can result from cancer and side effects of treatment. We initially focus on describing the impact of appearance changes involving weight, scarring from surgery, hair loss or change, ascites, and lymphedema. We then consider the degree to which patient demographics and treatment-related variables are associated with levels of appearance distress within an oncology setting. Finally, we present a comprehensive framework of psychological adjustment to living with a range of visible differences that has been extensively studied and is directly applicable to patients with cancer.

Throughout this chapter, the terms "disfigurement," "altered appearance," and "visible difference" are used to refer to changes to appearance that result in a person looking different in any way to what is generally considered to be "the norm." We use these terms interchangeably in order to limit repetition, although we acknowledge the concerns expressed about the pejorative use of the former. We specifically avoid the use of vocabulary such as "deformed," "abnormality," or "ugly" and encourage clinicians and researchers working in this field to do likewise.

WEIGHT CHANGES

Many people with cancer experience fluctuations in their weight—some cancers and treatments are associated with weight loss, others with weight gain. The detrimental physical (e.g., reduced strength) and psychosocial consequences (e.g., anxiety, distress, concerns about a possible cancer recurrence) associated with changes in weight are well documented[6,9] and can have implications for body image.[10] Indeed, both weight gain and loss have been linked with body dissatisfaction, embarrassment with the altered body, and psychological distress among patients at different stages of diagnosis and treatment.[6,9,11]

Weight gain can be a result of hormonal changes, the effect of steroid treatment and chemotherapy, and/or lower levels of physical activity. Among breast cancer patients, weight gain has been linked to disturbances in body image.[12] Vance and colleagues[13] reported that 50% to 96% of women with breast cancer experienced weight gain during treatment, and some (including those whose weight had remained stable throughout treatment) continued to gain weight over subsequent months and years [13] Women have described the experience of weight gain as living in an alien body,[14] together with practical issues (including the discomfort of ill-fitting clothes and the financial impact of needing to replace clothes with larger sizes) that affect how they view themselves and lead to feelings of embarrassment and impact negatively on self-esteem and quality of life.[6, 13–15]

Loss of weight can be attributed to diminished appetite, early satiety, alterations to the sense of taste and smell of food and drink, or nausea and vomiting as a consequence of chemotherapy.[16] Many patients note the physical impact of weight loss. For example, one study reported that the majority of postsurgery pancreatic cancer patients discussed weight loss in terms of reduced strength and being unable to walk long distances, in addition to changes in body image—one woman compared her appearance to that of "elderly ladies."[16] Physiological changes such as problems with swallowing (i.e., for laryngeal cancer patients) can result in difficulty eating, which can lead to decreased nutritional intake and weight loss. Psychosocial consequences can include patients avoiding eating in public due to feeling uncomfortable or embarrassed by their appearance and/or the need to use feeding tubes.[6] Such experiences and concerns can lead to feeling socially isolated.[6]

Cachexia is defined by malnutrition and physical wasting due to the effects of cancer (see Figure 7.1). In a qualitative study exploring the impact of cachexia on body image, Hinsley and Hughes[17] reported that patients felt less sexually desirable and attractive and avoided situations and environments that drew attention to their body, such as shopping for clothes and looking in a mirror. The authors also reported that patients felt they had to protect their partners from seeing their changed bodies and described their emaciated body as a constant and distressing reminder of the advanced stage of their disease.[17]

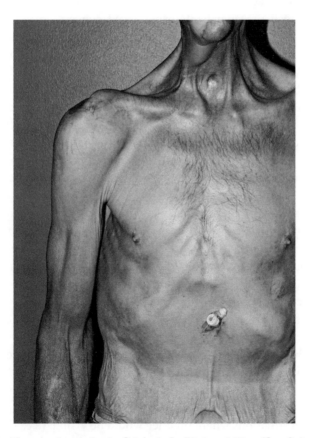

FIGURE 7.1: Patient with cachexia, required a G-tube to facilitate nutrition. (See Color Insert)

ALTERED APPEARANCE AFTER SURGERY

Surgical procedures invariably result in scarring to a greater or lesser degree, which may or may not be visible to others. Some scars may only be visible during intimacy. The extent, visibility, and appearance of scarring depends on the particular procedure and the individual's physiology and genetic predisposition with some people more inclined to create raised, red (keloid or hypertrophic) scars whilst others heal with relatively minor scarring. It is important to recognize that scars will change, and in many cases will fade and flatten over time, but there will still be some visible indication of the original wound. Some forms of reconstructive surgery remove skin and/or muscle and other tissue and use it to reconstruct or reform another part of the body. For example, breast reconstruction can involve moving tissue from the upper back or abdomen to recreate a breast mound. In these instances, there will be scarring at both the primary and donor sites (see Figures 7.2 and 7.3). Some individuals perceive their scars as a symbol of what their body overcame; a sign of strength and survivorship, whilst others find the scars a distressing reminder of pain and trauma.

Surgery can have a profoundly negative impact on individuals' body image.[18] Patients may undergo numerous invasive procedures to resect tumors or invaded tissue in visible areas of the body. For example, in head and neck cancer the surgical removal of a tumor can lead to scarring and changes to the shape of the face, putting patients at a high risk of experiencing body image distress.[19] Indeed, one study reported that 75% of surgically treated head and neck cancer patients experienced concerns or embarrassment about bodily changes at some point during treatment.[20] Furthermore, anxiety and depression are typically experienced by approximately 30% to 40% of this patient group following treatment,[21] and anxiety can continue long after treatment ends.[22]

Women with breast cancer are often faced with decisions about invasive surgical procedures including lumpectomy, mastectomy, and breast reconstruction. Treatment can involve multiple surgical procedures, all with potential for scarring which, in the case of reconstructive procedures, can leave significant scarring around the breast, back, or abdomen and loss of skin sensation—all of which can lead to body image disruption. The recreated breast mound is unlikely to look and feel the same as it was before mastectomy and reconstructive surgery, and the patient might not have a nipple unless she chooses to preserve it or recreate it in some way after mastectomy (typically additional surgery or tattooing). In the case of partial or segmental mastectomy, the shape of the breast may be altered and may not be symmetrical with the other breast. Surgery on the contralateral breast to restore balance and symmetry requires further adjustment to body image. A sizeable body of research has shown the various surgical options can leave women with breast cancer feeling mutilated, unattractive, less womanly, and inadequate.[23,24]

Surgery can also lead to visible changes in function. Fauske and colleagues[25] found that the majority of their study participants who underwent extensive surgery for treatment of primary bone sarcoma developed a limp resulting in the need to use a crutch, cane, or wheelchair to help their mobility, which emphasized their visible difference. The surgery also affected the shape of some patients' legs (e.g., one being skinnier than the other), which resulted in patients feeling less attractive, wanting to hide their appearance and avoid situations where their leg would be visible (e.g., dressing rooms and saunas).[25]

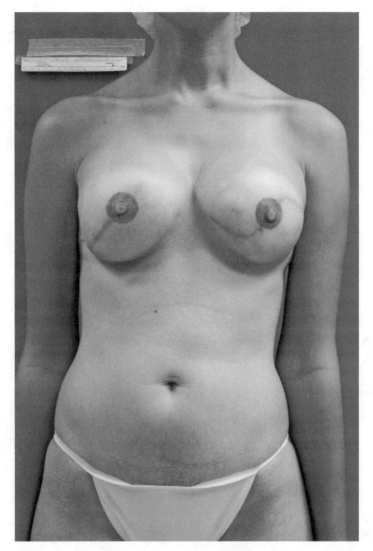

FIGURE 7.2: Patient with bilateral total mastectomy and implant-based breast reconstruction. (See Color Insert)

Some surgical procedures involve the removal or amputation of a body part (e.g., a limb, testicle, or breast) resulting in a very obvious change in appearance and the likelihood of emotional distress with implications for body image. Feelings of loss, shock, and comparisons with "damaged goods" have been reported by patients after such surgery.[24,26] For example, the removal of a testicle can lead to poorer body image, feelings of unease and shame due to the altered appearance, and a threat to masculinity with impacts on quality of life and intimacy.[27,28] In an interview study, body image, social relationships, ideas concerning what it means to be a man, and fears about self-image influenced men's decisions about testicular implants.[29]

Many patients engage in behaviors to avoid looking at the affected area of the body and attempt to hide or disguise it with clothes or the use of prostheses. For example, among women who do not undergo breast reconstruction, many choose to wear a breast prosthesis

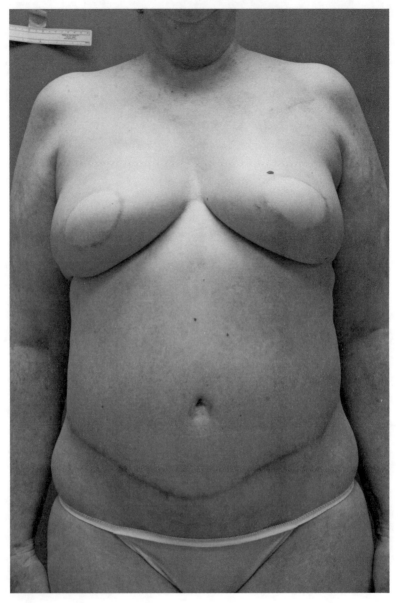

FIGURE 7.3: Patient with bilateral skin sparing mastectomy with autologous flap breast reconstruction using transverse rectus abdominis myocutaneous (TRAM) flap. (See Color Insert)

to gain symmetry and a sense of "wholeness" following mastectomy. However, there are numerous challenges and considerations involved in wearing a prosthesis; they have been described as inconvenient, a foreign object, and potentially embarrassing. Black and South Asian women have reported the difficulty of finding a prosthesis to match their skin tone.[30,31] Similar to the experience of extreme weight changes and hair loss, wearing a prosthesis can also be a painful reminder of cancer and mortality.

The decision to replace a surgically removed body part with a prosthesis or restore it with reconstructive surgery can be complex, and many patients choose not to do so

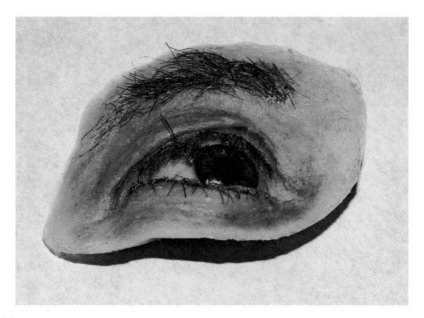

FIGURE 7.4: Example of eye prosthesis created for a patient. (See Color Insert)

(see Figure 7.4). One study found only 26.9% of testicular patients opted to have an implant,[27] mirroring acceptance rates found in similar studies (24% reported by Skoogh et al.[32]; 30% reported by Adshead et al.[33]). In a national audit of women undergoing mastectomy with or without breast reconstruction in England,[34] 21% of 16,485 women who underwent mastectomy also chose to undergo immediate reconstruction, whereas Flitcroft et al.[35] reported that 23% of 51 Australian women with locally advanced breast cancer chose *not* to have reconstructive surgery. Studies[35-37] have found that women who choose reconstruction do so predominantly to feel normal and to avoid a prosthesis, whereas those who decide not to have reconstruction believe it is not necessary for their psychological or physical well-being. Rates of contralateral prophylactic mastectomy (CPM; removing both breasts during surgery—that which contains the cancer in addition to the healthy breast) have been increasing in the United States and the United Kingdom.[38] In a recent review, cosmesis and the desire for breast symmetry were identified as key factors influencing women's decision to undergoing CPM.[39] Moreover, issues with body image and appearance following surgery influence women's satisfaction with the procedure.[39]

In some instances, for example treatment for rectal, anal, bowel, and urinary cancers, surgery can result in the need for a temporary or permanent stoma (see Figure 7.5).[40] The stoma and related scarring can alter the function and appearance of the affected area, with skin dehiscence (when surgical wound closures reopen instead of healing), rashes around the area of the stoma, and noises and odor associated with a stoma being significant concerns.[19] Patients have described the stoma bag itself as a "foreign object" that looks "unnatural," and it is perhaps not surprising that negative impacts on body image and sexuality have been reported. Feeling self-conscious, embarrassed, and sexually undesirable can lead to problems with intimacy and a reduction in sexual activity.[41]

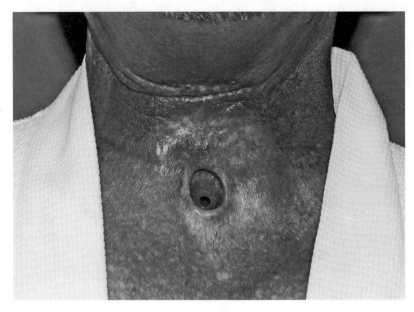

FIGURE 7.5: Patient with stoma after radiation and laryngectomy. (See Color Insert)

HAIR LOSS OR CHANGE

Approximately 65% of patients are affected by hair loss caused by the chemicals used in chemotherapy.[7,23] This is often considered to be one of the most distressing and feared side effects of treatment for women.[42,43] Indeed, 47% of gynecological cancer patients reported hair loss as the most traumatic side effect of their chemotherapy,[44] and a qualitative study focusing on women with tubo-ovarian cancer found alopecia to be the worst physical feature of cancer and its treatment.[45]

For many people, hair plays a significant role in defining their identity and thoughts about their appearance. Consequently, hair loss puts them at risk for negative body image (see Figure 7.6). Alopecia can be associated with a loss of self-confidence, identity, sexuality, attractiveness, and individuality and feelings of trauma, anger, sadness, shame, fear, and embarrassment.[7,46] For some, however, baldness due to cancer treatment is a symbol of pride and courage.[46] Although uncommon, some patients contemplate or outright refuse chemotherapy because their distress at the prospect of losing their hair (and gaining weight) is so profound.[47,48] Some women with breast cancer have described hair loss as being more traumatic than losing a breast[49] and a threat to their sense of femininity and womanhood.[45] The visible and physical loss of hair (e.g., holding clumps of hair in one's hand) can serve as a reminder to patients of the reality of their cancer and mortality, whilst also impacting on their ability to conceal their illness.[45,49–51] Moreover, hair can grow back with a different color or texture (e.g., that which was previously straight might grow back curly, and it is not uncommon for hair to appear more grey than it had been before chemotherapy), resulting in a continued and potentially long-lasting impact of chemotherapy-induced alopecia and the need to make further adjustments to an altered appearance and body image.[45]

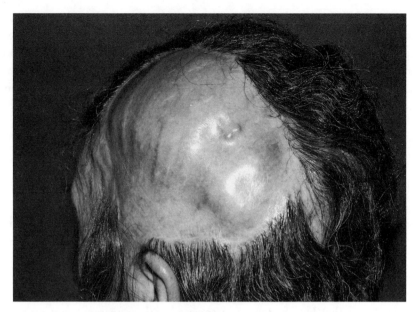

FIGURE 7.6: Patient with alopecia after scalp cancer and free flap. (See Color Insert)

Only a handful of studies have examined how men and women differ in the way they respond to hair loss.[7] Earlier studies found that women experienced greater levels of self-consciousness, appearance dissatisfaction, distress, and social anxiety in comparison to men who considered hair loss to be a normal and inevitable side effect of cancer treatment.[50,52] In contrast, Hilton and colleagues[51] found that men and women reacted in a similar way; both struggled to adjust to hair loss and to the reactions of others and felt that it portrayed them as a "cancer patient." One noticeable difference, however, was that women focused on the loss of hair from the head and above the eyeline, whereas men discussed losing hair from other areas of the body.

Whilst most research in this area has focused on the loss of hair from the scalp, hair loss affecting other parts of the body can also impact on patients' overall well-being and sense of self. For example, the loss of nasal hair increases dripping of mucus from the nose, which can result in people mistakenly treating patients as if they were ill,[46] and the loss of eyebrows can contribute to a sense of loss of self.[45]

Whilst the experience of hair loss is traumatic for many cancer patients, others view it positively.[7] Indeed, some patients begin to appreciate qualities that are unrelated to appearance whilst others appreciate the little things that they had once taken for granted.[48,53] For some patients, the regrowth of hair signifies life, hope, and renewal.[53]

ASCITES

Ascites refers to the "accumulation of fluid in the abdominal cavity, which results in swelling that can develop gradually over a few weeks or rapidly over a matter of days."[54] It can be a consequence of numerous cancers including ovarian, breast, bowel, stomach, pancreatic, lung, liver, womb, and mesothelioma in the peritoneum. A single qualitative study exploring the experiences of patients with ascites secondary to cancer found that both men and women described feeling pregnant, which caused embarrassment.[55] The authors also noted that patients appeared to be feel "disempowered" and "inadequate" due to the impact of ascites on their body. Further research is needed to explore the specific impact of ascites on body image.

LYMPHEDEMA

Lymphedema (swelling in the body's tissues) is a potential side effect of radiation therapy and surgery which can cause substantial changes to an individual's appearance including facial asymmetry, swelling, and pigmentation. Lymphedema can occur during or after treatment (see Figure 7.7). For example, 75.3% of 81 head and neck cancer patients experienced some form of late effect (three months or longer posttreatment) lymphedema.[56] Numerous studies have shown that lymphedema is associated with appearance concerns and body image distress [57] and is a particularly significant issue for women with breast cancer. Indeed,

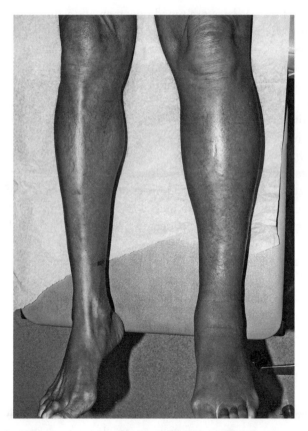

FIGURE 7.7: Patient with lower extremity lymphedema. (See Color Insert)

a qualitative study found that patients felt self-conscious as a result of the appearance of the lymphedema-affected area or compression garments, resulting in feelings of distress and an increase in social avoidance.[57] Lymphedema and body image are considered, in detail, in Chapter 10.

In summary, patients are likely to experience a variety of changes to their appearance (often simultaneously, such as concurrent weight changes, hair loss, and scarring) as a consequence of cancer and its treatment. An extensive body of research has shown that an altered appearance can negatively impact patients' body image, with serious physical and psychosocial consequences from the point of diagnosis to treatment and beyond. The following section considers whether an altered appearance affects some patients more than others.

WHO IS AFFECTED?

The evidence presented here and elsewhere in this text clearly demonstrates that body image and appearance-related concerns are potentially serious issues affecting a sizeable proportion of patients at some point during and/or after their cancer diagnosis and treatment. However, many patients manage the challenges they face as a consequence of an altered appearance very well, and they are not a significant issue for them. This section considers who is affected, in terms of whether any particular demographic or treatment-related factors are associated with increased or lower levels of appearance-related distress.

It is often assumed that patients with particular demographics are more susceptible to poor body image and appearance-related concerns. Such beliefs are particularly relevant in societies that place importance on appearance and promote the belief that "what is beautiful is good" and that meeting society's exacting standards of an idealized appearance is the key to a happy and fulfilling life. For example, it is commonly believed that changes to appearance will be more distressing for women than men, that older people place less importance on appearance and are thereby somewhat protected from the negative ramifications of treatment on appearance, and that changes that are more extensive, permanent, and visible to others are more upsetting than those that are limited, temporary, and/or hidden from view. Beliefs such as these could influence health professionals' interaction with their patients. For example, believing that appearance is no longer a concern for older people may mean that some women who are due to undergo mastectomy are not offered the option of breast reconstruction because it is assumed they would not be interested in having the additional surgery, yet older women still want to consider this option if it is offered.[58] The following section considers research evidence that supports or refutes these stereotypical views or "beauty myths."

GENDER

A commonly held view is that appearance is a more important issue for women than for men, and, therefore, women will be more detrimentally affected by changes to how they look. For many years, the broader body image and appearance research literature has examined in detail the psychological impact of women's high levels of dissatisfaction with their bodies and appearance. In recent years, increasing attention has also been given to the reports of dissatisfaction amongst men and the pressures that they feel to meet gender-based ideals of a perfect, yet usually unattainable, muscular and lean body. However, most body image research within psycho-oncology still centers around women, particularly those with early stage breast cancer, where the psychological impact of changes to appearance and body image are now well documented.[59,60] In contrast, relatively little research focuses specifically on men's experiences of altered appearance due to cancer. Refer to Chapter 14 for a discussion on body image and men.

Where comparisons have been made between male and female cancer patients, women and girls have tended to report higher levels of appearance-related distress (e.g., Liu's study of adult head and neck cancer patients[61] and Wu an Chin's study of children undergoing chemotherapy[62]). However, research that has specifically examined men's experiences still highlights the significance to them of changes to body image and appearance, with impacts on quality of life, sexual functioning, feelings of masculinity, and sense of identity. This has been reported amongst men with breast cancer,[63–66] as well as those with cancers specific to men (penile,[67] testicular,[28,68] and prostate[69,70]).

Chemotherapy-induced alopecia might be seen as more of an issue for women since hair loss (male pattern baldness) is considered acceptable or even "normal" for men. However, as discussed earlier in this chapter, qualitative data concluded that both men and women had similar negative experiences of hair loss.[51] Both had been made aware of their vulnerability and visibility as a "cancer patient," were shocked by it, and experienced negative reactions from other people. Interestingly, men did not describe the extent of pressures that were reported by women to try to prevent or disguise their hair loss, but they did talk more about losing hair from across their body whilst women only discussed loss of hair from their head. Similarly, a study by Can et al. concluded that alopecia is a difficult issue for both male and female cancer patients in Turkey.[71]

Research to date therefore challenges assumptions that men with cancer are not vulnerable to the impact of changes to their appearance. Some issues and experiences will be similar for both men and women, whilst there may also be distinct differences. Hilton and colleagues[51] emphasized the need for health professionals to understand men's experiences of hair loss in order that they can best support their patients in this situation. We support Can et al.[71] suggest that health professionals should be aware of the potential impact of hair loss for all their patients, both male and female, and extend this suggestion to apply to any changes to appearance, not only hair loss.

AGE

It is widely assumed that, regardless of the presence of any health condition, appearance is a more important issue for younger adults and adolescents and less of a concern for older people. Studies of patients who are undergoing or have completed a range of cancer treatments have explored the relationship between age and body image. A sizeable body of literature within breast cancer has concluded that younger women are more likely to report a negative impact on quality of life compared with their older counterparts (see a review by Howard-Anderson et al. [72]). Regarding surgery, one study found a significant negative relationship between age and body image disturbance amongst women undergoing nipple-sparing mastectomy with immediate breast reconstruction.[73] Similarly, a further study reported higher levels of body image dissatisfaction (assessed with three items from the Cancer Rehabilitation Evaluation System) amongst younger women (in this instance, women under the age of 40).[11] Regarding patients who are undergoing adjuvant treatments, a survey of 638 patients undergoing chemotherapy also reported a negative correlation between age and the degree of distress due to changes to appearance, so that older patients reported more favorable outcomes.[1]

However, it would be short-sighted to conclude that body image and appearance are not concerns for older adults and those in mid-life. Figueiredo et al.[74] studied a cohort of 563 women aged 67 or over with early-stage breast cancer, with data collection up to two years after surgery. They concluded that levels of appearance-related distress or body image concerns in this group were similar to younger patients, confirming the importance of appearance to this group when making decisions about treatment. The authors specifically remind clinicians not to rely on assumptions about the importance of appearance to older patients. Chapter 13 in the book further discusses body image in older adults.

Appearance takes on particular importance and significance during adolescence, as young people often become acutely aware of their bodies during this time of rapid physical, social, and sexual development. Looking "different" in any way during this time can be particularly difficult, so it might be assumed that young people undergoing cancer treatment will be significantly negatively affected by appearance changes. A study of 118 Chinese children undergoing chemotherapy found that those aged 14 to 18 years reported lower levels of body image satisfaction than younger children (aged 6 to 9 years).[62] However, Williamson et al.[48] and Wallace et al.[75] found that although an altered appearance due to cancer could be distressing for young people, some had successfully managed the particular challenges they faced. These studies support the view that appearance is a very important issue for young people but challenge any assumption that they would be unable to deal positively with an altered appearance. For further discussion on body image in pediatrics, see Chapter 12.

THE EXTENT OF APPEARANCE CHANGES

Another common assumption is that larger, more severe, and extensive differences or changes to appearance are more distressing than those that are smaller. This assumption has been examined within the broader visible difference literature where subjective assessments of the noticeability and severity of the difference are better predictors of psychological distress and adjustment to appearance than objective measures (such as the size of a scar).[76–78]

However, some studies within the cancer literature have shown more extensive scarring and changes to appearance to be more distressing and/or have a more negative impact on body image. For example, an aspect of cancer treatment that has perhaps received the most attention from psycho-oncology researchers interested in body image issues is the impact of mastectomy (with or without reconstructive surgery) compared with more conservative, less extensive surgical procedures (wide local excision or lumpectomy). Twenty years ago, a meta-analysis of literature at that time concluded that the more radical procedure (mastectomy) had a more negative impact on body image compared with breast-conserving operations (although the impact in terms of other psychosocial outcomes such as anxiety and depression was less consistent).[79] Härtl and colleagues drew a similar conclusion in a study involving 274 breast cancer patients.[80] More recent research has agreed that women who had undergone breast conservation reported greater satisfaction with appearance of the chest area and fewer body image concerns in the short term.[11,81]

However, one study found that at two year follow-up there were no significant differences between those women who had undergone breast conservation or mastectomy with or without reconstructive surgery.[81] A further study also found that body image did not differ significantly between these three surgical groups at two-year follow-up, although the severity of side effects did impact on body image in the first 12 months after surgery.[60] These studies highlight the importance of considering changes over time, and both short-term and longer term outcomes, although it would still be useful to explore the impact of the extent of surgery at longer follow up (e.g., 5 or 10 years). Similarly, a study reported no significant difference in body image between women electing to undergo mastectomy with or without breast reconstruction at one-year follow-up.[82] These studies are reminders that women who try to minimize the extent of scarring and other changes to the appearance of their breast(s) by choosing to undergo less extensive surgery (lumpectomy) or reconstructive surgery are not immune to appearance concerns and body image issues and that reconstructive surgery is not a panacea for the distress of mastectomy. An important issue that has received relatively little attention within the breast reconstruction literature is the impact of scarring elsewhere on the body when autologous procedures that involve transferring a woman's own body tissue (e.g., from the abdomen or back) in order to create a breast mound are carried out. Exceptionally, Abu-Nab and Grunfeld reported how some women had unrealistic expectations about the aesthetic outcome of breast reconstruction, particularly regarding the appearance of scarring at the donor site.[83]

VISIBILITY OF APPEARANCE CHANGES

It might also be assumed that changes to appearance that are more visible or noticeable by other people would be more distressing than those which are hidden from view. However, the relationship between visibility of differences and distress is complex.[84] Much of the broader visible difference literature has failed to show a clear relationship between appearance-related distress and the visibility of the aspect of appearance that is in some way different to "the norm."[76-78] However, the largest study to date of adults with a variety of visible differences including those associated with head and neck cancer, melanoma, skin conditions, burns, cleft lip and palate, and ocular prosthetics found that higher levels of distress were reported by participants who considered their "difference" was not visible to others in everyday situations.[3] One explanation for this is that people with differences that are permanently on view or harder to disguise (such as scarring, asymmetry, and loss of function affecting the face or hands) must develop strategies to deal with the (possibly predictable) reactions of other people. Failing to do so makes everyday social interactions difficult, raising fears of being judged negatively by others and increasing the likelihood of social avoidance and withdrawal.[85]

Changes to appearance that are not ordinarily visible to others might be exposed when in an intimate relationship, giving rise to potentially high levels of stress about how and when to reveal the difference to partners for the first time and anxiety around their subsequent reactions. Such issues have been identified within a range of studies including patients with testicular cancer,[68] abdominal stoma,[41,86] lower limb amputations,[87] those who have undergone mastectomy,[88] and those who are using wigs to disguise chemotherapy-induced alopecia.

Again, the common assumption is not supported by the research literature, and it should not be presumed that differences that are normally hidden from view will not be a source of distress, nor that those that are always on show will necessarily have a negative impact on those affected.

PERMANENT VERSUS TEMPORARY CHANGES TO APPEARANCE

It can be tempting to believe that changes to appearance that might be temporary (either because they are expected to "remedy" themselves naturally, e.g., hair that should regrow after chemotherapy has ended, or because the option of surgical intervention such as reconstructive surgery is available) are less distressing than those that are permanent (e.g., amputation of a limb). The literature around the psychosocial impact of hair loss due to chemotherapy treatment challenges this view that temporary changes are not so distressing. Both qualitative[53] and quantitative studies[43] have demonstrated the negative impact of hair loss on body image and psychosocial well-being. For example, in a cross-sectional survey of 168 breast cancer patients in Korea, 93 women who self-reported high levels of alopecia-associated distress were more likely to have poorer body image than those reporting low levels of distress associated with hair loss.[89] Again, most of the research has focused on the experiences of women treated for breast cancer, and the experiences of men have received far less attention, possibly because hair loss is deemed more acceptable for men than women.[51] However, alopecia is still a significant and distressing experience for many men (as described earlier in this chapter).

STAGE OF DISEASE

A sizeable body of research now demonstrates that early-stage invasive breast cancer often has a negative impact on body image. However, the impact of preinvasive and advanced diseases on body image and patients' thoughts and feelings about their appearance have received much less consideration. Studies of the preinvasive condition ductal carcinoma in situ have shown that, despite being reassured their condition is not life-threatening, some women reported ongoing body image distress and found it hard to adjust to their altered appearance (e.g., scarring was a reminder of extensive surgery which they had found hard to comprehend when there was no threat from invasive cancer).[90,91]

It might be assumed that patients with advanced, terminal disease are no longer invested in appearance and that their priorities lie elsewhere. Yet a small number of studies examining patients with advanced cancer (including women with metastatic breast cancer) have reported their distress about changes to appearance including hair loss, scars, weight gain, and lymphedema, demonstrating how appearance issues can still be a concern and an important aspect of quality of life for women facing the challenge of noncurative disease.[92–95] Similarly, Williamson and Rumsey reported that 87% of health professionals working in a pediatric oncology setting believed appearance was a concern for their patients but expressed surprise to hear that appearance-related concerns were an issue for young people at every stage of their cancer diagnosis and treatment, including when they were terminally ill.[96] The relevance of appearance for patients with other types of advanced disease, and the best ways of meeting their needs, warrants further research and consideration.

TIME

The adage that "time is a great healer" would suggest that the ramifications of an altered appearance become easier to manage over the years. Yet the numbers of patients seeking reconstructive procedures at a later date suggest otherwise. For example, despite an increase in the numbers of women seeking immediate breast reconstruction, a national audit in England reported that 1,731 women underwent delayed reconstruction, from a total of 16,485 who underwent mastectomy in the same period.[34] Previous research has shown that dissatisfaction with postmastectomy appearance and poor body are prime motivations for delayed reconstruction.[35] For many patients, their initial focus is on their survival and the treatment of the cancer, so that issues of appearance are less of a priority at that stage, but become more pertinent as they begin to resume their previous roles and lifestyle (e.g., returning to work). It would therefore be naïve to assume that those who do not report concerns about their appearance early on will not be adversely affected by them in due course. Likewise, neither should it be assumed that those who are bothered by changes initially will continue to be so indefinitely. This reflects the dynamic nature of body image.

In summary, it is clear that clinicians must be mindful not to let assumptions about age, gender, disease factors, or the severity and visibility of an altered appearance influence their interactions with patients and the choices they offer them for treatment that might impact on their appearance. Rather, the lack of equivocal findings regarding who is negatively affected by visible differences supports the call for clinicians to discuss appearance and body image issues with all their patients, when doing so is possible within the confines of busy clinic settings.[97] Creating an ethos of care in which appearance and body image concerns can be openly and easily discussed is key to being able to direct patients towards appropriate supportive care and interventions (these are considered in Chapter 4).

ADJUSTMENT TO CHANGES
TO APPEARANCE

As noted throughout this chapter, not everyone will be equally affected by an altered appearance. Whilst some find it profoundly distressing, others cope effectively with changes. It is important to understand what factors help to buffer an individual against the potential negative effects of an altered appearance so that efforts can be made to identify and support those at higher risk for distress. This section draws on relevant theory and evidence to examine the factors shown to predict adjustment to an altered appearance.

A MODEL OF ADJUSTMENT

A variety of models have been developed to explain adjustment to an altered appearance (see Thompson for a review).[98] Since body image is a complex, multifactorial concept, it is unsurprising that researchers have stressed different factors in understanding individual responses. Consequently, Thompson suggests that no single model encapsulates all the different dimensions.[98] When considering different models, it is also important to note that adjustment is dynamic, and even those who appear to have adjusted well over long periods of time can still find it difficult to cope with the ongoing challenges and strain it can put on them. Life events and milestones such as attending a new school, the break-up of a relationship, or seeking new employment are potential trigger points, even for those who have previously managed very well but now worry that their appearance will have negative repercussions.

Newell's model focuses on avoidant and confrontational responses, with the latter associated with more adaptive adjustment to an altered appearance.[85] Avoidant responses are prompted by the expectation of negative outcomes and fear which are considered to mediate poor body image. In line with this model, research suggests that some patients with cancer reduce or avoid social activities and situations out of fear that people will treat them differently as a result of their altered appearance.[7]

White proposed a cognitive-behavioral model which focuses on the feelings, beliefs, and behavior that shape an individual's response.[99] This model stipulates that ineffective coping strategies, negative thoughts, and psychological distress are more likely to occur amongst individuals whose cancer affects a valued body part and who place increased importance on their appearance. White suggests this model as a practical heuristic for explaining the variability in individual response.[99] Similarly, Kent offers a model based on cognitive behavioral principles and suggests that appearance anxiety is caused when an individual is faced with an anxiety inducing situation (e.g., being invited to a party).[100] As a result, they employ coping strategies that reduce anxiety in the short term (e.g., avoidance or concealment) but which are likely to reinforce appearance anxiety over time.

Drawing on multiple models and theories within this field, the Appearance Research Collaboration (ARC) developed and tested a framework of adjustment (see Figure 7.8) with individuals with a range of visible differences ($N = 1,265$).[3,98] This framework incorporated

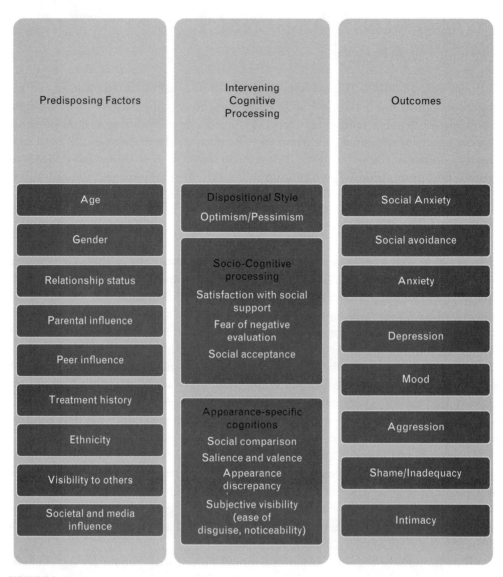

FIGURE 7.8: Research framework devised by the Appearance Research Collaboration.

From Appearance Research Collaboration. Factors and processes associated with psychological adjustment to disfiguring conditions. In Clarke A, Thompson AR, Jenkinson E, Rumsey N, Newell R, eds. CBT for Appearance Anxiety: Psychosocial Interventions for Anxiety due to Visible Difference. *Oxford: John Wiley, 2013: 194–271.*

predisposing factors (including demographic factors and physical aspects such as the cause and visibility of any difference), intervening cognitive processes (including perceptions of social support and acceptance and appearance-related beliefs and schemas such as the salience of appearance and tendency to make comparisons on the basis of looks), and measurable outcomes (including social avoidance, social anxiety, mood, and shame) to examine the impact of disfigurement.

Whichever model or framework one chooses to work with, the purpose of using them (i.e. to understand the patient perspective and provide a systematic approach to managing any problems) remains the same. Without a systematic approach, intervention lacks an evidence base and alternative management approaches are potentially inconsistent.[99] An underlying model is also essential so that the rationale for potential treatment can be discussed with the patient.

FACTORS THAT PREDICT ADJUSTMENT TO CHANGES IN APPEARANCE

Understanding what factors protect or predispose individuals to appearance-related distress is crucial in informing the development and use of appropriate interventions. Findings from the broader visible difference literature suggest that family support, social skills, the extent to which an individual is invested in his or her appearance, sense of self, humor, determination, and networking all influence how people cope with an altered appearance.[2] The study conducted by the ARC[3] (outlined earlier) found that four key factors accounted for the variance in determining appearance-related distress.[3] Whilst the media, society, and culture contributed to pressure on those vulnerable to appearance concerns, as documented in previous research and outlined earlier in this chapter, severity, cause, or type of the objective condition was unrelated to adjustment.[76] Instead, adjustment was confirmed as being multifactorial and influenced by dispositional style (optimism/pessimism) and cognitive processes (such as fear of negative evaluation by others, perceived social acceptance), appearance-specific cognitions (including salience of appearance), and appearance-related self-discrepancies (differences between how individuals *think* they look, how they would *like* to look, and how they feel they *should* look).

Whilst this section focuses on modifiable factors (i.e., ones that can be changed) that predict adjustment to changes in appearance, when developing and using interventions it is important to consider factors which are not amenable to change but can impact individual's adjustment. For example, ethnicity and culture can influence how individuals adjust to a diagnosis of cancer and its treatment and to changes to their appearance.[101,102] As such, it is vital to explore the manner in which appearance alterations due to cancer affect patients from different backgrounds. With respect to the impact on body image, a study conducted in the United Kingdom examining the experiences of women who were between six months and five years post–breast cancer diagnosis found that black and South Asian women reported higher levels of body image concerns than white women.[101] Previous research has also demonstrated that wigs, skin-colored breast prostheses, and lymphoedema sleeves are harder to access for black and minority ethnic women, which are likely to contribute to women's body image concerns.[31,101] Given these differences, health professionals must be aware that culture and ethnicity can have a significant impact on the healthcare outcomes, experiences, and needs of black and minority ethnic patients. An understanding of the values and beliefs of ethnic minority groups (i.e., in relation to body image and an altered appearance) is essential.[102] The following section outlines some of the key modifiable factors that play a role in adjustment:

INVESTMENT IN APPEARANCE

Appearance investment is recognized to be comprised of two appearance-specific cognitive processes: (a) individuals' efforts to engage in behaviors to enhance their attractiveness (motivational salience) and (b) the importance they place on their appearance in defining their self-worth (self-evaluative salience). For example, in a sample of Portuguese breast cancer patients, investment in appearance helped to distinguish women who adjusted poorly to breast cancer from those who adjusted well.[103] Specifically, motivational salience was found to be a protective factor. The authors noted that making an effort to be or feel attractive provided women with a sense of control over their appearance changes, and consequently this was associated to more positive outcomes (e.g., improved quality of life). In contrast, self-evaluative salience (i.e., believing that appearance is an important element of self-esteem) was associated with poorer outcomes. Findings from this study mirror those from an earlier study which found that increased investment in appearance resulted in higher appearance-related distress prior to surgery and during the following year for women with breast cancer.[104]

SOCIAL SUPPORT

Social support is generally associated with better quality of life and well-being among cancer patients. Higher levels of perceived social support have been correlated with higher levels of body satisfaction among women treated for breast cancer.[105] For adolescents with cancer, social support is particularly important in regards to helping them adjust to their altered appearance.[106,107] For example, peer support helped young people manage the negative reactions of others. Previous research within the broader visible difference literature has also highlighted the value of supportive friends and family, by increasing feelings of acceptance and helping individuals cope with other people's reactions to their appearance.[108,109]

DISPOSITIONAL STYLE

The largest study to date of factors and processes that predict adjustment amongst adults with a visible difference identified the significance of dispositional style, with those with an optimistic outlook on life faring better than those with a more negative, problem-focused view of the world.[3] Similarly, qualitative research with adults who self-identified as having adjusted positively to their appearance concluded that they had a very positive outlook on life, were optimistic and forward thinking, and viewed their experience in terms of the personal growth that had come from it.[109] Strategies that seemed to work well for them included pragmatism and "getting on with it" in the face of challenges, acceptance and determination, and engaging with problems and difficulties rather than avoiding them.

PREOCCUPATION WITH APPEARANCE

Some patients pay far more attention to their altered appearance than others, seeming to constantly monitor it and other people's reactions and fearing that they will be judged

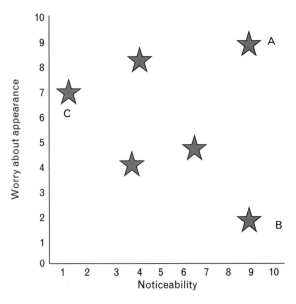

FIGURE 7.9: Self-assessment of appearance by patients (indicated by stars) on a 0 to 10 scale of noticeability and worry.

Reproduced with permission from Appearance Research Collaboration. Factors and processes associated with psychological adjustment to disfiguring conditions. In Clarke A, Thompson AR, Jenkinson E, Rumsey N, Newell R, eds. CBT for Appearance Anxiety: Psychosocial Interventions for Anxiety due to Visible Difference. *Oxford: John Wiley, 2013: 194–271.*

negatively by them. It is typically the patients' subjective view of the perceived change in appearance that determines their psychological well-being. Indeed, health professionals are sometimes surprised by the level of distress experienced by a patient with minimal changes to his or her appearance. Figure 7.9 illustrates how individuals may respond to their altered appearance and the aim of surgical and psychological interventions.

The horizontal axis in the figure represents the extent that the patient's appearance differs from the norm, assessed by them on a scale of 0 (not significantly) to 10 (extremely), whilst the vertical axis represents the degree to which they are preoccupied or worried about appearance. Surgical interventions to improve appearance of a defect or disfigurement directly change people's physical appearance in order to change their perception of how unusual or noticeable it is to themselves and others. In contrast, psychological interventions do not target physical appearance but aim instead to change the impact of how appearance is experienced by modifying cognitions and behaviors. Thus a successful surgical intervention aims to reduce the patient's score on the vertical axis (worry) by targeting the horizontal axis (noticeability) whilst a psychological intervention aims to directly reduce the score on the vertical axis. Interestingly, both kinds of intervention have the ultimate goal of reducing body image anxiety.

Each star in Figure 7.9 represents a different patient, each of whom has made a self-assessment of his or her appearance and the extent to which he or she is worried by it. Consider the following case examples.

Adele (patient at point A), aged 42, had recently undergone a mandibulectomy (i.e., surgery to remove a portion of the lower jaw) and bilateral neck dissection to treat a malignancy in her oral cavity with metastasis to lymph nodes. She had also lost a significant amount of weight in the last few months, at first because she was eating poorly due to the pain in her mouth and later because of issues surrounding tube feeding while in the hospital. She rated the changes in her appearance as being highly noticeable (rated 10/10) and is particularly fixated on the resulting asymmetry of her jaw and not looking like her usual self. She is experiencing high body image anxiety about seeing her friends or other people she knows (rated at 9/10) and rarely leaves her home.

Bernard (patient at point B), aged 73, recently underwent an orbital exenteration to treat an ocular melanoma in his left eye. He recognizes that wearing his eye patch whenever he goes out draws the attention of others and that it makes his appearance very noticeable (rated 9/10). It took some adjusting to the stares, especially from young children; however, he now experiences a low level of concern or worry about his appearance changes (rated 2/10). In fact, he relishes making up pirate stories for children when asked about his eye.

Cory (patient at point C), aged 43, recently had a surgery to treat bowel cancer and had a placement of an ileostomy bag. Although he verbalizes that his outward appearance changes are unremarkable (rated 1/10), he is nonetheless very preoccupied and worried by the possibility that he looks different (7/10). He discarded all his close-fitting shirts and now only wears shirts that are baggy or loose so that the "bulge" under his clothing is less obvious.

In terms of predisposing factors and intervening cognitive processes, it is likely that Bernard is less invested in appearance as a component of his self-worth or has a more robust social support network, lower fear of negative evaluation, better strategies for managing the interest and curiosity of others, and/or other cognitions and behaviors associated with positive adjustment. As we have stressed elsewhere in this chapter, severity or extent of a visible difference does not predict distress, so Adele and Cory are similar in terms of anxious preoccupation with appearance despite the fact that Cory accepts that his appearance is far less noticeable than Adele's.

Treatment options are different for patients Adele, Bernard, and Cory. Adele is the only one for whom elective reconstructive surgery may offer benefits, depending on the surgeon's assessment of whether further reconstructive procedures are possible. However, surgical intervention alone is not expected to fully address her body image distress. Adele will have limitations in the degree to which her appearance can be restored with surgical intervention and will need psychological intervention to target intervening cognitive processes that are contributing to highly negative psychological outcomes from appearance changes.

Bernard may be an appropriate candidate for reconstructive intervention, (i.e., placement of a prosthetic eye), but given that he is relatively unconcerned about his appearance, it is arguable that there is little to be gained by further procedures. In Bernard's case, there does not appear to be a need for psychological intervention aimed at reducing body image anxiety. However, should he be considering whether to undergo additional surgery for placement of a prosthesis, psychological intervention could help facilitate treatment decision-making about trade-offs for undergoing additional procedures to enhance his body image. Cory's body image distress can only be addressed via psychological intervention. Further surgical intervention cannot enhance the appearance of his stoma, which he recognizes is not necessarily noticeable to others. For Cory, psychological intervention offers the opportunity to explore the underlying cognitive processes involved in his poor adjustment to appearance changes from cancer.

These examples further illustrate how surgeons need to work together with psychologists and other mental health professionals to determine the relative contributions that each can make to ensure the best outcomes for patients whose appearance has been changed by cancer and its treatment. Surgeons need to be equipped to facilitate referrals for psychological services for patients struggling with changes to appearance regardless of location or extent of disfigurement. Treatment decision-making regarding whether to undergo surgical revision to enhance appearance can be a complex process that also warrants co-management of patients. Surgeons are understandably invested in achieving the best possible physical outcome for their patients; however, there is also an important balance to strike so as to avoid a series of revisions or minor procedures that deliver diminishing returns whilst risking overinvestment in surgery as a means to psychological equilibrium.

In summary, factors that are key to successful adjustment to an altered appearance are those that are amenable to psychosocial intervention (in contrast to demographic and physical/biological factors). Understanding individual responses to an altered appearance is important for the whole oncology team, not just mental health specialists working in a one-to-one setting. The essence of working successfully with cancer patients who are experiencing an altered appearance is to acknowledge the variability in individuals' responses and to recognize the high levels of distress that can be experienced by those who value appearance highly as a component of their self-concept.

LOOKING AHEAD

As the broader visible difference literature continues to develop, it is important that both researchers and practitioners working within oncology contribute to and learn from the advances being made in our understanding of individuals' experiences of an altered appearance and the best ways to meet their needs through appropriate supportive care and interventions (see Chapter 4). To date, most research on altered appearance and visible difference after diagnosis of cancer has centered on women with breast cancer, with a sizeable yet much smaller literature on the experiences of head and neck cancer patients. There is still a need to explore in greater detail the unique issues facing patients with rarer diseases (e.g., penile cancer) and treatment side effects that have so far received relatively little attention from body image researchers (e.g., ascites; see previous discussion) or the experiences and needs of populations that have been underrepresented in this area of research to date (e.g., older people and those from different racial, ethnic, and cultural backgrounds, such as black and minority ethnic groups).

Given that concern with appearance is a global issue affecting individuals across the lifespan, it is important to ensure that research examining the impact of cancer on appearance and body image is inclusive. Most work in this field has focused on adjustment amongst adults, and the psychosocial factors and processes that influence young people's adjustment to an altered appearance still warrant exploration. Furthermore, most research examining the impact of an altered appearance due to cancer has been conducted in developed, high-income countries, such as the United States, Australia, and the United Kingdom, with some being conducted in East Asian countries such as China and Korea. Looking ahead, more research is needed to examine how individuals in low-income countries experience and manage an altered appearance after cancer treatment, so that effective and appropriate care and interventions can be developed that meet their needs within the specific, challenging confines of limited and competing resources.

As new treatments, including advances in surgical techniques, continue to be developed at a considerable pace, it is important for researchers and clinicians to consider the impact of these new interventions on body image. Additionally, they must ensure that patients who are increasingly offered a choice of complex procedures are sufficiently supported in making the decision that is best for them, in line with their individual values and goals. Managing the consequences of changes to appearance continues to be an important issue beyond the end of treatment. Whilst the longer term impact of breast cancer on body image has been explored, the longer term implications of other cancers still needs to be investigated. Indeed, Rhoten et al. have called for longitudinal studies of body image amongst head and neck cancer patients.[110] The increasing focus on survivorship within the cancer agenda has prompted longitudinal cohort studies with patients with various cancer diagnoses, which offer an opportunity to learn more about the longer term consequences of an altered appearance and body image, how and when the importance of appearance changes, and how patients' adjustment shifts or remains constant over time. This would very usefully inform the development and evaluation of appropriate interventions.

Finally, Hefferon and colleagues note that overcoming the adverse effects of chemotherapy helped some survivors to appreciate their bodies.[14] As a result, they positively reconnected with the bodies that had once frightened and shocked them. Further research into positive body image (defined as the love and acceptance of one's body and appreciation of its uniqueness and the functions it performs)[111] amongst people who have been diagnosed and treated for cancer would provide a more comprehensive understanding of their experiences compared with the current tendency to focus on problems and negative body image. The findings of such research could usefully inform the development and provision of information and interventions in the future.

CONCLUSION

In summary, this chapter has demonstrated the importance of altered appearance and body image amongst people treated for cancer of any sort, highlighting the need to avoid assumptions based on demographic-, disease-, or treatment-related factors. Instead, an evidence-based, theoretical psychosocial approach needs to be encompassed within oncology services in order to facilitate the development and evaluation of appropriate care and interventions that will best support those patients whose lives are negatively affected by changes to their appearance.

REFERENCES

1. Nozawa K, Shimizu C, Kakimoto M, Mizota Y, Yamamoto S, Takahashi Y, Ito A, Izumi H, Fujiwara Y. Quantitative assessment of appearance changes and related distress in cancer patients. *Psychooncology.* 2013;22(9):2140–2147.

2. Rumsey N, Harcourt D. Body image and disfigurement: issues and interventions. *Body Image.* 2004;1(1):83–97.

3. Appearance Research Collaboration. Factors and processes associated with psychological adjustment to disfiguring conditions. In: Clarke A, Thompson AR, Jenkinson E, Rumsey N, Newell R, eds. *CBT for Appearance Anxiety: Psychosocial Interventions for Anxiety due to Visible Difference.* Oxford: John Wiley; 2013:194–271.

4. Bullen TL, Sharpe L, Lawsin C, Patel DC, Clarke S, Bokey L. Body image as a predictor of psychopathology in surgical patients with colorectal disease. *J Psychosom Res.* 2012;73(6):459–463.

5. Lam WW, Shing YT, Bonanno GA, Mancini AD, Fielding R. Distress trajectories at the first year diagnosis of breast cancer in relation to 6 years survivorship. *Psychooncology.* 2012;21(1):90–99.

6. Stamataki Z, Burden S, Molassiotis A. Weight changes in oncology patients during the first year after diagnosis: a qualitative investigation of the patients' experiences. *Cancer Nurs.* 2011;34(5):401–409.

7. Dua P, Heiland MF, Kracen AC, Deshields TL. Cancer-related hair loss: a selective review of the alopecia research literature. *Psychooncology.* 2017;26(4):438–443. doi:10.1002/pon.4039

8. Lehmann V, Hagedoorn M, Tuinman MA. Body image in cancer survivors: a systematic review of case-control studies. *J Cancer Survivor.* 2015;9(2):339–348.

9. Halbert CH, Weathers B, Esteve R, Audrain-McGovern J, Kumanyika S, DeMichele A, Barg F. Experiences with weight change in African-American breast cancer survivors. *Breast J.* 2008;14(2):182–187.

10. Brunet J, Sabiston CM, Burke S. Surviving breast cancer: women's experiences with their changed bodies. *Body Image.* 2013;10(3):344–351.

11. Rosenberg SM, Tamimi RM, Gelber S, et al. Body image in recently diagnosed young women with early breast cancer. *Psychooncology.* 2013;22:1849–1855.

12. Raggio GA, Butryn ML, Arigo D, Mikorski R., Palmer SC. Prevalence and correlates of sexual morbidity in long-term breast cancer survivors. *Psychol Health.* 2014;29(6):632–650.

13. Vance V, Mourtzakis M, McCargar L, Hanning R. Weight gain in breast cancer survivors: prevalence, pattern and health consequences. *Obesity Rev.* 2011;12(4):282–294.

14. Hefferon K, Grealy M, Mutrie N. Transforming from cocoon to butterfly: the potential role of the body in the process of posttraumatic growth. *J Human Psychol.* 2009;50(2):224–247.

15. DeGeorge D, Gray JJ, Fetting JH, Rolls BJ. Weight gain in patients with breast cancer receiving adjuvant treatment as a function of restraint, disinhibition, and hunger. *Oncol Nurs Forum.* 1989;17(3):23–28.

16. Cooper C, Burden ST, Molassiotis A. An explorative study of the views and experiences of food and weight loss in patients with operable pancreatic cancer perioperatively and following surgical intervention. *Support Care Cancer.* 2015;23(4):1025–1033.

17. Hinsley R, Hughes R. "The reflections you get": an exploration of body image and cachexia. *Int J Palliat Nurs.* 2007;13(2):84–89.

18. Fingeret MC, Teo I, Goettsch, K. Body image: a critical psychosocial issue for patients with head and neck cancer. *Curr Oncol Rep.* 2015;17(1):1–6.

19. Williamson H, Wallace M. When treatment affects appearance. In: Rumsey N, Harcourt D, eds. *The Oxford Handbook of the Psychology of Appearance.* Oxford: Oxford University Press; 2012:414–427.

20. Fingeret MC, Yuan Y, Urbauer D, Weston J, Nipomnick S, Weber R. The nature and extent of body image concerns among surgically treated patients with head and neck cancer. *Psychooncology* 2012;21(8):836–844.

21. Semple CJ, Sullivan K, Dunwoody L, Kernohan WG. Psychosocial interventions for patients with head and neck cancer: past, present, and future. *Cancer Nurs.* 2004;27(6):434–441.

22. Dropkin, MJ. Anxiety, coping strategies, and coping behaviors in patients undergoing head and neck cancer surgery. *Cancer Nurs.* 2001;24(2):143–148.

23. Helms RL, O'Hea EL, Corso M. Body image issues in women with breast cancer. *Psychol Health Med.* 2008;13(3):313–325.

24. Ussher JM, Perz J, Gilbert E. Changes to sexual well-being and intimacy after breast cancer. *Cancer Nurs.* 2012;35(6):456–465.

25. Fauske L, Lorem G, Grov EK, Bondevik H. Changes in the body image of bone sarcoma survivors following surgical treatment—a qualitative study. *J Surg Oncol.* 2015;113:229–234.

26. Sjodahl G, Gard G, Jarnlo GB. Coping after trans-femoral amputation due to trauma or tumour—a phenomenological approach. *Disabil Rehabil.* 2004;26(14–15):851–861.

27. Dieckmann KP, Anheuser P, Schmidt S, et al. Testicular prostheses in patients with testicular cancer—acceptance rate and patient satisfaction. *BMC Urol.* 2015;15(1):16. doi: 10.1186/s12894-015-0010-0

28. Rossen P, Pedersen AF, Zachariae R, von der Maase H. Sexuality and body image in long-term survivors of testicular cancer, *Eur J Cancer.* 2012;48(4):571–578.

29. Chapple A, McPherson A. The decision to have a prosthesis: a qualitative study of men with testicular cancer. *Psychooncology.* 2004;13(9):654–664.

30. Maguire P. Psychological aspects of surgical oncology. In U. Veronesi, B. Arnesjø, I. Burn, L. Denis, & F. Mazzeo (Eds.): *Surgical Oncology.* Berlin: Springer; 1989:272–281.

31. Patel G, Harcourt D, Naqvi H, Rumsey N. Black and South Asian women's experiences of breast cancer: a qualitative study. *Divers Equal Health Care.* 2014;11(2):135–149.

32. Skoogh J, Steineck G, Cavallin-Ståhl E, et al. Feelings of loss and uneasiness or shame after removal of a testicle by orchidectomy: a population-based long-term follow-up of testicular cancer survivors. *Int J Androl.* 2011;34(2):183–192.

33. Adshead J, Khoubehi B, Wood J, Rustin G. Testicular implants and patient satisfaction: a questionnaire-based study of men after orchidectomy for testicular cancer. *BJU Int.* 2001;88:559–562.

34. Jeevan R, Cromwell DA, Browne JP, et al. Findings of a national comparative audit of mastectomy and breast reconstruction surgery in England. *J Plast Reconstr Aesthet Surg.* 2014;67(10):1333–1344.

35. Flitcroft K, Brennan M, Costa D, Wong A, Snook K, Spillane A. An evaluation of factors affecting preference for immediate, delayed or no breast reconstruction in women with high-risk breast cancer. *Psychooncology.* 2016;25(12):1463–1469.

36. Denford S, Harcourt D, Rubin L, Pusic A. Understanding normality: a qualitative analysis of breast cancer patients' concepts of normality after mastectomy and reconstructive surgery, *Psychooncology.* 2011;20:553–558.

37. Reaby LL. Reasons why women who have mastectomy decide to have or not to have breast reconstruction. *Plast Reconstr Surg.* 1998;101:1810–1818.

38. Boughey JC, Attai DJ, Chen SL, et al. Contralateral prophylactic mastectomy consensus statement from the American Society of Breast Surgeons: additional considerations and a framework for shared decision making. *Ann Surg Oncol.* 2016;23(10):3106–3111.

39. Ager B, Butow P, Jansen J, Phillips KA, Porter D, Group CDA. Contralateral prophylactic mastectomy (CPM): a systematic review of patient reported factors and psychological predictors influencing choice and satisfaction. *Breast.* 2016;28:107–120.

40. Benedict C, Rodriguez VM, Carter J, Temple L, Nelson C, DuHamel K. Investigation of body image as a mediator of the effects of bowel and GI symptoms on psychological distress in female survivors of rectal and anal cancer. *Support Care Cancer.* 2016;24(4):1795–1802.

41. Brown H, Randle J. Living with a stoma: a review of the literature. *J Clin Nurs.* 2005;14:74–81.

42. Batchelor D. Hair and cancer chemotherapy: consequences and nursing care—a literature study. *Eur J Cancer Care.* 2001;10(3):147–163.

43. Lemieux J, Maunsell E, Provencher L. Chemotherapy-induced alopecia and effects on quality of life among women with breast cancer: a literature review. *Psychooncology.* 2008;17:317–328.

44. Münstedt K, Manthey N, Sachsse S, Vahrson H. Changes in self-concept and body image during alopecia induced cancer chemotherapy. *Support Care Cancer.* 1997;5(2):139–143.

45. Jayde V, Boughton M, Blomfield P. The experience of chemotherapy-induced alopecia for Australian women with ovarian cancer. *Eur J Cancer Care.* 2013;22(4):503–512.

46. Boehmke MN, Dickerson SS. Symptom, symptom experiences, and symptom distress encountered by women with breast cancer undergoing current treatment modalities. *Cancer Nurs.* 2005;28(5):382–389.

47. Fawzy NW, Secher L, Evans S, Giuliano AE. The Positive Appearance Center: an innovative concept in comprehensive psychosocial cancer care. *Cancer Pract.* 1994;3(4):233–238.

48. Williamson H, Harcourt D, Halliwell E, Frith H, Wallace M. Adolescents' and parents' experiences of managing the psychosocial impact of appearance change during cancer treatment. *J Paediatr Oncol Nurs.* 2010;27(3):168–175.

49. Freedman TG. Social and cultural dimensions of hair loss in women treated for breast cancer. *Cancer Nurs.* 1994;17(4):334–341.

50. Rosman S. Cancer and stigma: experience of patients with chemotherapy-induced alopecia. *Patient Educ Counsel.* 2004;52(3):333–339.

51. Hilton S, Hunt K, Emslie C, Salinas S, Ziebland S. Have men been overlooked? A comparison of young men and women's experiences of chemotherapy-induced alopecia. *Psychooncology.* 2008;17(6):577–583.

52. Weitz R. *Rapunzel's Daughters: What Women's Hair Tells Us about Women's Lives.* New York: Macmillan; 2004.

53. Kim IR., Cho JH, Choi EK, et al. Perception, attitudes, preparedness and experience of chemotherapy-induced alopecia among breast cancer patients: a qualitative study. *Asian Pac J Cancer Prevent.* 2012;13(4):1383–1388.

54. Cancer Research UK, 2016. http://www.cancerresearchuk.org/about-cancer/coping-with-cancer/coping-physically/fluid-in-the-abdomen-ascites/about-fluid-in-abdomen. Accessed December 12, 2016.

55. Day R, Mitchell T, Keen A, Perkins P. The experiences of patients with ascites secondary to cancer: a qualitative study. *Palliat Med.* 2013;27(8):739–746.

56. Deng J, Ridner SH, Dietrich MS, et al. Prevalence of secondary lymphedema in patients with head and neck cancer. *J Pain Symptom Manage.* 2012;43(2):244–252.

57. Rhoten BA, Radina ME, Adair M, Sinclair V, Ridner SH. Hide and seek: body image-related issues for breast cancer survivors with lymphedema. *J Womens Health Issues Care.* 2015;4:2.

58. Hamnett KE, Subramanian A. Breast reconstruction in older patients: a literature review of the decision-making process. *J Plast Reconstr Aesthet Surg.* 2016;69(10):1325–1334.

59. Rosenberg SM, Tamimi RM, Gelber S, et al. Body image in recently diagnosed young women with early breast cancer. *Psychooncology.* 2013;22:1849–1855.

60. Collins KK, Liu Y, Schootman M, Aft R, Yan Y, Dean G, Eilers M, Jeffe DB. Effects of breast cancer surgery and surgical side effects on body image over time. *Breast Cancer Res Treat.* 2011;126(1):167–176.

61. Liu HE. Changes of satisfaction with appearance and working status for head and neck tumour patients. *J Clin Nurs.* 2008;17(14):1930–1938.

62. Wu LM, Chin CC. Factors related to satisfaction with body image in children undergoing chemotherapy. *Kaohsiung J Med Sci.* 2003;19:217–224.

63. France L, Michie S, Barrett-Lee P, Brain K, Harper P, Gray J. Male cancer: a qualitative study of male breast cancer. *Breast J.* 2000;9:343–348.

64. Donovan T, Flynn M. What makes a man a man? The lived experience of male breast cancer. *Cancer Nurs.* 2007;30(6):464–470.

65. Pituskin E, Williams B, Au HJ, Martin-McDonald K. Experiences of men with breast cancer: a qualitative study. *J Mens Health Gender.* 2007;4(1):44–51.

66. Brain K, Williams B, Iredale R, France L, Gray J. Psychological distress in men with breast cancer. *J Clin Oncol.* 2006;24(1):95–101.

67. Bullen K, Edwards S, Marke V, Matthews S. Looking past the obvious: experiences of altered masculinity in penile cancer. *Psychooncology.* 2010;19:933–940.

68. Carpentier MY, Fortenberry JD. Romantic and sexual relationships, body image, and fertility in adolescent and young adult testicular cancer survivors: a review of the literature. *J Adolesc Health.* 2010;47(2):115–125.

69. Harrington J. Implications of treatment on body image and quality of life. *Semin Oncol Nurs.* 2011;27:290–299.

70. Taylor-Ford M, Meyerowitz BE, D'Orazio LM, Christie KM, Gross ME, Agus DB. Body image predicts quality of life in men with prostate cancer. *Psychooncology.* 2013;22:756–761.

71. Can G, Demir M, Erol O, Aydiner A. A comparison of men and women's experiences of chemotherapy-induced alopecia. *Eur J Oncol Nurs.* 2013;17:255–260.

72. Howard-Anderson J, Ganz PA, Bower JE, et al. Quality of life, fertility concerns, and behavioral health outcomes in younger breast cancer survivors: a systematic review. *J Nat Cancer Instit.* 2012;5:386–405.

73. Sherman KA, Woon S, French J, Elder E. Body image and psychological distress in nipple-sparing mastectomy: the roles of self-compassion and appearance investment. *Psychooncology.* 2017;26(3):337–345. doi: 10.1002/pon.4138

74. Figueiredo MI, Cullen J, Hwang YT, Rowland JH, Mandelblatt JS. Breast cancer treatment in older women: does getting what you want improve your long-term body image and mental health? *J Clin Oncol.* 2004;22(19):4002–4009.

75. Wallace M, Harcourt D, Rumsey N. Managing appearance changes resulting from cancer treatment: resilience in adolescent females. *Psychooncology.* 2007;16(10):1019–1027.

76. Ong JJ, Clarke A, Johnson M, White P, Withey S, Butler PE. Does severity predict distress? The relationship between subjective and objective measures of severity in patients treated for facial lipoatrophy. *Body Image.* 2007;4:239–248.

77. Moss T. The relationship between objective and subjective ratings of disfigurement severity and psychological adjustment. *Body Image.* 2005;2:151–159.

78. Brown BC, Moss TP, McGrouther DA, Bayat A. Skin scar preconceptions must be challenged: importance of self-perception in skin scarring. *J Plast Reconstr Aesthet Surg.* 2010;63:1022–1029.

79. Moyer A. Psychosocial outcomes of breast-conserving surgery versus mastectomy: a meta-analytic review. *Health Psychol.* 1997;16(3):284–298.

80. Härtl K, Janni W, Kästner R, Sommer H, Strobl B, Rack B, Stauber M. Impact of medical and demographic factors on long-term quality of life and body image of breast cancer patients. *Ann Oncol.* 2003;14(7):1064–1071.

81. Parker PA, Youssef A, Walker S, Basen-Engquist K, Cohen L, Gritz E, Wei QX, Robb GL. Short-term and long-term psychosocial adjustment and quality of life in women undergoing different surgical procedures for breast cancer. *Ann Surg Oncol.* 2007;14(11):3078–3089.

82. Harcourt DM, Rumsey NJ, Ambler NR, et al. The psychological effect of mastectomy with or without breast reconstruction: a prospective, multicenter study. *Plast Reconstr Surg.* 2003;111(3):1060–1068.

83. Abu-Nab Z, Grunfeld EA. Satisfaction with outcome and attitudes towards scarring among women undergoing breast reconstructive surgery. *Patient Educ Counsel.* 2007;66(2):243–249.

84. Moss T, Rosser B. Psychosocial adjustment to visible difference. *Psychologist.* 2008;21(6):492–495.

85. Newell R. *Body Image & Disfigurement Care.* London: Routledge; 2000.

86. Fucini C, Gattai R, Urena C, Bandettini L. Quality of life among five-year survivors after treatment for very low rectal cancer with or without a permanent abdominal stoma. *Ann Surg Oncol.* 2008;15(4):1099–1106.

87. Mathias Z, Harcourt D. Dating and intimate relationships of women with below-knee amputation: an exploratory study. *Disabil Rehabil.* 2014;36(5):395–402.

88. Fallbjörk U, Rasmussen BH, Karlsson S, Salander P. Aspects of body image after mastectomy due to breast cancer—a two-year follow-up study. *Eur J Oncol Nurs.* 2013;17(3):340–345.

89. Choi EK, Kim I, Chang O, et al. Impact of chemotherapy-induced alopecia distress on body image, psychosocial well-being, and depression in breast cancer patients. *Psychooncology.* 2014;23:1103–1110.

90. Kennedy F, Harcourt D, Rumsey N. The challenge of being diagnosed and treated for ductal carcinoma in situ (DCIS). *Eur J Oncol Nurs.* 2008;12:103–111.

91. Kennedy F, Harcourt D, Rumsey N, White P. The psychosocial impact of ductal carcinoma in situ (DCIS): a longitudinal prospective study. *Breast.* 2010;19:382–387.

92. Mosher CE, Johnson C, Dickler M, Norton L, Massie MJ, DuHamel K. Living with metastatic breast cancer: a qualitative analysis of physical, psychological, and social sequelae. *Breast J.* 2013;19(3):285–292.

93. McClelland SI, Holland KJ, Griggs JJ. Quality of life and metastatic breast cancer: the role of body image, disease site, and time since diagnosis, *Qual Life Res.* 2015;24(12):2939–2943.

94. Rhondali W, Chisholm GB, Daneshmand M, et al. Association between body image dissatisfaction and weight loss among patients with advanced cancer and their caregivers: a preliminary report. *J Pain Symptom Manage.* 2013;45(6):1039–1049.

95. Rhondali W, Chisholm GB, Filbet M, Kang DH, Hui D, Fingeret MC, Bruera E. Screening for body image dissatisfaction in patients with advanced cancer: a pilot study. *J Palliat Med.* 2015;18(2):151–156.

96. Williamson H, Rumsey N. The perspectives of health professionals on the psychosocial impact of an altered appearance among adolescents treated for cancer and how to improve appearance-related care. *J Psychosoc Oncol.* 2017;33(1):47–60.

97. Fingeret MC, Teo I, Epner DE. Managing body image difficulties of adult cancer patients: lessons from available research. *Cancer.* 2014;120:633–641.

98. Thompson AR. Researching appearance: models, theories and frameworks. In: Rumsey N, Harcourt D, eds. *The Oxford Handbook of the Psychology of Appearance.* Oxford: Oxford University Press; 2012: 91–110.

99. White C. Body image dimensions and cancer: a heuristic behavioural model. *Psychooncology.* 2000;9:183–192.

100. Kent G, Thompson, A. The development & maintenance of shame in disfigurement: implications for treatment. In: Gilbert P, Miles J, eds. *Body Shame.* Hove: Brunner-Routledge; 2002:103–116.

101. Patel-Kerai G, Harcourt D, Rumsey N, Naqvi H, White P. The psychosocial experiences of breast cancer amongst black, South Asian and white survivors: Do differences exist between ethnic groups? *Psychooncology.* 2016;26:515–522.

102. Naqvi H, Saul K. Culture and ethnicity. In: Rumsey N, Harcourt D, eds. *The Oxford Handbook of the Psychology of Appearance.* Oxford: Oxford University Press; 2012:203–216.

103. Moreira H, Silva S, Canavarro MC. The role of appearance investment in the adjustment of women with breast cancer. *Psychooncology.* 2010;19(9):959–966.

104. Carver C, Pozo-Kaderman C, Price A et al. Concern about aspects of body image and adjustment to early stage breast cancer. *Psychosom Med.* 1998;60(2):168–174.

105. Aguilar Cordero M, Neri Sánchez M, Mur Villar N, Gómez Valverde E. Influencia del contexto social en la percepción de la imagen corporal de las mujeres intervenidas de cáncer de mama. *Nutr Hosp.* 2013;28(5):1453–1457.

106. Larouche SS, Chin-Peuckert L. Changes in body image experienced by adolescents with cancer. *J Pediatr Oncol Nurs.* 2006;23(4):200–209.

107. Fan SY, Eiser C. Body image of children and adolescents with cancer: a systematic review. *Body Image.* 2009;6(4):247–256.

108. Thompson AR, Broom L. Positively managing intrusive reactions to disfigurement: an interpretative phenomenological analysis of naturalistic coping. *Divers Health Care.* 2009;6:171–180.

109. Egan K, Harcourt D, Rumsey N, Appearance Research Collaboration. A qualitative study of the experiences of people who identify themselves as having adjusted pos.itively to a visible difference. *J Health Psychol.* 2011;16:739–749.

110. Rhoten BA, Murphy B, Ridner SH. Body image in patients with head and neck cancer: a review of the literature. *Oral Oncol.* 2013;49(8):753–760.

111. Tylka TL, Wood-Barcalow NL. What is and what is not positive body image? Conceptual foundations and construct definition. *Body Image.* 2015;14:118–129.

CHAPTER 8

BODY IMAGE AND FUNCTIONAL LOSS

Melissa Henry and Ali Alias

This chapter addresses the implications of limb and sensory loss in pediatric and adult oncology patients alongside its impact on body image. First, we present the World Health Organization's (WHO) International Classification of Functioning, Disability and Health (ICF) and propose how the body image construct can be understood within this model. Second, we present an overview of the scientific literature on limb and sensory loss, emphasizing what is known about its broader impact on psychological distress and, more specifically, on body image. Other important functional losses such as sexual dysfunction/infertility as well as speech and swallowing impairments are covered in Chapters 9 and 11, respectively. Finally, we propose future areas of scientific inquiry as well as implications for clinical practice in the area of body image and functional loss with illustrative case examples.

CONCEPTUAL FRAMEWORK OF FUNCTIONING AND HOW IT RELATES TO BODY IMAGE

The WHO's ICF is a model that describes impact on functioning of a health condition, whether it be a disorder or a disease (see Figure 8.1).[1] The model posits the integration of three intersectional levels of impact on functioning: on body functions and structure, on activity, and on participation. "Functioning [is considered] at the level of body or body part, the whole person, and the whole person in a social context. Disability therefore involves dysfunction at one or more of these same levels: impairments, activity limitations and participation restrictions."[1] The notion of disability is not defined by medical terms alone

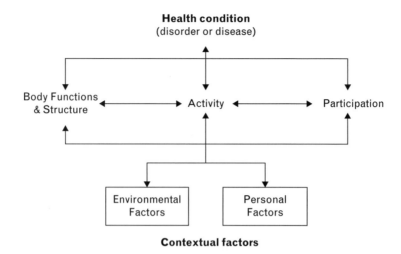

Health condition
(disorder or disease)

Body Functions & Structure ↔ Activity ↔ Participation

Environmental Factors

Personal Factors

Contextual factors

FIGURE 8.1: World Health Organization's International Classification of Functioning, Disability and Health.

Reprinted with permission from the World Health Organization, Towards a common language for functioning, disability and health: ICF (The International Classification of Functioning, Disability and Health), *p. 9. Retrieved March 25, 2018, from http://www.who.int/classifications/icf/training/icfbeginnersguide.pdf.*

(i.e., the direct impact of the health condition on physiological functions of the body) but includes the integration of the loss of function within a system that considers the patient's perception and experience of the change, as well as its impact within the broader context of patients' lives, both in terms of activity and participation in society. This broader conceptualization is person-centered in that it corresponds to what is central to and valued by patients themselves.[2,3] It also recognizes barriers and facilitators on both individual and environmental levels, which expand or limit a person's potential for functionality or disability on a continuum ranging from a strictly internal response (e.g., depression, social anxiety) to one that is exclusively externally driven (e.g., social stigma, lack of adapted resources). In this sense, both functioning and disability can be defined objectively with a corresponding normative assessment, as well as subjectively experienced and measured through patient-reported outcomes.[4] Dysfunction on one level can influence the other domains and compromise adaptation following the loss of function, leading to further compromise of function and, ultimately, deterioration of the health condition that caused the loss of function in question.[1,5]

Body image is defined as a subjective and dynamic concept, encompassing one's perceptions, thoughts, feelings, and behaviors toward the body. While there has been much emphasis in the scientific literature on appearance-based research leading to conceptualizations of conditions such as anorexia and bulimia, the construct of body image in oncology has been less studied and is generally understood as comprising both appearance- and function-based changes.[6-8] This is in line with a recent concept analysis of body image disturbances defining three attributes of the concept in oncology:[9] (a) self-perception of a change in appearance and lack of satisfaction with the alteration (or sense of alteration), (b) self-perception of a decline in an area of function, and (c) psychological distress regarding changes in appearance and/or function. One caveat to integrating body image into the ICF's model is the complex task of distinguishing between the adaptational challenges related to a change in function (e.g., the impact of a change in function on levels of anxiety, depression, and anger) and the more pervasive negative effects of these changes on one's self-image as it relates to the body. This being said, body image encompasses body image satisfaction (i.e., the extent to which one is content with one's physical and functional features) and investment (i.e., the value placed on a feature and the measures taken to maintain its value),[6,10] and it is influenced by a plethora of individual and environmental factors, including personal (e.g., personality and self-esteem), interpersonal (e.g., family, peers, colleagues, the public), biological (e.g., genetic and overall health), cultural (e.g., social values and norms, media messages), and developmental (e.g., life experiences) factors.[11] Hence, body image disturbances arise when one's identity has been breached due to an altered characteristic on which considerable importance is placed.

Consequently, the integration of the body image and functioning constructs can be highlighted via use of the ICF model alongside the three key attributes of body image disturbances (see Figure 8.2).[1,9] This intersectional perspective provides an overview of objective medical domains of functioning and embodiment combined with the subjective patient-centered analysis of key outcomes in response to the health-related domains, as proposed by the ICF. The key change from the ICF model is the refinement of underlying psychological mechanisms at play in the context of impairments, disability, and restrictions. The addition of body image disturbances to the understanding of functioning seeks to delineate more explicitly the psychosocial repercussions of the various health-related domains in light of the condition of cancer and cancer-related treatment side effects, an undertaking which, to our knowledge, has not been replicated in current bodies of literature. The patient-centered perspective highlighted by this model seeks to further promote a multidimensional understanding in response to an illness, gaining importance in understudied areas of functional loss in oncology, such as limb and sensory loss.

LIMB AND SENSORY LOSS IN ONCOLOGY

LIMB LOSS IN ONCOLOGY

Limb loss objectively refers to the amputation of one (or several) of the lower extremities and/or upper extremities,[12] further subdivided into two types: (a) major (transhumeral or transtibial) and (b) minor (the wrist or digits) amputations.[13] The incidence of limb amputation in oncology is rare and mainly arises in primary bone and soft-tissue sarcomas (e.g., osteosarcomas and Ewing sarcomas).[14–17] Tumor resection is performed either through amputation of the affected area or, more commonly, through limb-sparing surgery (LSS).[18,19] LSS is the initially preferred treatment course as it maximizes physical function, stability, and ambulation in the affected limb.[20] The procedure entails resection of malignant tissue with a portion of the surrounding healthy tissues.[21] Despite the benefits of LSS, secondary amputations may be necessary when complications arise (e.g., limb shortening, impaired healing, and infection).[17,20]

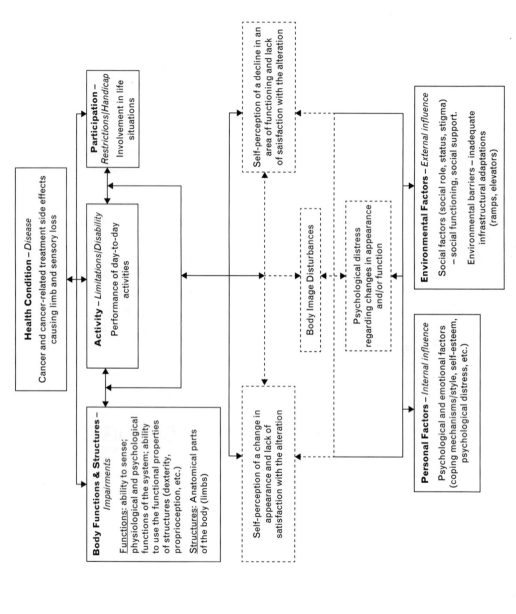

FIGURE 8.2: World Health Organization's International Classification of Functioning, Disability, and Health with an integrated body image construct.

Adapted with permission from the World Health Organization, Towards a common language for functioning, disability and health: ICF (The International Classification of Functioning, Disability and Health), p. 9. Retrieved March 25, 2018, from http://www.who.int/classifications/icf/training/icfbeginnersguide.pdf.

Postsurgical quality of life typically declines following amputation and LSS, especially in areas of physical function, physical role performance, social function, and pain.[14,17] Amputation is often accompanied by multiple challenges for the patient, and its level of impact on psychological well-being is often assessed through time-dependent depression.[22] Furthermore, despite the acquisition of compensatory functional abilities, self-confidence and overall well-being often fail to return to pre-amputation levels.[23] According to previous studies, the occurrence of depression among lower-limb amputees ranges between 13% and 30%,[24] with a high risk of the depressive episode recurring or persisting even years after the amputation.[22,25] This risk may even be present following completion of an initial rehabilitation program in which the patient regains functional independence.[25] Depression and anxiety in amputees have been linked to psychological factors such as a negative coping style that includes catastrophizing, a traumatic context surrounding the amputation, the existence of medical comorbidities, and poor social support.[25,26] These same variables have also been associated with patients' decreased motivation and adherence to a rehabilitation program, which have ultimately been found to compromise recovery in function and autonomy.[24]

Additionally, readjustment to the loss of limb has been associated with the extent of physical impairment and disability; the value given to appearance, to the lost body part, and to its function; the self-awareness of impairment and self-identification with being "impaired"; the process of adjusting to assistive devices; the degree of pain experienced (e.g., nociception, phantom limb pain, prosthesis-related); and contextual factors such as age, gender, pre-existing psychiatric conditions, patient's level of general health, and sociocultural appraisal of health and disability.[10,14,17,18,23,24,27] All of these variables would need to be assessed before and after the amputation procedure, as these conditions may alter the perception and coping of patients in response to their amputation.[14,24]

Additionally, normal feelings of loss and grief can emerge as patients are slowly readjusting their expectations or self-ideals to their new reality. The cosmetic appearance and physical sensation of the amputated site, the use of prosthetics and assistive devices along with deviations from normal body mechanics (e.g., modified gait cycle and performance of activities of daily living [ADLs]), can be constant reminders of a changed body and of its meaning as tied to cancer.[20,23,28] Difficulties arise when the loss of limb becomes a sense of total loss, permeating the patients' whole sense of self to the point of feeling their self to be impaired, damaged, or even crippled.[22] This transient and, in severe cases, pervasive state risks, in turn, contribute to further deterioration, limiting ADLs and restricting participation in previously meaningful life roles, ultimately feeding the cycle of emotional turmoil and disability.

Beyond the normative levels of functioning, amputation can also affect sexual functioning.[29] The self-perception of disability may generate embarrassment and confusion between patients and their partners due to misconceptions or miscommunications, difficulties in body positioning, impairments in balance and movement, sensations of phantom limb pain, anxiety around sexual performance, and feelings of diminished masculinity or femininity, which may further heighten their perception of differences.[30,31]

Patients can also face an extensive amount of explicit and/or implicit stigma associated with their socially visible difference, which can further reinforce their ideal-self discrepancy and, in turn, impact their readjustment.[32] This is likely to affect the patients' satisfaction, as their capacity for self-fulfillment is limited not only by physical disability but also by societal demands and constraints.[3] These constraints can take the form of environmental barriers in the face of an impairment in independent functional mobility (e.g., bilateral transfemoral amputation, important balance impairments), as patients rely on wheelchairs and/or other assistive devices for ambulation. This dependency necessitates the environment to be wheelchair-friendly and accessible (e.g., access to ramps, elevators, large doorways), requiring adequate adaptations for the proper and independent participation of the patient in their daily life activities.[33,34]

In face of these biopsychosocial adversities, patients will consequently undergo a process of identity adjustment due to the change in their status from a healthy individual to one living with a functional impairment.[32] In light of our model, body image disturbances in the context of limb loss are an understudied area in oncological care. The health condition of general amputation has relevant evidence-backing implications with respect to the overarching health-related domains of the ICF (e.g., implications for activity and participation arising from balance impairments; implications for the re-education of the locomotor system) alongside the process of adaptation to the condition and the prosthesis in question, which are ultimately dependent of patient factors such as time of fitting of the prosthesis, the coping mechanisms at play, the pre-amputation status of patients, and the patients' contextualization of their own condition. Little is known with respect to conclusive adaptation trends and developmental patterns among amputees from musculoskeletal malignancies, in part due to limited research on the role of the body image construct. However, we are seeing an important shift in understanding of the body image construct along with an interest in transcending the objective construct of physical functioning, as reflected in recent articles assessing sexual functioning and highlighting patient experience.[3,32] However, the importance of analyzing psychological difficulties and distress arising from changes in appearance and/or function needs to be further studied in order to accurately depict and understand attributes of body image disturbances relevant to the oncological population. This knowledge also requires a longitudinal framework to highlight the process of biopsychosocial adaptation following the loss of limb due to cancer. Such a methodology will highlight key individual and environmental factors that act either as facilitators or barriers during the post-amputation adaptation process, identifying key markers for future clinical practice in terms of cancer survivorship interventions.

SENSORY LOSS IN ONCOLOGY

Types of sensory loss, including auditory, visual, olfactory, gustatory, and somatosensory loss, are considered separately. Given their different etiologies, studies have tended to focus on these issues independently.

AUDITORY LOSS

Hearing loss is categorized on a continuum reflecting severity (mild to severe, temporary to permanent) and type of hearing loss (conductive, sensorineural, and mixed hearing loss).[35]

Generally speaking, conductive hearing losses result from pathologies affecting the outer or middle ear, whereas sensorineural hearing losses arise from pathologies affecting the cochlea and auditory nervous system.[35–38]

In oncology, hearing impairments arise in the context of ototoxicity, which can present as hearing loss and/or tinnitus (i.e., perception of noise or ringing in the ear).[39] Ototoxicity appears more often in relation to antineoplastic therapies, including platinum chemotherapy, radiation, and surgery involving the ear, auditory nerve, sensorial pathways, and integration sites.[36,39] Auditory loss can have substantial repercussions on an individual's quality of life, largely depending on its extent and permanency.[36,40,41]

Cancer treatment–related hearing loss has been associated with child-related cancers such as neuroblastomas and central nervous system (CNS) tumors, given that the neuronal pathways and auditory structures of children are in the process of maturation, rendering them vulnerable to the late side effects of cancer treatment.[35,42] Due to the tonotopic organization of the cochlear hair cells, the initial damage of ototoxicity impairs the perception of high-frequency sounds before impacting low-frequency sounds. This has strong implications for pediatric cancer survivors. High-frequency sounds ensure proper acquisition of language and communication skills, and impaired perception may have repercussions on the child's future academic performance and social functioning.[35,39] In a similar condition seen in adults, hearing impairments may generate work-related and financial difficulties, and the presence of tinnitus may impair social attainment.[43,44] Thus, these patients require timely identification and delivery of audiology services posttreatment to avoid detrimental developmental and functional consequences.

While hearing aids and cochlear implants have been medically successful in restoring auditory function, patients may experience discontinuity and a lack of satisfaction as these devices do not restore hearing to its original form but rather enhance hearing and speech comprehension by amplifying sounds.[35] A spectrum in the quality of such hearing aids, largely determined by finance and health coverage, may influence the degree of a patient's satisfaction.[35,41]

Additionally, the use of hearing devices may be socially perceived as a direct physical manifestation of disability. The attached stigma can be imbued with ageist connotations, with important implications for adult cancer survivors.[40,41] In addition to this stigma, the presence of phantom noises may further diminish patients' quality of life by heightening impairments in their physical and social functioning.[45] Consequently, patients can experience an identity conflict requiring the remodeling of their sense of being an able-bodied individual in light of the functional impairment.[40] This breach in their self-schema can generate important emotional distress ranging from anxiety or anger to depressive episodes, potentially creating more triggers to remind patients of their impairment. These biopsychosocial repercussions can generate important disturbances, whose impact has been found to depend largely on such variables as age and extent of functional loss, along with the late ototoxic effects arising from anti-cancer treatment.[9,39]

In the domain of auditory loss, the etiology of the loss (i.e., specific anti-cancer protocol, cancer site, and affected site of treatment), the body structures impaired (i.e., auditory apparatus), and the repercussion on participation restrictions (e.g., academic achievement, social interactions) are well documented in the literature. However, the development of the body image disturbance construct needs to be further considered, given that the pediatric oncological population is at high risk for development of auditory loss. Recent evidence encourages prompt identification of hearing loss to mitigate the developmental consequences arising from inadequate management of treatment side effects.[35] It is also important to understand how children view this loss and the satisfaction related to the management of the auditory loss and use of hearing devices. A longitudinal framework is indicated in this context to properly appreciate the process of postauditory loss adaptation, especially in future years (e.g., adolescence, adulthood). Such an understanding has direct benefits for the immediate provision of care and future implications, if any, to support the young patients who become cancer survivors in later stages of life. These findings may have further implications for public administration. A proper understanding of the use of hearing aids within the pediatric oncological context may justify the remodeling of health coverage.

VISUAL LOSS

Vision loss refers to partial blindness (i.e., a limited vision in one or more of the visual fields) or complete blindness (more specifically, a legally blind person possesses either (a) a visual acuity of 20/200 or less even with correction or (b) a field of vision so restricted that it subtends an angle of 20 degrees or less even with correction).[46] As in the case with other sensory networks, maintenance of visual acuity requires integrity of the visual network (e.g., visual receptors, optic nerve and other pathways near the integrative sites). As most of these structures are anatomically near the eyes and the cerebrum, malignancies impacting these areas (e.g., retinoblastoma and optic glioma, malignancies of the CNS) have the highest potential of causing vision loss.[47] The loss in question may happen suddenly during or following the termination of curative treatment.[38,47]

Studies have focused on assessing visual losses in the pediatric cancer population, as survivors of pediatric malignancies are at risk for late side effects that may impair their visual acuity.[47] In this population, the important risk factors for development of these late side effects include exposure to radiation, cisplatin, or glucocorticoids and a young age upon cancer diagnosis, along with long-term neurocognitive and psychosocial sequelae.[47] The concept of losing the ability to see may be particularly distressing in children, who are often described, in developmental terms, as relying on visual stimulation to directly and concretely appreciate their environment. Consequently, the repercussions on a child's self-esteem are important, in a period where children are themselves grasping firsthand the concept of disability.[47,48]

Adjustment difficulties are further exacerbated by the potential for social stigma around visual impairment.[38,49] Common misconceptions of the public toward the pediatric oncological population revolve around the use of a cane for independent mobility during physical rehabilitation, with patients' perception of self-worth and satisfaction weighing against their capacity to adapt.[50] The dependency on family members for ADLs and financial issues arising from the condition can challenge family roles and dynamics.[50] These issues will fluctuate with time as the child develops and faces new milestones (e.g., advent of adolescence, seeking employment, achieving independence). Consequently, the possibility of functional decline and of adjustment issues alongside the uncertainty of the cancer prognosis raises challenges for this population due to the changing nature of the disability in question. This sense of instability may have important repercussions on the patient's sense of identity and level of satisfaction.[51]

The period of adjustment for children and adolescents with visual impairments may be marked by pervasive and intense anxiety, frustration, aggression, and depression, which may be underlying an overtly defensive attitude.[52,53] Additionally, the literature on irreversible vision loss in adults has demonstrated high levels of depression during adjustment to the visual impairment, and depressive symptoms seem to remain over time.[46] Furthermore, vision loss arising from orbital exenteration (i.e., removal of the entire contents of the orbit) and from the loss of actual eye and eye structures can cause important functional repercussions, as well as cause facial disfigurement, which may further impact patients' social interactions and affect their sense of embodiment.[54,55] In this context, it can be beneficial to consider orbital reconstruction procedures (e.g., orbital prosthesis, free flap reconstruction) to minimize the psychosocial difficulties that patients can experience post-exenteration.[54] However, recognition of the complications that can arise in the context of reconstruction is important, ultimately requiring an understanding of the value the patient attributed to the lost (and newly replaced) feature alongside the patient's level of satisfaction in light of this reconstruction. Thus, facial disfigurement is another aspect that needs to be assessed in the context of psychosocial oncology due to the importance of the facial region for one's self-concept and communication (verbal and nonverbal).[54,55] The topic of disfigurement is further covered in Chapter 7.

Consequently, in the context of malignancies affecting the eyes and the CNS, the implications of functioning together with the attached emotional turmoil related to the patient's dysfunction and disfigurement can further heighten disturbances during the cancer survivorship period, especially in domains of physical, role, emotional, and social functioning.[38,48] Further inquiry into the psychological and socioeconomic repercussions should be encouraged, in part due to the late effects following anti-cancer treatment.[47] An appreciation of the long-term adaptation process highlighting stage- and patient-dependent psychosocial and physical interventions for cancer survivors may benefit patients in terms of adjusting their self-image to include their new impairment, supporting their efforts to adequately resume their ADLs and reintegrate into their daily lives.

OLFACTORY AND GUSTATORY LOSS

Olfaction (i.e., the capacity to smell) and gustation (i.e., the capacity to taste) are senses that can also be impaired temporarily or completely lost following cancer treatments such as radiotherapy or chemotherapy. Olfaction is the ability to detect and identify an odor and to discriminate between odors, whereas gustation is the ability to sense the chemical reaction of a substance with receptors located on taste buds in the oral cavity. The sensation of gustation includes five established basic tastes: sweetness, sourness, saltiness, bitterness, and savory. Both olfaction and gustation require the physical and physicochemical integrity of the structures involved for proper sensation and perception of both modalities (i.e., from the olfactory mucosa and taste buds to the central nervous pathways).[56]

In oncology, olfactory and gustatory losses (OGL) mostly occur in head and neck cancers (HNC), as they concern the anatomical sites involved in the sensation, transmission, and integration of both modalities. In HNC, patients often undergo intensive radiotherapy, which increases the potential of acute and long-term side effects, including xerostomia (i.e., dryness in the mouth), dental issues, and impairments in mastication (i.e., capacity to use the jaw and teeth to crush and grind food), deglutition (i.e., process of swallowing), and taste.[57] More specifically, OGLs can be defined as either (a) a total (or partial) and permanent (or temporary) absence of taste and/or smell (b) an alteration of one's sensitivity to these stimuli, (c) a distortion of the sensation of taste and/or smell, or (d) the presence of phantom taste and/or odor.[56] As in visual losses, olfactory or gustatory dysfunctions may be conductive or sensorineural,[58] where conductive problems arise from mechanical obstruction of the upper nasal cavity, and sensorineural disorders arise following deficits in sensory receptors, nerve fibers, and/or defects within the integrative sites.[58,59]

Seen through our proposed model, the implications of a loss in function along with the lack of satisfaction arising from this alteration may bring important repercussions in terms of body image disturbances, especially as these losses often appear in the highly burdened context of patients with HNC (e.g., disfigurement, alteration in basic functions such as eating and speech). The loss of these basic sensations, with concurring side effects such as xerostomia and dysphagia, may not only interfere with the patients' ADLs and overall levels of functioning due to immediate repercussions on food enjoyment and nutritional intake but can also heighten the well-documented psychological toll in this oncological population. It can, for example, further stimulate the patient's sense of embodiment, particularly since the subjective perception of taste and smell alterations has been seen to endure following termination of curative treatment.[57,58,60,61] Ultimately, in the clinical care of cancer survivors, it is important to acknowledge the significance and diversity of OGLs along with the hedonic experience of foods, since valuing and normalizing the patient's loss can ultimately benefit adaptation.[56,62] Lastly, the impact on quality of life of the sensorineural impairments also depends on the value or importance placed on the function as well as the degree to which the function is temporarily or permanently altered (e.g., temporary altered sense of smell or taste during chemotherapy, permanent olfactory loss after radiation therapy).[57,58]

SOMATOSENSORY LOSS

Somatosensation refers to the CNS's ability to assess physical and other types of sensations applied to the skin (e.g., pressure, vibration, and temperature), along with its ability to sense movement within joints and joint positioning in space (e.g., proprioception and kinesthesia). Physiologically speaking, the capacity to sense, perceive, and react to a stimulus requires the integrity of the three-neuron complex: namely, the receptors (e.g., mechano-, chemo-, thermo-receptors), afferent and efferent neurons, and the integration sites. Thus, a somatosensory loss would arise within the context of impairment in these structures, potentially associated with radiation, surgery, lymphedema, or neuropathy. Despite the absence of evidence to support the implications of this loss, we may apprehend them by considering repercussions in terms of functional abilities like gait, ambulation, and balance, which can portray a sense of impairment and hence, impact one's self-schema.[37,63]

With respect to our proposed model, many health-related domains need to be further explored considering the sparse literature covering implications of somatosensory losses in oncology. For this purpose, further appreciation and understanding of somatosensation is required, mainly to comprehend specific etiologies in connection with the respective consequences of the loss (e.g., neuropathic pain, impairments in the locomotor and balance apparatus). This could also result in enhanced support and interventions developed in response to limitations of activity and restrictions in participation.

CLINICAL APPLICATIONS

In summary, just as cancer can generate definite changes in appearance and in function, limb and sensory losses can further impact the patient's sense of integrity due to visible losses as well as breaches in basic human functioning (e.g., gait, nutritional intake, social interactions, ADLs). From this presentation on limb and sensory loss in oncology, many clinical implications and future perspectives in terms of clinical inquiry and provision of healthcare services can be identified.

First, the sparse oncological literature in both domains of functional loss limits the adequate understanding of their impact on body image in clinical practice. It would be worthwhile to further study this impact using a conceptual model such as the ICF, given that the construct of body image has often been generalized to a noticeable (or even perhaps perceived) impairment in bodily structure.[18,64,65] Additionally, one may want to contextualize body image through the basis of validated frameworks of health and disability, an intersection that has not been to our knowledge previously elucidated in the body image literature.[66,67] As the outlook of the ICF stresses the all-encompassing understanding of health and functioning with respect to the various spheres of the individual (i.e., body structures/functions, activity, and participation, along with mediating and moderating personal and environmental factors), it becomes valuable to view body image, through an integrated understanding of the intersection of these spheres, in order to accurately target physical, psychological, and/or social impairments that heighten the disturbance in body image. For this matter, we proposed a model combining the ICF with attributes of body image disturbances relevant to the oncological context (see Figure 8.2).[1,9] The intent was to propose a standard model for defining, assessing, and addressing body image disturbances following cancer and cancer-related treatment, one that incorporates elements of human functioning, disability, and health that have an intersectional and reciprocal influence on the sense of self.

Another key point relates to the loss of limb and of senses and their impact on body image. Although they are considered separately in this chapter, it is important to contextualize the loss of functioning and its impact on body image as a dynamic system, in which each functional loss potentially acts synergistically as a trigger for body image disturbances. Within this framework, it appears necessary to incorporate cancer- and population-specific factors (e.g., late neurocognitive effects, implications of the cancer prognosis, and recurrences) to appreciate the burden of the losses and the remedial process of physically and psychologically adapting to the impairments in question.

This contextualization of the ICF requires a thorough review of the WHO's methodology of assessing functioning, in order to ensure standardization of terminologies and principles.[65] This methodology can easily be clinically appreciated through the structural perspective of Steiner et al.'s Rehab-CYCLE and their Rehabilitation Problem-Solving Form.[68] Despite their physical rehabilitation framework, the key elements of both models are noteworthy and adaptable to this area of inquiry. The Rehab-CYCLE possesses five sequential and cyclic key elements that highlight the process of rehabilitation by identifying the patient's problems and viewing them through an interdisciplinary framework to address the objective medical problems by relaying them to the patient's subjective concerns (see Figure 8.3).

With respect to the Rehab-CYCLE, the first element to be considered is *the identification of the problems and needs*. This step seeks to appreciate the current understanding of the patient's state of functioning and disability in terms of body structure and/or function in relation to activity limitations and participation restrictions, alongside acknowledging the patient's main concerns and short- and long-term goals.

The second element to be considered is *the relation of the problems to modifiable and limiting factors*. This step seeks to appreciate the individual and environmental factors that are mediating the effects of the impairments, limitations, and restrictions.

The third element to be considered is *the definition of target problems and target mediators and/or moderators alongside the selection of appropriate measures*. This step seeks to develop an objective clinical perspective considering the results of the previous steps. It comprises of interprofessional discourse between healthcare professionals (HCPs) and patients or proxies, which serves in aligning the patient's concerns and goals with the objective medical standards of the interdisciplinary team (e.g., markers of quality of life, scales to assess

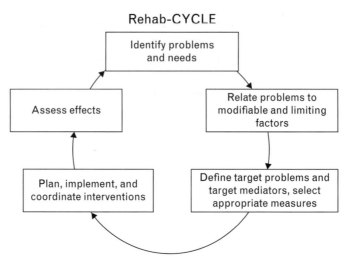

FIGURE 8.3: Steiner et al.'s Rehab-CYCLE.

Reprinted from Steiner W, Ryser L, Huber E, Uebelhart D, Aeschlimann A, Stucki G. Use of the ICF model as a clinical problem-solving tool in physical therapy and rehabilitation medicine. Physical Therapy. *2002;82(11):1100, by permission of Oxford University Press.*

This figure is an adaptation of the Rehabilitation Cycle developed by Stucki and Sangha[69]; the original figure was published in Rheumatology *(2nd ed.) Stucki G, Sangha O, Principles of rehabilitation, 11.1–11.14, Copyright Elsevier (1998).*

biopsychosocial functioning [e.g., mobility, strength, depression, anxiety, coping, social integration]). This process ensures that patients understand and agree with the proposed therapeutic protocol.

The fourth element within this framework is *the planning, implementation, and co-ordination of interventions*. This step seeks to address physical and psychosocial problems through the basis of interventions that directly and/or indirectly affect the functioning of individuals in their activities and/or participation (e.g., patient and proxy education, cognitive-behavioral therapy, physical rehabilitation).

The fifth element consists of *the assessment of the effects of the interventions*. This step seeks to re-assess the patient postintervention, combining the patient's subjective perception and selected measures to determine the results of the interventions. The endpoint of this framework consists of *successful problem resolution and/or achievement of goals*. However, if problems persist or new problems arise, the HCPs would reassess the patient, considering his or her current health status, and consequently revisit the Rehab-CYCLE.

The following example is presented to fully apprehend the Rehab-CYCLE along the lines of functional loss and body image. Following a limb loss (and/or the insertion of a prosthesis), a patient is required to adapt to the new biomechanics of his or her own body and potentially to the mechanical constraints of the prosthesis. This period of adaptation may require time and effort for the patient to be able to perform meaningful occupations. During this period of physical adaptation, the patient may exhibit negative psychological responses, such as difficulties with coping, anxiety, and depression, which may exacerbate feelings of shame and further depreciate one's self-image. In this case example, the use of the Rehab-CYCLE may allow the provision of interprofessional and multimodal services to ensure adequate physical and psychological rehabilitation. The first step in the Rehab-CYCLE involves delineating the repercussions in body impairments (e.g., limb loss) and activity limitations/participation restrictions (e.g., inability to perform meaningful occupations in the same manner such as work and leisure) and to explicitly acknowledge the patient's goals. The second step highlights the interplay of patient-specific (biopsychosocial factors; i.e., the patient's medical, psychological, and social status) and environmental (external influences; e.g., access to materials and services) facets of the problem. The third step seeks to ensure common ground between patients and therapists where there is presentation of the thera-peutic regimens (e.g., physical and occupational rehabilitation with psychosocial treatments such as antidepressants, cognitive-behavioral therapy involving work on irrational thoughts, negative schemas, relaxation, and social skills training) alongside the clinical objectives that will be monitored throughout the rehabilitative period (e.g., markers of physical function such as the ability to perform a given task [range of motion and fine motor skill assessments, etc.]) and levels of measured psychological state (such as depression, anxiety, and levels of body image disturbances). This step requires strong patient–therapist alliance and com-munication, as well as an alignment between the patient's and therapist's goals. The fourth step consists of the execution of the treatment protocol, and the fifth step consists of the reassessment of the patient following the plan's implementation.

Furthermore, steps 1, 2 and 5 of the Rehab-CYCLE can benefit from a template such as the Rehabilitation Problem-Solving Form, which is a clinical tool based on the ICF's health-related domains and cumulates the patient's subjective perspective alongside the HCP's ob-jective understanding in combination with domains of activity limitations, participation

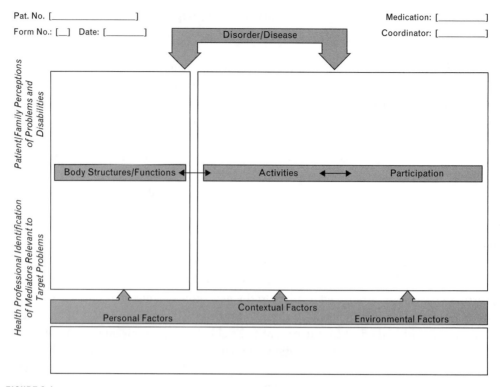

FIGURE 8.4: Steiner et al.'s Rehabilitation Problem-Solving Form.

Reprinted from Steiner W, Ryser L, Huber E, Uebelhart D, Aeschlimann A, Stucki G. Use of the ICF model as a clinical problem-solving tool in physical therapy and rehabilitation medicine. Physical Therapy. 2002;82(11):1101, by permission of Oxford University Press.

restrictions, and patient-dependent individual and environmental factors to further tailor treatment (see Figure 8.4).

The use of both frameworks ensures a broader evaluation of functioning, disability, and health, paving the way toward enhanced healthcare provision and understanding of the intersection between bodily dysfunction and body image. Consequently, satisfaction is not viewed as purely medically driven, based on objective physical results, but with consideration for the patient's subjective perspective of the loss.[70] One needs to pay careful attention in this evaluation to the balance between what is achievable in terms of functional adaptation and what would help patients adjust their expectations to the reality of limitations.[71,72] This evaluation is important to direct supportive services accordingly, including attention to the redefinition of body image following dysfunction.

Application of the ICF is essential in oncology for many reasons. First, in light of the complex needs that arise from limb and sensory losses, often involving specialized services for both physical (e.g., adaptation to assistive devices) and psychosocial (e.g., grief, coping with the loss, anxiety about the future) rehabilitation, some, if not all, patients may benefit from appropriate services before the initiation of the treatment protocol.[22,73] This period should inform patients and their proxies about long-term survivorship issues and seek to project the patients' functional needs to prepare them in light of these functional limitations and the ensuing psychosocial turmoil.[21] These services may also prepare patients to face social interactions in the transition from being perceived as an able-bodied individual to being perceived as one living with an impairment. Continuity from prehabilitative services throughout survivorship is key to sustain both physical and psychosocial functioning, ultimately requiring strong care pathways between hospitals and community settings.[3,42] All of this while keeping in mind that objective outcomes are often uncertain before treatment commences and that one needs to sustain hope in patients, if not in functional recovery then in their capacity to readjust. Second, the value placed on a patient-centered perspective commands thorough assessment of the various health-related domains throughout the cancer trajectory. This requires interdisciplinary collaboration as a *sine qua non* as well as proper communication, enabling the delivery of time-appropriate and efficient services.

The following clinical cases outline how the proposed frameworks can help in the assessment and treatment of functional losses alongside the implications for body image.

Clinical Vignette 1: Limb Loss

Mr. L., a 52-year-old patient recently diagnosed with soft-tissue sarcoma affecting his right distal calf, has undergone a LSS, followed by postoperative chemotherapy. The operation went well, and Mr. L. was quickly transferred to a rehabilitation unit. However, Mr. L.'s recovery has been slower than expected.

Mr. L. is a construction worker who lives with his wife, a housewife, on the third floor of an apartment building. They have one son that is currently in his last year of high school. The patient has taken some time off work to receive his treatments. Mr. L. is a regular jogger and enjoys biking during the summer.

From the moment of receiving the news of his cancer diagnosis, Mr. L. and his wife appeared very anxious and preoccupied. Mr. L. specifically demonstrated concerns regarding his postsurgical ability to return to work and perform his leisure activities. The wife expressed further concerns involving finances, employment, and uncertainty about the future, specifically worrying about the financing of their son's expenses for higher education. After additional probing, Mr. L. revealed feeling afraid of losing his "fight against cancer" considering that he lost his own mother to breast cancer. Mr. L. further disclosed that he was raised in a setting where men were thought to be the breadwinners and therefore feared that he would fail in supporting his family and in securing his son's future.

Due to the slow recovery, instead of going directly home, Mr. L. following discharge from acute care was transitioned to a community rehabilitation setting. He was demonstrating a lack in physical capacity (e.g., endurance, mobility), experienced constant fatigue, was often agitated, and experienced pain despite receiving an adequate pain control regimen. The patient was noncompliant with the treatments proposed by rehabilitation specialists. While medical doctors ordered tests and confirmed that he was stable on a physical and biochemical level, Mr. L. insisted that he was still ill, was pessimistic about the future, constantly complained about his functioning, and showed anger upon assistance by healthcare providers or by his wife and son, which further impaired his postoperative healing, caused muscle atrophy, ankle joint stiffening, and overall deconditioning. After several weeks, the team decided to send a consultation request to the attending psychologist.

The psychologist concluded that Mr. L. was presenting with an adjustment disorder with depressed mood. The clinical understanding was that Mr. L. experienced lowered self-esteem and self-worth, as well as feelings of shame arising from feeling physically incapable. These feelings translated into anger and resentment at any help, reinforcing this negative self-image. The sense of incapacity was fueled by Mr. L.'s sense of previous importance derived from work-related pursuits, jogging, and biking, as well as his role of provider for the family. Mr. L. mentioned feeling vulnerable and having lost the essence of who he was.

The psychologist initiated a treatment regimen focused on Mr. L.'s sense of loss and negative body image, which included cognitive-behavioral therapy and interpersonal therapy. His sense of value and self-worth eventually increased, and he was able to engage more proactively in his rehabilitation. He was offered Intensive Functional Rehabilitation and was discharged from the community rehabilitation setting two weeks after. The patient continued to be followed by a physiotherapist as an outpatient and continuous support was provided by a liaison nurse.

Clinical Vignette 2: Sensory Loss

Miss V., a seven-year-old girl and neuroblastoma cancer survivor, is currently followed by rehabilitation specialists for residual chemotherapy side effects. She is experiencing learning difficulties secondary to changes in audition and cognition. She has also shown a lack of balance, probably attributable to impaired equilibrium reactions.

Miss V. lives with her two parents in a two-floor bungalow. Both parents are elementary school teachers. Healthcare professionals have noted that the parents continuously express anxiety and frustration since their child's cancer diagnosis. Upon recent assessment, there are apparent changes in the family dynamics, secondary to financial demands and due to the parents' fears about the child's future prospects. The father increased his alcohol intake and has become increasingly absent, furthering the mother's feelings of helplessness and depression.

Miss V. reported fear and high levels of anxiety in response to the current family environment upon discussion with healthcare professionals. Her perception of her parents' actions have had important repercussions on her sense of self-worth and overall well-being. This was expressed in her social isolation, based on a profound fear of rejection from others, shame, and sense that she was not functioning at the same level as peers of her age. Her refusal to go to the park and her preference to stay inside was understood as an expression of inhibition related to poor self-esteem largely attributable to family conflicts. Her social isolation and devalued self impacted her capacity to adequately develop her auditory perception and to cognitively perform.

This understanding of the impact of her functional limitations on her sense of self and body image led to the broadening of the interdisciplinary team from a liaison nurse, audiologist, and physiotherapist to including a social worker, psychologist, and occupational therapist. It was initially important to prioritize addressing family dynamics around anxiety and difficulties coping, since these were modifiable barriers to optimal functioning for the child. The interdisciplinary team was eventually able to alleviate financial strain, improve parental communication, and increase their optimism toward the future. This work ensured gradual social reintegration of the parents into their meaningful activities and emphasized the benefit of their presence as support for their child. The inclusion of Miss V.'s parents in rehabilitation not only allowed to decrease anxiety and shame in her but also gradually increased her perception of self-worth. Concomitantly, Miss V. was able to benefit from audiology, speech language therapy, and physical rehabilitation.

While this chapter focuses primarily on exploring the impact of losses of limb and sensation, many other losses need to be considered in oncology with respect to body image. Functional losses that can be experienced in relation to physical symptoms (e.g., pain, fatigue, and nausea), decline in physical functioning, changing social (e.g., family and relationship dynamics) and living situations (e.g., necessity of temporary or prolonged hospitalizations), and the implications of services ranging from ambulatory and emergency care to palliative care have important contexts that need to be further appreciated. Their implications for health-related domains of functioning are crucial, and their intersection with body image and body image disturbances can become substantial if not properly addressed. In addition, the value of ascertaining the degree of overlap and influence of constructs such as depression, demoralization,[74] dignity,[75] and body image in relation to appearance and functioning is considerable, especially with respect to the various stages of the illness (e.g., diagnosis, posttreatment, survivorship, recurrence, and end of life). As outlined by the previous frameworks on the assessment of functioning, this intersectional framework further requires the understanding of the patient as a dynamic entity whose perceptions, beliefs, and values may change during the different stages of the illness.[71] This perspective may permit better distinctions between psychological dysfunction and body image, along with a better understanding of individual and environmental factors that may influence body image disturbances following a loss in function. Expanding our knowledge and conceptual frameworks in this field of inquiry can only lead to enhanced healthcare provision and better quality of life for our patients.

REFERENCES

1. World Health Organization. *Towards a Common Language for Functioning, Disability and Health: ICF.* Geneva: World Health Organization; 2002.

2. Henry M, Bdira A, Cherba M, et al. Recovering function and surviving treatments are primary motivators for health behavior change in patients with head and neck cancer: Qualitative focus group study. *Palliat Support Care.* 2016;14(4):364–375.

3. Furtado S, Briggs T, Fulton J, et al. Patient experience after lower extremity amputation for sarcoma in England: a national survey. *Disabil Rehabil.* 2017;39(12):1171–1190.

4. Garcia SF, Cella D, Clauser SB, et al. Standardizing patient-reported outcomes assessment in cancer clinical trials: a patient-reported outcomes measurement information system initiative. *J Clin Oncol.* 2007;25(32):5106–5112.

5. Tucker CA, Cieza A, Riley AW, et al. Concept analysis of the Patient Reported Outcomes Measurement Information System (PROMIS(R)) and the International Classification of Functioning, Disability and Health (ICF). *Qual Life Res.* 2014;23(6):1677–1686.

6. Cash TF, Smolak L. *Body Image: A Handbook of Science, Practice, and Prevention.* New York: Guilford Press; 2011.

7. DeFrank JT, Mehta CC, Stein KD, Baker F. Body image dissatisfaction in cancer survivors. *Oncol Nurs Forum.* 2007;34(3):E36–E41.

8. Henry M, Ho A, Lambert SD, et al. Looking beyond disfigurement: the experience of patients with head and neck cancer. *J Palliat Care.* 2014;30(1):5–15.

9. Rhoten BA. Body image disturbance in adults treated for cancer—a concept analysis. *J Adv Nurs.* 2016;72(5):1001–1011.

10. White CA. Body image dimensions and cancer: a heuristic cognitive behavioural model. *Psychooncology.* 2000;9(3):183–192.

11. Rhondali W, Chisholm GB, Filbet M, et al. Screening for body image dissatisfaction in patients with advanced cancer: a pilot study. *J Palliat Med.* 2015;18(2):151–156.

12. Varma P, Stineman MG, Dillingham TR. Epidemiology of limb loss. *Phys Med Rehabil Clin N Am.* 2014;25(1):1–8.

13. Paul K, Deirdre MD, Laura C, et al. *Limb Amputation.* Oxford: Oxford University Press; 2012.

14. Furtado S, Grimer RJ, Cool P, et al. Physical functioning, pain and quality of life after amputation for musculoskeletal tumours: a national survey. *Bone Joint J.* 2015;97B(9):1284–1290.

15. Richardson A, Addington-Hall J, Amir Z, et al. Knowledge, ignorance and priorities for research in key areas of cancer survivorship: findings from a scoping review. *Br J Cancer.* 2011;105(Suppl. 1):S82–S94.

16. Dillingham TR, Pezzin LE, MacKenzie EJ. Limb amputation and limb deficiency: epidemiology and recent trends in the United States. *South Med J.* 2002;95(8):875–883.

17. Eiser C, Darlington AS, Stride CB, Grimer R. Quality of life implications as a consequence of surgery: limb salvage, primary and secondary amputation. *Sarcoma.* 2001;5(4):189–195.

18. Furtado S, Errington L, Godfrey A, Rochester L, Gerrand C. Objective clinical measurement of physical functioning after treatment for lower extremity sarcoma—a systematic review. *Eur J Surg Oncol.* 2017;43(6):968–993.

19. Ozger H, Bulbul M, Eralp L. Complications of limb salvage surgery in childhood tumors and recommended solutions. *Strategies Trauma Limb Reconstr.* 2010;5(1):11–15.

20. Kadam D. Limb salvage surgery. *Indian J Plast Surg.* 2013;46(2):265–274.

21. Robert RS, Ottaviani G, Huh WW, Palla S, Jaffe N. Psychosocial and functional outcomes in long-term survivors of osteosarcoma: a comparison of limb-salvage surgery and amputation. *Pediatr Blood Cancer.* 2010;54(7):990–999.

22. Washington ED, Williams AE. An exploratory phenomenological study exploring the experiences of people with systemic disease who have undergone lower limb amputation and its impact on their psychological well-being. *Prosthet Orthot Int.* 2016;40(1):44–50.

23. Desteli EE, Imren Y, Erdogan M, Sarisoy G, Cosgun S. Comparison of upper limb amputees and lower limb amputees: a psychosocial perspective. *Eur J Trauma Emerg Surg.* 2014;40(6):735–739.

24. Senra H. How depressive levels are related to the adults' experiences of lower-limb amputation: a mixed methods pilot study. *Int J Rehabil Res.* 2013;36(1):13–20.

25. Singh R, Ripley D, Pentland B, et al. Depression and anxiety symptoms after lower limb amputation: the rise and fall. *Clin Rehabil.* 2009;23(3):281–286.

26. Coffey L, Gallagher P, Horgan O, Desmond D, MacLachlan M. Psychosocial adjustment to diabetes-related lower limb amputation. *Diabet Med.* 2009;26(10):1063–1067.

27. Jowsey-Gregoire SG, Kumnig M, Morelon E, Moreno E, Petruzzo P, Seulin C. The Chauvet 2014 Meeting Report: Psychiatric and psychosocial evaluation and outcomes of upper extremity grafted patients. *Transplantation.* 2016;100(7):1453–1459.

28. Clerici CA, Ferrari A, Luksch R, et al. Clinical experience with psychological aspects in pediatric patients amputated for malignancies. *Tumori.* 2004;90(4):399–404.

29. Verschuren JE, Geertzen JH, Enzlin P, Dijkstra PU, Dekker R. Sexual functioning and sexual well-being in people with a limb amputation: a cross-sectional study in the Netherlands. *Disabil Rehabil.* 2016;38(4):368–373.

30. Verschuren JE, Geertzen JH, Enzlin P, Dijkstra PU, Dekker R. People with lower limb amputation and their sexual functioning and sexual well-being. *Disabil Rehabil.* 2015;37(3):187–193.

31. Shell JA, Miller ME. The cancer amputee and sexuality. *Orthop Nurs.* 1999;18(5):53–57, 62–64.

32. Fauske L, Lorem G, Grov EK, Bondevik H. Changes in the body image of bone sarcoma survivors following surgical treatment—a qualitative study. *J Surg Oncol.* 2016;113(2):229–234.

33. Smith EM, Sakakibara BM, Miller WC. A review of factors influencing participation in social and community activities for wheelchair users. *Disabil Rehabil Assist Technol*. 2016;11(5):361–374.

34. Frost KL, Bertocci G, Stillman MD, Smalley C, Williams S. Accessibility of outpatient healthcare providers for wheelchair users: pilot study. *J Rehabil Res Dev*. 2015;52(6):653–662.

35. Bass JK, Knight KR, Yock TI, Chang KW, Cipkala D, Grewal SS. Evaluation and management of hearing loss in survivors of childhood and adolescent cancers: a report from the children's oncology group. *Pediatr Blood Cancer*. 2016;63(7):1152–1162.

36. van As JW, van den Berg H, van Dalen EC. Different infusion durations for preventing platinum-induced hearing loss in children with cancer. *Cochrane Database Syst Rev*. 2016;8:CD010885.

37. Bair WN, Prettyman MG, Beamer BA, Rogers MW. Kinematic and behavioral analyses of protective stepping strategies and risk for falls among community living older adults. *Clin Biomech*. 2016;36:74–82.

38. de Blank PM, Fisher MJ, Lu L, et al. Impact of vision loss among survivors of childhood central nervous system astroglial tumors. *Cancer*. 2016;122(5):730–739.

39. Landier W. Ototoxicity and cancer therapy. *Cancer*. 2016;122(11):1647–1658.

40. Hindhede AL. Negotiating hearing disability and hearing disabled identities. *Health*. 2012;16(2):169–185.

41. Aurelio FS, Silva SP, Rodrigues LB, Kuniyoshi IC, Botelho MS. Satisfaction of patients fit with a hearing aid in a high complexity clinic. *Braz J Otorhinolaryngol*. 2012;78(5):69–77.

42. Liberman PH, Goffi-Gomez MV, Schultz C, Novaes PE, Lopes LF. Audiological profile of patients treated for childhood cancer. *Braz J Otorhinolaryngol*. 2016;82(6):623–629.

43. Oliveira PF, Oliveira CS, Andrade JS, Santos TF, Oliveira-Barreto AC. Cancer treatment in determination of hearing loss. *Braz J Otorhinolaryngol*. 2016;82(1):65–69.

44. Lasak JM, Allen P, McVay T, Lewis D. Hearing loss: diagnosis and management. *Prim Care*. 2014;41(1):19–31.

45. Dille MF, Konrad-Martin D, Gallun F, et al. Tinnitus onset rates from chemotherapeutic agents and ototoxic antibiotics: results of a large prospective study. *J Am Acad Audiol*. 2010;21(6):409–417.

46. Senra H, Barbosa F, Ferreira P, et al. Psychologic adjustment to irreversible vision loss in adults: a systematic review. *Ophthalmology*. 2015;122(4):851–861.

47. Saha A, Salley CG, Saigal P, et al. Late effects in survivors of childhood CNS tumors treated on Head Start I and II protocols. *Pediatr Blood Cancer*. 2014;61(9):1644–1652; quiz 1653–1672.

48. Sato I, Higuchi A, Yanagisawa T, et al. Impact of late effects on health-related quality of life in survivors of pediatric brain tumors: motility disturbance of limb(s), seizure, ocular/visual impairment, endocrine abnormality, and higher brain dysfunction. *Cancer Nurs*. 2014;37(6):E1–E14.

49. Avery RA, Hardy KK. Vision specific quality of life in children with optic pathway gliomas. *J Neurooncol*. 2014;116(2):341–347.

50. Khan F, Amatya B. Factors associated with long-term functional outcomes, psychological sequelae and quality of life in persons after primary brain tumour. *J Neurooncol*. 2013;111(3):355–366.

51. Pinquart M. Body image of children and adolescents with chronic illness: a meta-analytic comparison with healthy peers. *Body Image*. 2013;10(2):141–148.

52. Ishtiaq R, Chaudhary MH, Rana MA, Jamil AR. Psychosocial implications of blindness and low vision in students of a school for children with blindness. *Pak J Med Sci*. 2016;32(2):431–434.

53. Bhuvaneswari M, Immanuel Selvaraj C, Selvaraj B, Srinivasan T. Assessment of psychological and psycho-physiological problems among visually impaired adolescents. *Iran J Psychiatry Behav Sci*. 2016;10(1):e3895.

54. Kuiper JJ, Zimmerman MB, Pagedar NA, Carter KD, Allen RC, Shriver EM. Perception of patient appearance following various methods of reconstruction after orbital exenteration. *Orbit*. 2016;35(4):187–192.

55. Ackuaku-Dogbe EM, Biritwum RB, Briamah ZI. Psycho-social challenges of patients following orbital exenteration. *East Afr Med J*. 2012;89(12):385–389.

56. Alvarez-Camacho M, Gonella S, Ghosh S, et al. The impact of taste and smell alterations on quality of life in head and neck cancer patients. *Qual Life Res*. 2016;25(6):1495–1504.

57. Badr H, Lipnick D, Gupta V, Miles B. Survivorship challenges and information needs after radiotherapy for oral cancer. *J Cancer Educ*. 2017;32(4):799–807.

58. Riva G, Raimondo L, Ravera M, et al. Late sensorial alterations in different radiotherapy techniques for nasopharyngeal cancer. *Chem Senses*. 2015;40(4):285–292.

59. Garzaro M, Pezzoli M, Landolfo V, Defilippi S, Giordano C, Pecorari G. Radiofrequency inferior turbinate reduction: long-term olfactory and functional outcomes. *Otolaryngol Head Neck Surg*. 2012;146(1):146–150.

60. Tribius S, Raguse M, Voigt C, et al. Residual deficits in quality of life one year after intensity-modulated radiotherapy for patients with locally advanced head and neck cancer: results of a prospective study. *Strahlenther Onkol*. 2015;191(6):501–510.

61. Janssens GO, Langendijk JA, Terhaard CH, et al. Quality-of-life after radiotherapy for advanced laryngeal cancer: results of a phase III trial of the Dutch Head and Neck Society. *Radiother Oncol*. 2016;119(2):213–220.

62. Belqaid K, Tishelman C, McGreevy J, et al. A longitudinal study of changing characteristics of self-reported taste and smell alterations in patients treated for lung cancer. *Eur J Oncol Nurs*. 2016;21:232–241.

63. Ko SU, Simonsick EM, Deshpande N, Studenski S, Ferrucci L. Ankle Proprioception-associated gait patterns in older adults: Results from the Baltimore Longitudinal Study of Aging. *Med Sci Sports Exerc*. 2016;48(11):2190–2194.

64. Halliwell E. Future directions for positive body image research. *Body Image*. 2015;14:177–189.

65. Stucki G, Kostanjsek N, Ustun B, Cieza A. ICF-based classification and measurement of functioning. *Eur J Phys Rehabil Med*. 2008;44(3):315–328.

66. Rhoten BA, Murphy B, Ridner SH. Body image in patients with head and neck cancer: a review of the literature. *Oral Oncol*. 2013;49(8):753–760.

67. Liu J, Peh CX, Mahendran R. Body image and emotional distress in newly diagnosed cancer patients: the mediating role of dysfunctional attitudes and rumination. *Body Image*. 2016;20:58–64.

68. Steiner WA, Ryser L, Huber E, Uebelhart D, Aeschlimann A, Stucki G. Use of the ICF model as a clinical problem-solving tool in physical therapy and rehabilitation medicine. *Phys Ther*. 2002;82(11):1098–1107.

69. Klippel JH, Dieppe P. *Rheumatology*. London; Philadelphia: Mosby; 1998.

70. Schaeffeler N, Pfeiffer K, Ringwald J, et al. Assessing the need for psychooncological support: screening instruments in combination with patients' subjective evaluation may define psychooncological pathways. *Psychooncology*. 2015;24(12):1784–1791.

71. Brinksma A, Tissing WJ, Sulkers E, Kamps WA, Roodbol PF, Sanderman R. Exploring the response shift phenomenon in childhood patients with cancer and its effect on health-related quality of life. *Oncol Nurs Forum*. 2014;41(1):48–56.

72. von Blanckenburg P, Seifart U, Conrad N, Exner C, Rief W, Nestoriuc Y. Quality of life in cancer rehabilitation: the role of life goal adjustment. *Psychooncology*. 2014;23(10):1149–1156.

73. Daigeler A, Lehnhardt M, Khadra A, et al. Proximal major limb amputations—a retrospective analysis of 45 oncological cases. *World J Surg Oncol*. 2009;7:15.

74. Clarke DM, Kissane DW. Demoralization: its phenomenology and importance. *Aust N Z J Psychiatry*. 2002;36(6):733–742.

75. Chochinov HM. Dignity and the eye of the beholder. *J Clin Oncol*. 2004;22(7):1336–1340.

CHAPTER 9

SEXUALITY, FERTILITY, AND CANCER

Kristen M. Carpenter and Lora L. Black

Advances in cancer screening and treatments have resulted in an increase in the number of cancer survivors, necessitating a greater focus on issues of survivorship.[1–4] Concerns related to sexuality and fertility are among the most common and distressing sequelae of cancer diagnosis and treatment.[5–8] Further, many of these problems persist late into survivorship, even after other side effects have diminished or resolved.[9,10] Survey data indicate that providers and patients agree that sexuality and fertility are important survivorship issues[11–13]; unfortunately, discussions related to sexuality and fertility are rare.[14–20] In this chapter, we provide a broad overview of concerns related to sexual function and fertility among cancer survivors. First, we review sexuality, sexual function concerns, and related treatment recommendations by problem area (e.g., desire, arousal, orgasm, pain). Second, we review the impact of cancer treatments on fertility and provide an overview of fertility preservation options by gender. In both sections, we provide information on special considerations for working with pediatric cancer survivors.

BODY IMAGE AND SEXUAL FUNCTION

Body image is a multifaceted concept that involves people's thoughts, feelings, and attitudes regarding their satisfaction/dissatisfaction about the way they look, as well as the importance and sense of self one derives from their physical appearance.[21,22] Research has consistently shown that body image impacts sexual function in both cancer and non-cancer populations.[23–27] High dissatisfaction and investment in one's physical appearance can lead to self-consciousness and avoidance of body exposure during sexual activity, which can have downstream effects on sexual function.[28] Poor body image is associated with a variety of poor sexual outcomes, including lower desire,[21,29,30] diminished arousal,[21,31] less frequent sexual activity,[21,29,32] infrequent or absent orgasm,[21,29,32] and lower satisfaction.[25,33]

As is covered throughout this volume, cancer patients and survivors suffer from body image disruption. Direct effects of treatment vary widely (e.g., hair loss,[26,34] urostomy/colostomy placement[35]) and negatively impact body image. Disfiguring surgeries are a common experience for cancer patients. For instance, vulvectomy (treatment for vaginal or vulvar cancer) or penectomy (treatment for penile cancer) can result in external genitalia that appear and function differently than "normal" and serve as a deterrent to sexual activity.[27,36,37] Similarly, women who undergo mastectomy report significantly more problems with sexual function compared to healthy controls or those undergoing breast conserving treatment.[38–41] The research concerning the impact of breast reconstruction on body image and sexual function in this population is mixed; some researchers have found no beneficial effect of breast reconstruction on sexual function,[27,42,43] while others have found that patients undergoing reconstruction actually have poorer sexual outcomes.[44,45]

Body image disruption can also occur due to indirect effects of cancer treatments, which can be both physical and emotional. Cachexia (i.e., significant loss of muscle mass or body weight) is a common experience of pancreatic, gastrointestinal, lung, and head and neck cancers.[46] Weight gain is also a common experience of survivors (e.g., breast[34]), which is contrary to lay notions of a "cancer patient." In any event, increases and decreases in body weight can negatively impact body image.[34,47] These experiences can be transient in some cases, but many patients and survivors report that their bodies "never" return to baseline form or function.[48] Disease and treatment often results in loss of functional capacity among cancer survivors,[47] furthering dissatisfaction with their bodies. The inability to engage in previously enjoyed activities due to functional loss or the feeling that their body is no longer able to serve a reproductive role can also impact a survivor's sense of masculinity or femininity. Given the relationship between body image and sexuality, it is important to assess body dissatisfaction in cancer survivors and incorporate elements of this as appropriate into treatment for sexual difficulties.

SEXUAL DYSFUNCTION/DIFFICULTY

Sexuality, like body image, is multifaceted. It follows that sexual difficulty, or sexual *morbidity* in the context of illness, takes many forms. Cancer survivors experience a variety of changes to their sexual lives—alterations to behavior (i.e., less frequent or absent sexual activity, more restricted sexual repertoire), function (i.e., less frequent/intense or absent desire, arousal, orgasm), satisfaction (i.e., reduced subjective sense of pleasure or enjoyment of sexual contact), and/or psychological distress related to sexual difficulties (e.g., guilt over lack of interest, sadness about lack of pleasure, anxiety about the possibility of pain). The data suggest that most cancer survivors will experience some level of sexual difficulty.[6–8] The most commonly reported problems among cancer survivors are loss of desire in both women and men, problems with lubrication and pain during intercourse in women, erectile disorder (ED) in men, and difficulties with orgasm.[49,50] These problems can result from hormonal, vascular, neurologic, psychological, and surgical changes associated with cancer treatments, including medications.[27,49,51] The type and extent of cancer treatment appears to be one factor that impacts sexual function in cancer survivors. For example, sexual problems tend to be worse among breast cancer patients who have undergone mastectomies and reconstructive surgery (vs. breast-conserving surgery).[42,44,52] Regardless of gender or disease site, individuals undergoing chemotherapy report nausea, weakness, pain, depression, and fatigue—all of which can impact sexual function.[27]

The most recent iteration of the *Diagnostic and Statistical Manual of Mental Disorders* (fifth edition [DSM-5])[51] separates sexual dysfunction diagnoses by gender and specifies seven disorders within the class.[a] Each carries unique features, but most share several general criteria: (a) symptoms must persist for at least six months; (b) they must cause significant distress in the patient; and (c) symptoms cannot be better accounted for by another symptom disorder, severe relationship distress, other significant stressors, or the effects of a substance or other medical condition. Other diagnostic specifiers include lifelong versus acquired, generalized versus situational, and severity (mild vs. moderate vs. severe). Because DSM-5 is a relatively recent development, much of the existing research is based on outdated criteria. For instance, hypoactive sexual desire disorder (HSDD), female sexual arousal disorder, and sexual aversion disorder in women have been collapsed under the broader diagnostic category of female sexual interest/arousal disorder. For the purposes of this chapter, we discuss issues of sexual desire, arousal, orgasm, and pain. It is important to note that many cancer survivors report sexual difficulties at "subclinical" levels, but regardless of whether subjective sexual difficulties experienced by cancer patients and survivors meet DSM-5 criteria, they are associated with significant psychological distress and reduced quality of life.[11-13] It follows that comprehensive cancer care must address patients' sexual concerns, during active treatment and well into survivorship. If this is to occur, providers must have an understanding of the range and complexity of sexual difficulties. It is also important to note that sexual difficulties might be longstanding, often preceding a patient's cancer diagnosis and treatment; however, providers seldom discuss sexual concerns with their patients[15-17,19,20] and this conversation might be a patient's first opportunity to do so. The recommendations throughout this chapter apply regardless of onset or duration.

ASSESSMENT AND TREATMENT OF SEXUAL DIFFICULTIES

Masters and Johnson[53] provided the first conceptualization of physiologic sexual response as a process that proceeds through phases of excitement (arousal), plateau, orgasm, and resolution. Kaplan[54] introduced a triphasic model that introduced a psychological component, sexual desire. More recently, Basson has expanded on these conceptualizations by integrating intimacy-based sexual motivations and rewards.[55] This integrated model outlines multiple pathways through which desire and arousal can be enhanced (e.g.,

---

[a]As is the case throughout the DSM-5, there are also categories for substance/medication-induced sexual dysfunction and for sexual difficulties that do not meet full criteria for another disorder in the class (e.g., other specific sexual dysfunction; unspecified sexual dysfunction).

seeking out sexual experiences; modification of negative processing of sexual stimuli) and suggests target outcomes (e.g., sexual responsiveness, satisfaction).[55] Such a conceptualization is particularly relevant to cancer survivors, as many treatment-related physiologic changes (e.g., vaginal shortening, numbness) will not remit. Indeed, a number of evidence-based treatments for sexual problems incorporate components implied by this model.[56,57]

The DSM-5 diagnostic criteria can serve as a useful starting point for assessment of sexual problems (see Table 9.1). It is important for sexual health providers to take a thorough sexual and medical history prior to addressing sexual concerns. There are a number of available questionnaires to assess sexual function, but there is no "gold standard." In 2004, consensus guidelines and a screening checklist were developed to evaluate sexual dysfunction in men and women within medical settings.[58] The version developed for women has also been adapted to address the unique needs of female cancer survivors (see Figure 9.1).[59] These checklists can be used as self-report screeners or as a way to start conversations about sexual concerns with cancer survivors. While there are unique aspects to sexual problems

TABLE 9.1: **DSM-5 and DSM-IV-TR Diagnostic Categories for Sexual Dysfunctions**

DSM-IV-TR	DSM-5[a]	Changes from DSM-IV-TR to DSM-5
Female		
Female Sexual Arousal Disorder	Female Sexual Arousal/ Interest Disorder	Sexual desire and arousal disorders combined in DSM-5
Sexual Aversion Disorder		Male and female sexual arousal disorders separated in DSM-5
Hypoactive Sexual Desire Disorder		
Female Orgasmic Disorder	Female Orgasmic Disorder	Addition of reduced intensity symptom
Dyspareunia	Genital-Pelvic Pain/ Penetration Disorder	Combination of dyspareunia and vaginismus
Vaginismus		Addition of fear or anxiety symptom
Men		
Hypoactive Sexual Desire Disorder	Male Hypoactive Sexual Desire Disorder	Male and female sexual desire disorders separated in DSM-5
Sexual Aversion Disorder		
Erectile Disorder	Erectile Disorder	No major changes
Male Orgasmic Disorder	Delayed Ejaculation	Terminology changed from orgasm to ejaculation in DSM-5
Premature Ejaculation	Premature Ejaculation	Addition of time specification (1 minute)

Note: DSM-5 = *Diagnostic and Statistical Manual of Mental Disorders* (5th ed.); DSM-IV-R = *Diagnostic and Statistical Manual of Mental Disorders* (4th ed., text rev.).
[a]In the DSM-5, all diagnoses require that the symptoms have persisted for a minimum duration of approximately six months. Aside from genito-pelvic pain/penetration disorder and male hypoactive sexual desire disorder, symptoms must also be experienced on all or almost all (approximately 75%–100%) of sexual activity.

Please answer the following questions about your overall sexuall function:

1. Are you satisfied with your sexual function? ☐ Yes ☐ No

2. Do you have any concerns about vaginal health? ☐ Yes ☐ No

   If not satisfied with sexual function AND/OR concerns about vaginal health, please continue.

2. Do you experience any of the following sexual problems or concerns?

☐ Little or no interest in sex

☐ Decreased sensation (or loss of sensation)

☐ Decreased vaginal lubrication (dryness)

☐ Difficulty reaching orgasm

☐ Pain during sex

☐ Vaginal or vulvar pain or discomfort (not during sex)

☐ Anxiety about having sex

☐ Other Problem or Concern: _____

[TIP: Some patients will respond that they are not having these problems or concerns because they stopped having sex altogether. The provider should reassure the patient, let her know that she is not alone, and ask if she can recall what kinds of problems or concerns she was having that led her to stop having sex.]

3. Would you like more information, resources, and/or would you like to speak with someone about these issues?

☐ Yes ☐ No

FIGURE 9.1: Sexual symptom checklist for women after cancer.

Reprinted from Bober SL, Reese JB, Barbera L, Bradford A, Carpenter KM, Goldfarb S, Carter J. How to ask and what to do: a guide for clinical inquiry and intervention regarding female sexual health after cancer. Current Opinion in Supportive and Palliative Care. *2016;10(1):46. Copyright 2016 Wolters Kluwer Health. Reprinted with permission.*

among cancer survivors, it is recommended that symptoms be treated in a manner similar to those without a cancer history.[60] There are relatively few trials of psychosexual interventions for cancer patients, but most incorporate elements of the models described here. Intimacy is an important component of sexuality that is often overlooked and should be evaluated when assessing for sexual dysfunctions among cancer survivors.[61] Targeted treatment for specific problems, such as vaginal dryness and erectile dysfunction, can easily be incorporated into multicomponent interventions. Treatment approaches are discussed within each section of specific sexual concerns.

SEXUAL PROBLEMS AMONG WOMEN

PROBLEMS WITH DESIRE

Sexual desire, or libido, refers to an individual's interest, drive, and/or motivation for sex and receptivity to sexual stimuli. Lack of desire is the most common clinical complaint among women seeking help for sexual problems in the United States and around the world.[62–67] Not surprisingly, it is one of the most common complaints among female cancer survivors as well.[12,49,60] DSM-5 defines female sexual interest/arousal disorder as a lack of or significant reduction in sexual interest or arousal, manifest by at least three of the following symptoms: absent/reduced sexual interest, absent/reduced sexual thoughts, no/reduced initiation of sexual activity, absent/reduced sexual excitement or pleasure during all or almost all sexual encounters, absent/reduced sexual interest or arousal in response to sexual cues, or absent/reduced genital or nongenital sensations in all or almost all sexual encounters.[51] Because prior iterations of the DSM separated disorders of desire and arousal, we discuss these issues separately. Prevalence studies of desire disorders in the general population suggest a wide range, from 10% to 46% among adult women, with rates higher among postmenopausal women.[64] A recent epidemiologic study suggests a prevalence of approximately 38%.[68] Cancer treatments, especially those that induce early menopause, are also associated with decreased sexual desire in some female cancer survivors.[20,27,69–72] For example, individual studies have reported problems with sexual interest or desire in 23% to 64% of female breast, bladder, and colorectal cancer survivors.[60,73] In addition, desire may continue to be impacted long after treatment has ended. One study found that 77% of women who underwent radical hysterectomy for gynecologic cancer reported low or little interest in sex five weeks after surgery, with 57% continuing to report this problem two years after surgery.[74]

Low/absent desire can arise from physical, physiological, psychological, and/or relationship factors.[60,75] Post-cancer sexual experiences that were painful or uncomfortable can reduce desire and increase anxiety related to sexual activity in female cancer survivors. For this reason, it is important to identify associated physical factors such vaginal dryness, vulvar discomfort, and pain with sexual activity in the sexual history. Significant alterations in hormones (e.g., estrogen, progesterone, testosterone) can further contribute to loss of desire in addition to causing changes in vaginal health. Androgen depletion deserves special mention in a conversation about sexual desire. Androgens, notably testosterone, appear to play a role in sexual desire among women.[76,77] Women who have undergone natural or iatrogenic menopause via oophorectomy, pelvic radiation, or chemotherapy lose approximately 50% of bioavailable testosterone.[78,79] There has been a great deal of interest in androgen supplementation as a treatment for HSDD,[80] and results from several randomized, controlled trials of androgen and/or androgen-estrogen replacement have suggested that testosterone supplementation can increase sexual desire (for reviews, see Amato and Buster[81], and David and Braunstein[82]); however, the benefits seem to occur only at supraphysiologic doses and appear to be lost without concurrent estrogen replacement,[83,84] and long-term safety data are not available.[85] Of particular concern in this context is the potential for increased breast and other cancer risk with such therapies.[86–91] To date, testosterone has not been approved by the U.S. Food and Drug Administration (FDA) for treatment of HSDD in women—cancer survivors or otherwise—though there are extensive reports and clinical examples of off-label use.[80]

A number of commonly prescribed psychiatric drugs have sexual side effects, such as low libido, including antipsychotics (including many anti-emetic agents, e.g., Compazine, Zofran), benzodiazepines, monoamine oxidase inhibitors, selective serotonin reuptake inhibitors (SSRIs), and tricyclic antidepressants.[92] Among the antidepressants, bupropion produces fewer sexual side effects, improves sexual function when substituted for an SSRI, and can be used as an adjunct to reduce sexual dysfunction induced by other (typically serotonergic) medications among depressed patients. Moreover, several studies have suggested bupropion is an effective standalone treatment for HSDD (see Mol and Brown[93] for a review). In August 2015, the FDA approved Addyi™ (flibanserin), a non-hormonal pill (developed as an antidepressant—5-HT$_{1A}$ agonist and 5-HT$_{2A}$ antagonist), for the treatment of acquired, generalized HSDD in premenopausal women.[94] It should be noted that flibanserin has only been approved for premenopausal women and has not been studied in cancer populations; uptake of the medication has also been exceedingly low.[95]

In any event, psychotherapy remains treatment of choice for low desire. Cognitive-behavioral therapy, specifically identifying and modifying maladaptive thoughts, expectations, and behaviors that contribute to/maintain low desire, has been efficacious,[96–98] as have behavioral sex therapy techniques, such as communication skills training and sensate focus,[99–101] often used in combination. Treatments that reduce sexual pain have also resulted in improvements in sexual desire.[102–104]

PROBLEMS WITH AROUSAL

Sexual arousal refers to the mental excitement and bodily sensations (e.g., increase in heart rate, increased sensitivity in breasts, muscle tension, genital engorgement, etc.) that occur in response to sexual stimuli, both physical and imaginal. Similar to desire, sexual arousal in females is complex; previous studies have noted at least 20 distinct genital and nongenital changes that occur when a women becomes aroused.[105] Genital changes include engorgement/vasocongestion, constriction and relaxation of smooth muscles of the vagina; vaginal lubrication response; increases in lactic acid, glycerol, and higher-molecular-weight lipids in vaginal fluid; and concomitant increase in vaginal pH, as well as increased heart rate, blood pressure, and respiration rate (see Meston[106] for a thorough overview of female sexual arousal). In some women, the physiological signs associated with arousal may or may not be correlated with subjective reports.[55,107] Some have suggested this is due to a tendency of some women to focus more on cognitive responses versus physiological sensations.[108] Indeed, previous research has shown that instructing women to attend to genital sensations increases concordance between physiological and subjective measures of arousal when viewing erotic stimuli.[109,110] A recent large-scale epidemiologic study ($N = 31,581$ American women 18 and older) suggested that 26% of healthy women reported current difficulties with sexual arousal.[68]

Reduced or absent sexual sensation during sexual activity arises from a number of physiologic, psychological, or hormonal factors.[51,111] Surgery for gynecologic, bladder, or colorectal cancer may involve extensive pelvic surgery and/or pelvic lymph node dissection that can result in vascular or lymphatic impairments. Such impairments in the genital region can reduce sensation and impact sexual function.[112] In addition, surgery and radiation therapy for breast cancer can also lead to reduced sensation or numbness in the breasts that may impact sexual function, especially if breasts were an important part of sexual activities prior to cancer.[27] As mentioned, current conceptualizations of female sexual response suggest that desire and arousal overlap.[113] In addition, the lack of relationship between subjective and physiologic arousal suggests that women's sexual behavior is more likely than men's to be contextually based (see Basson[114]) and driven by the need for emotional intimacy rather than physical arousal per se. There are no trials of psychological interventions specifically for arousal disorders, and thus psychotherapy strategies for desire and other disorders have been used. For example, one mindfulness-based cognitive-behavioral intervention for gynecologic cancer survivors was found to increase sexual function and self-reported arousal even though subjective measures of physiological arousal did not change.[115]

Vaginal lubrication during sexual activity is often regarded as an indicator of arousal. Prevalence rates for problems with lubrication range from 16% to 38% of women ages 40 to 80 worldwide, with 21% of American women reporting this problem.[116,117] Prevalence of lubrication issues range from 20% to 78% among female survivors, but when problems exist, they tend to be chronic.[74] Vaginal lubrication during sexual arousal is a result of vasocongestion (i.e., blood flow) to the genitals. The process depends on bioavailable estrogen. Difficulties with vaginal lubrication are commonly endorsed by female cancer survivors and are often attributable to menopause, whether natural or iatrogenic. Vaginal atrophy—thinning of the vaginal wall, loss of elasticity, impaired blood flow, and vaginal stenosis—can result from a variety of treatments, including surgery,[9,60,73,74] chemotherapy,[9,60,73] oral preventative agents (e.g., aromatase inhibitors, selective estrogen receptor modulators),[118–123] whole body radiation,[60] or pelvic radiation therapy.[60,124] Vaginal estrogen treatments can improve vaginal atrophy[125,126] but are contraindicated for a subset of women with breast or gynecologic cancers due to the risk of disease progression or recurrence. While there is preliminary evidence to suggest that use of estrogen may not increase breast cancer recurrence and mortality, there is a need for randomized control trials to assess safety.[126] Nonhormonal vaginal lubricants and moisturizers are available. Lubricants can be used to address acute dryness and pain during sexual activity.[120,127] Vaginal moisturizers, on the other hand, are used on a more regular basis and are meant to address day-to-day vaginal dryness and prevent sexual pain.[127–129] Moisturizers are recommended for sexual dysfunction treatment among cancer patients as a matter of routine care.[120,130] Use of other medications, such as PDE5 inhibitors, has not been found to be effective for treatment of low sexual arousal in postmenopausal women.[131,132]

PROBLEMS WITH ORGASM

A universal definition of female orgasm has eluded scientists, philosophers, and clinicians alike, though it is clearly characterized by a number of physiological reactions (e.g., myotonia, including rhythmic contractions of the vagina, uterus, and/or rectum) and subjective experiences (e.g., pleasure, altered consciousness) that vary both between and within individuals.[133,134] To complicate matters, an individual may herself be unable to determine whether she experienced orgasm during a given sexual experience.[133,135] Nevertheless, it is clear that orgasmic difficulties affect a substantial proportion of women at some point in their lives. DSM-5 defines female orgasmic disorder (FOD) as delay, infrequency, absence, or reduced intensity of orgasm in the majority of sexual experiences.[51] A review of prevalence studies between 1990 and 2000 found estimates ranging from 4% to 24% in general populations from the United States and Europe[64]; only one of these studies, however, utilized DSM criteria for the disorder. The distress criterion, in particular, is often omitted, which significantly affects prevalence estimates given that many women report infrequent or absent orgasms without experiencing associated distress. For example, a study of a nationally representative sample of Swedish women found that only about 60% of women who reported orgasmic problems found them distressing.[136] Data utilizing DSM-5 criteria are not yet available, but studies utilizing full DSM (fourth edition, text revision) criteria (including the distress criterion) and population-based samples suggest a more conservative prevalence estimate of 3% to 10% in the United States and Europe.[137–141] Rates of difficulties achieving orgasm range from 0% to 30% of colorectal,[142] 16% to 36% of breast,[60] 45% of bladder,[143] and 44% to 64% of bone marrow/lymphatic female cancer survivors.[144,145]

Although pharmacotherapy for female sexual dysfunctions has received an enormous amount of interest in recent decades,[146,147] cognitive and behavioral techniques remain the most effective and are recommended as first-line treatment for FOD by the International Society for Sexual Medicine.[148] Andersen's[149] review of FOD treatment trials beginning in the 1960s thoroughly documents the efficacy of directed masturbation, sensate focus, and systematic desensitization alone or in combination. These classic components remain essential tools in the treatment of FOD. Few studies specifically targeting FOD with behavioral treatments have been conducted since the 1980s; recent research has focused more on desire, arousal, and sexual dysfunction more broadly. However, reviews of the FOD treatment literature suggest that directed masturbation is the most effective of the three treatment components described and that adding sensate focus may enhance its effects.[149,150] More recent research indicates that the coital alignment technique may be helpful for partnered women particularly interested in experiencing orgasm during vaginal intercourse.[151] In addition to psychotherapies directly targeting sexual behavior, a number of evidence-based psychotherapies appear to improve orgasmic function among women or serve as valuable adjuncts to sex therapy. Many forms of couples therapy, for example, are effective in addressing problems within intimate relationships that can contribute to orgasmic dysfunction (see Lebow, Chambers, Christensen, and Johnson[152] for a review). In addition to its relation to FOD itself, as discussed previously, relationship satisfaction may interact with individual treatment targeting FOD to influence outcomes.[153]

Given pelvic floor involvement in orgasm, the pelvic musculature seems a natural target for intervention in FOD. Although Kegel exercises are widely recommended, there is no evidence of direct benefit for FOD.[154–156] That said, to the extent that Kegel exercises improve sexual arousal,[157,158] reduce anxiety/muscle tension, and/or improve a women's comfort during sexual activity, Kegels can serve as a beneficial adjunct to cognitive-behavioral therapy. More recently, interventions targeting pelvic muscle function have focused on women with urinary incontinence. These conditions are regularly treated with Kegel exercises or sacral neuromodulation, an electrical stimulation of the nerves that control the pelvic floor, urethral sphincter, and other pelvic muscles. Preliminary evidence supports the use of pelvic floor muscle training,[159,160] sacral neuromodulation,[161,162] or a combination of these interventions[163] to improve orgasmic function in women with incontinence, but no randomized trials exist and more evidence is needed. The Eros Therapy™ device is an FDA-approved clitoral vacuum that increases blood flow and engorgement.[164] Although it has not been tested in women with FOD, it has been found to improve orgasmic function in small samples of healthy controls, women with unspecified female sexual dysfunction, and women with sexual dysfunction following radiation therapy for cervical cancer.[164–166]

Case Example: Mary

Mary was a married, Caucasian female in her early 60s. She and her husband had been married 40 years; he had been her only lifetime sexual partner. She identified as Roman Catholic. One year prior to presentation, Mary had been diagnosed and treated for ovarian cancer. Treatment included total abdominal hysterectomy, bilateral salpingo-oophorectomy, and pelvic and para-aortic lymph node sampling. She received eight cycles of intravenous chemotherapy over the subsequent six months. Mary had been postmenopausal (~eight years) at the time of her cancer diagnosis; medical history was remarkable for hypothyroidism, which was well-managed.

Mary reported intercourse frequency of two to four times per week throughout her marriage. Mutual manual and oral stimulation were typical in their sexual routine. She reported she had not masturbated at any point in her life due to religious beliefs and feeling it was "unnecessary" given her rich sexual life with her husband. She reported a pre-cancer history of satisfactory sexual interest, arousal during sexual activity, and a history of orgasm "almost always" with sexual contact. She stated she had begun to experience mild vaginal dryness and concomitant discomfort with penetration at the time of menopause but that she and her husband used water-based lubricants with perceived benefit. Mary and her husband abstained from sexual intercourse for several months following her surgery and resumed sexual activity during chemotherapy on off-cycle weeks. She described her partner as loving, patient, and supportive. She described feelings of closeness and was satisfied with the emotional connection she felt to her husband during sexual activity.

When Mary presented to clinic, she and her husband engaged in sexual activity one to three times per week; she continued to report satisfactory interest and arousal but absent orgasm. Her Female Sexual Function Inventory total score was 27 (in the clinical range), her Female Sexual Distress Scale score was 13 (slightly below the clinical cut-off score of 15, with higher scores indicating more distress), and she rated her sexual satisfaction as "somewhat inadequate." Depressive and anxious symptoms were low outside the context of her sexual life. Mary felt her relationship with her partner was beginning to suffer because she would "shut down" during sexual activity if she did not feel she was moving closer to orgasm. She reported that she would become distressed to the point of "sobbing" during and following sexual encounters. Under DSM-5, Mary met criteria for FOD (acquired, generalized, severe). We recommended a course of cognitive-behavioral therapy, with the goals of reducing distress associated with sexual difficulties, increasing orgasmic capacity, and improving relationship functioning.

SEXUAL PAIN

DSM-5 defines genito-pelvic pain/penetration disorder as persistent or recurrent difficulty with vaginal penetration, vulvovaginal or pelvic pain during intercourse, fear or anxiety about pain related to vaginal penetration, or tensing/tightening of pelvic floor muscles during attempted vaginal penetration.[51] There are currently no prevalence rates for genito-pelvic pain/penetration disorder, as this is a significant modification from previous iterations of the DSM. However, recent studies have suggested that approximately 15% of women in North America and 9-% to 31% of women globally report experiencing pain with sexual activity (previously referred to as dyspareunia in the DSM).[116,117] Reports of pain during sexual activity are exceedingly common among female cancer survivors: 35% to 38% for breast,[12] 6% to 60% for colorectal,[12] 35% to 61% for bone marrow/lymphatic,[12] and 29% to 40% for gynecologic cancer.[19,74,112,124,167] While pain during intercourse in female cancer survivors is often associated with vaginal dryness, other treatment sequelae contribute. For example, chemotherapy-induced immunosuppression can lead to vaginal thrush or infections that result in persistent vulvar pain.[27] In addition, chemotherapy and bone marrow transplants can cause graft versus host disease, which affects the genitals in 25% to 35% of female cancer survivors. This complication may result in scar tissue and narrowing of the vagina that can exacerbate dyspareunia.[168,169] Fear or anxiety related to pain during or following vaginal penetration is a common report from female cancer survivors.[170] Another potential source of pain is fibrosis or atrophy related to pelvic radiation or surgery. Vaginal dilators are often recommended for women who have undergone these treatments. Dilation is believed to increase vaginal comfort during penetrative sex and improve pelvic floor muscle control[171]; however, there is limited research to show the beneficial effects of regular dilator use for preventing stenosis or improving quality of life.[172] It is unclear whether the treatment mechanism for dilator use is the stretching of vaginal tissue or stimulating oxygenated blood flow, calling into question the possible utility of alternative methods.[49]

Psychotherapy can help to address fear of pain, reduce pain catastrophizing, and teach skills for pain prevention/reduction. Behavioral strategies, such as using alternative sexual positions and/or using supports (e.g., pillows), can ease discomfort during sexual activity.[59] In addition, one study has shown decreases in dyspareunia and distress in breast cancer survivors when using topical lidocaine on the vulva prior to sexual activity.[173] However, this is a small study in which few survivors had ever used vaginal moisturizers to help with pain associated with vulvovaginal dryness. Additional research is needed to assess any beneficial effects of lidocaine above and beyond regular use or moisturizers and/or lubricants.

SEXUAL PROBLEMS IN MEN

PROBLEMS WITH DESIRE

In contrast to the diagnosis of female sexual interest/arousal disorder, the DSM-5 does not collapse disorders of desire and arousal for males. DSM-5 defines male hypoactive sexual desire disorder as persistently/recurrently deficient or absent sexual thoughts or fantasies and desire for sexual activity.[51] As this definition does not provide specific symptoms, it is difficult to compare rates of desire disorders between males and females. Community-based studies indicate prevalence rates of 0% to 3% among healthy men, with incidence rates increasing with age[64]; however, other studies have shown rates as high as 6% among men 18 to 24 years old and 44% among men 66 to 74 years old.[141] While decreased desire is reported by some men, it has received far less attention among male cancer survivors compared to female survivors.

As with women, low desire among men is multifactorial and arise from physical,[174] hormonal,[175] psychological,[176] and/or relationship issues.[175,177] In non-cancer populations, lower sexual desire is seen among individuals with higher levels of depression,[178] anxiety, and anger.[177] In cancer survivors, uncertainties about prognosis, fear of recurrence and/or treatment, reduced quality of life, and impairment in physical function can all negatively impact sexual desire. Body image concerns following treatment for prostate, penile, and testicular cancer can also impact sexual desire in these populations.[179] Management of psychological conditions though medication and/or psychotherapy may help to improve distress, which can have a positive impact on sexual desire. Further, targeted psychosexual interventions or psychoeducation may be helpful in resolving relationship factors or other sexual problems that impact sexual desire.[174]

Serum testosterone level is a well-established correlate of sexual desire among men with and without a cancer diagnosis.[175,180,181] Several studies investigating desire in male prostate cancer survivors have shown an association between androgen deprivation therapy and decreased levels of sexual interest and arousal, as well as poorer overall sexual function.[182–185] Reduction in sexual interest has been reported among testicular cancer survivors as well.[186] Many studies show success with testosterone replacement in healthy men, although there is concern about the use of such treatment among prostate cancer survivors, as exogenous testosterone can stimulate the growth of some prostate cancer cells and increase risk of recurrence.[179,187] The benefit of such interventions is unclear, as the primary outcome of studies of hypogonadism (diminished output of the gonads, resulting in low serum testosterone levels)[187] among prostate cancer survivors has been serum testosterone level (vs. discrete sexual symptoms, such as desire). Most studies do note incidental increases in libido,[188–190] erectile function,[188,189] and sexual performance[190] in the majority of patients; however, the samples are very small ($n = 5$–13), making it difficult to draw conclusions about efficacy or safety. To date, there have been no studies of psychosexual interventions targeted for low desire among male cancer survivors; however, one trial demonstrated an improvement in desire following a rehabilitation counseling intervention targeting erectile function in sample of prostate cancer survivors.[191] Thus there may be utility for psychosocial interventions targeting difficulties erectile functioning and sexual desire simultaneously.

PROBLEMS WITH AROUSAL/ERECTION

Erection is the principal sign of sexual arousal among men. Erections are produced by autonomic nerve activity that relaxes smooth muscle to increase arteriolar dilation and blood flow to the erectile tissue in response to genital or nongenital sexual stimulation.[192] ED is defined as a male experiencing marked difficulty obtaining or maintaining an erection during sexual activity and/or a decrease in erectile rigidity during all or almost all occasions of sexual activity.[51] Medical conditions, medications, and medical treatments that impact nerves or blood flow can disrupt this cascade of events, negatively affecting erectile function. Overall prevalence rates of ED in the general population range from 10% to 19%, with rates increasing with age.[116,193,194] A recent large-scale epidemiological study across 29 countries ($n = 13,618$) found that rates of ED increase from 2% of 30- 39-year-olds to 53% of 70- to 80-year-olds.[116] ED is one of the most common sexual complaints in non-cancer populations, and risk factors are similar to those for heart disease due to the role of vascular function in the process of erection.[116,195,196]

Recent studies have reported rates of ED in prostate,[12] testicular,[186,197,198] colorectal,[199] and bone marrow/lymphatic[144] cancer survivors ranging from 14% to 90%; however, studies vary widely in how they assess ED, making it difficult to ascertain true rates in this population.[12,198,200] The pathology causing postsurgical ED among prostate, testicular, and bladder cancer survivors is damage to the nerves that control erections. Studies have shown that patients undergoing nerve-sparing surgeries are more likely to regain erectile function than those undergoing traditional surgeries.[201–203] While nerve-sparing techniques can be used to reduce damage, preservation cannot be guaranteed[49,204] and other problems can arise. For instance, scar tissue can impair blood flow in the accessory pudendal arteries, leading to ED among prostate cancer survivors who have no apparent cavernous nerve damage.[204] Further, fibrosis in the soft tissue of the penis can build up after surgery, resulting in ED issues.[205] ED has also been reported in patients undergoing external beam radiation therapy and brachytherapy for prostate, testicular, or pelvic cancers; however, these rates are lower than those seen following radical prostatectomy.[206–209] The fibrosis associated with radiotherapy appears to be more gradual than that seen after surgery and thus presents as a more gradual onset of ED.[206,210] Further, post-radiation ED in cancer survivors is likely due to a combination of vascular changes in multiple penile structures (e.g., cavernous bodies,[211] neurovascular bundles,[212] and the penile bulb[213]), making it difficult to establish whether there are dose-response relationships related to individual anatomical structures.[60]

The majority of research on treating sexual dysfunction among men focuses on ED. Some of the strongest evidence in cancer samples has been found for oral phosphodiesterase type 5 (PDE5) inhibitors (e.g., tadalafil, sildenafil) following treatment for prostate cancer[214]; however, these medications are ineffective in the event of complete loss of erectile function following radical prostatectomy.[215] Recently, PDE5 inhibitors have been used prophylactically as part of a penile rehabilitation protocol following radical prostatectomy[216] and radiotherapy[217] for prostate cancer. However, large multicentered, placebo-controlled studies are still needed to assess therapeutic benefit and cost-effectiveness.[218] While the use of more invasive treatments (e.g., penile injections, prostheses) produces similar or better outcomes than oral medications, uptake of these treatment options is low, possibly due to their increased risk of side effects, inconvenience, and discomfort associated with more invasive treatments.[219,220]

Despite the availability of effective interventions, a number of cancer survivors do not seek treatment for ED. One study found half of the prostate cancer survivors surveyed were concerned with their sexual function posttreatment, but most had not trialed any medication or devices.[219] Possible explanations for this include patient reluctance to bring up ED concerns to healthcare professionals, as well as failure of providers to discuss these options with patients.[219] There are a limited number of studies investigating the effectiveness of psychotherapeutic treatments for ED. Available evidence is mixed regarding their effectiveness. Some studies show that group psychotherapy may improve erectile function among non-cancer populations, but only one has shown therapy to be superior to PDE5 inhibitors (see a meta-analysis of psychosocial interventions for ED[221]). In a recent review of available treatments for cancer survivors,[214] the only psychotherapeutic intervention found to improve sexual functioning among prostate cancer survivors was a psychoeducational intervention on impact of prostate cancer on sexual function. Interestingly, there was no difference whether the sessions were conducted with the patient alone or with a partner. A separate trial for prostate cancer survivors aimed to increase uptake of prostaglandin E1 intra cavernous injections yielded no improvements in sexual function.[214]

Case Example: John

John, age 58, was a married, African American male who presented to clinic with complaints of erectile difficulties following treatment for prostate cancer. He and his wife, who accompanied him to the appointment, had been married for 35 years and had one adult daughter. John was diagnosed with early-stage prostate cancer eight months prior and underwent a radical prostatectomy soon after diagnosis. John reported that he and his wife engaged in sexual intercourse approximately two to three times per month prior to his cancer treatment; he denied a history of sexual problems. John reported that he was able to achieve partial erections during partnered and individual sexual activity approximately half the time but stated that his erections were seldom sufficient for penetration. He reported that he was able to achieve orgasm most of the time. John reported significant frustration and reported he feels like "less of a man." John stated that he was informed of possible erectile difficulties following prostatectomy but did not think they would be this significant/distressing and now regrets the decision to undergo the procedure. John was initially prescribed sildenafil but had only a partial response; he received additional education regarding PDE5 inhibitors at his last urology visit and agreed to trial tadalafil.

At presentation, John reported attempting intercourse approximately once per month. He stated that he quickly becomes frustrated and ends the sexual encounter. John's wife reported that he will sometimes engage in manual and oral stimulation in an effort to "please (her)." John expressed concern that she will be unfaithful if he is unable to perform sexually; his wife reported that she tries to reassure him but that the ongoing conversation now leads to arguments. John's total score on the International Index of Erectile Dysfunction was 10 (severe erectile dysfunction). His score on the Beck Depression Inventory-II was 13 (minimal depressive symptoms); he stated that these symptoms are confined to his sexual concerns. Under DSM-5, John met criteria for male ED (acquired, generalized).

We recommended a course of cognitive-behavioral therapy with the goal of reducing distress and improving communication. We also recommended continued follow-up with urology; John planned to return for follow-up in one month to discuss the effectiveness of tadalafil, as well as the possibility of other treatment options, such as penile injections. John expressed some concerns about injections, including possible pain and awkwardness of self-administering injections before sexual encounters, but agreed to discuss this option with his urologist at the next appointment.

PROBLEMS WITH ORGASM/EJACULATION

Male orgasm is characterized by the rhythmic contractions of the bulbocavernosus and isehiocavernosus muscles, and the external urethral sphincter that result in ejaculation.[192] In the DSM-5, diagnoses related to orgasm in males include delayed ejaculation and premature (early) ejaculation. Delayed ejaculation occurs when males experience marked delay in or infrequency or absence of ejaculation in all or almost all partnered sexual activity.[51] Recent changes to the DSM make prevalence rates outdated. Prevalence of male orgasmic disorder in community-based studies suggest it has ranged from 0% to 3%,[64] with a recent large-scale epidemiological study in the United States showing a higher rate of 8%.[64,117] DSM-5 defines premature (early) ejaculation as persistent or recurrent ejaculation during partnered sexual activity that occurs within one minute of vaginal penetration and before the person wishes it.[51] Community-based studies suggest prevalence rates between 4% and 29% based on previous diagnostic criteria (e.g., did not include the one-minute time frame).[64] As premature ejaculation is not commonly endorsed by patients following cancer diagnosis or treatment, it is not discussed in this chapter. There are several other ejaculatory difficulties that are not specified in the DSM. For instance, dry ejaculation, in which semen passes into the bladder during orgasm, can result from surgery for prostate[27,222] and bladder cancer.[60] Climacturia, the inadvertent leakage of urine during orgasm, has also been reported by 20% to 100% of those undergoing surgery for prostate cancer.[222-226] While many studies found no baseline factors related to climacturia, one study found that those further from surgery were less likely to experience orgasm-associated urination[225] and another found that self-reported daytime incontinence, shortened penile length, and ED were related to climacturia.[226] While these side effects do not appear to impact the survivor's ability to achieve orgasm, sensations may be altered or diminished, and loss of urine can be embarrassing/distressing, which can lead to avoidance of sexual contact.[27,222]

While there are a number of recommended coping strategies and therapies, there are limited data regarding their effectiveness. Survivors may benefit from psychotherapy that addresses changes in sensations associated with orgasm or lack of ejaculation during orgasm.[222] Behavioral strategies can be helpful; for instance, men who experience urine leakage at orgasm are advised to empty their bladder before sexual activity[222,224,225] and to use condoms if they believe leakage would interfere with sexual contact.[225] The use of a variable tension loop (ACTIS™) placed around the base of the penis has also been shown to reduce climacturia in some patients.[224,225] There have been anecdotal reports in support of daily tricyclic antidepressant use; however, there are no trials or discernable analyses to support this practice.[225]

SPECIAL CONSIDERATIONS FOR PEDIATRIC CANCER SURVIVORS

Research on sexual development among pediatric cancer survivors clearly demonstrates that treatment for pediatric cancers impacts sexual function in adulthood. Rates of self-reported problems with sexual function range from 18% to 52% among survivors.[13,227,228] In a recent cohort study ($N = 291$ adult survivors of childhood cancers in the United States), Bober et al.[228] demonstrated that nearly one-third report two or more discrete sexual symptoms. Regarding particular issues, 30% reported they were not interested in sex and 23% reported difficulties with arousal. Further, 19% of men reported difficulties obtaining and/or maintaining an erection and 29% of females reported difficulties in achieving orgasm.[228] Another cross-sectional study ($N = 599$ adult pediatric cancer survivors in the

United States) showed that 12% report problems with arousal, 8% of men reported difficulty achieving/maintaining an erection, and 25% of women reported difficulty with orgasm.[227] A smaller study of 60 Dutch childhood cancer survivors found that 41% report almost no sexual desire.[13] Finally, a large study of US and Canadian male childhood cancer survivors ($n = 1,622$) found that 12% met criteria for ED (per scores on the International Index of Erectile Function). Interestingly, only 6% reported receiving treatment for ED.[229] Studies have consistently reported higher rates of sexual problems among female survivors compared to their male counterparts.[227,228] This stands to reason, as treatment for a subset of pediatric cancers can result in complete ovarian failure (i.e., iatrogenic menopause), which can lead to vaginal dryness and the many other concerns described earlier.[230] Unfortunately, there are no studies reporting rates of genito-pelvic pain/penetration disorder or dyspareunia among female childhood cancer survivors.

Treatment for sexual difficulties among survivors of childhood cancer mirror those for survivors of adult cancers. While discussions about sexuality may be difficult for pediatric oncologists to have with adolescent survivors, such discussions may help to identify concerns and prompt appropriate referrals as needed.[13] In addition, some studies have shown that sexual difficulties among pediatric cancer survivors do not appear to be associated with treatments that are known to cause gonadal toxicity or infertility. Thus, it is important for healthcare providers to address sexuality among pediatric cancer survivors and to avoid limiting this discussion to potential impact on fertility.

SUMMARY

Overall, a significant number of cancer survivors report difficulties with sexual function following their diagnosis and treatment. Anatomical, physiological, and hormonal changes from cancer treatments, as well as psychological and relationship changes, impact patients' sexual lives. In general, their problems should be treated in a similar fashion to those experienced in non-cancer populations. Research to date has shown that psychotherapy (e.g., mindfulness strategies, cognitive restructuring, etc.) and behavioral sex therapy can improve desire, arousal, sexual pain, and orgasmic function in female survivors. In addition, vaginal moisturizers and lubricants are recommended to help with inadequate vaginal lubrication and concomitant pain with sexual activity. Pelvic floor training (physical therapy) and sacral neuromodulation can improve orgasmic function among women. For men, research has shown that the most effective treatments for erectile difficulties are pharmacological or mechanical. Preliminary research has shown mixed evidence for psychosocial interventions among men, with the most robust evidence for couples-based treatments that incorporate elements of sex therapy. In spite of effective treatments for many of these difficulties, sexual problems are often not identified by medical professionals during routine cancer care. It is important to note that difficulties with sexuality in cancer survivorship also appear to generalize to pediatric cancer survivors, including low desire and difficulties with arousal. However, this area is largely understudied, and, while treatments may mirror those for adult cancers, limited work has been done in this area.

FERTILITY

Infertility is defined as the inability to conceive after one year of intercourse without contraception by the Committee for Monitoring Assisted Reproductive Technology and the World Health Organization.[231] The loss or compromise of reproductive potential is a worry for many cancer survivors of child-bearing age.[232] In many ways, survivors are no different than others suffering with infertility. Affective responses include distress,[11,49,233] depression,[11] and grief[234] and is a source of relationship distress.[18,234] Perhaps unique to the cancer context, many survivors worry about the possible impact of cancer treatments on the health of their future children.[18] Generally, infertility in cancer survivors can be the result of hormonal or anatomical changes as well as the gonadotoxic effects of radiation and/or chemotherapy.[232,234] Chemotherapy agents with high to intermediate risk of gonadotoxicity include cyclophosphamide, cholarambucil, melphalan, busulfan, nitrogen mustard, procarbazine, cisplatin, and adriamycin.[235] Many of these agents are used in combination therapy for ovarian, breast, and testicular cancer, as well as Hodgkin's disease.[236] Rates of permanent infertility following cancer treatment vary and are dependent on many factors. Azoospermia (i.e., absence of sperm in ejaculate) and amenorrhea (i.e., the absence of menstruation) can result from radiotherapy or chemotherapy treatments. External beam radiation that includes the testes or ovaries in the radiation field and high doses of alkylating agents are particularly gonadotoxic. More advanced stages of disease often require more extensive treatment and can increase the chances of infertility. Older age at time of treatment is associated with an increased risk of infertility following treatment. Further, premorbid fertility is also a predictor of posttreatment fertility, though this is best documented among men.[232,234]

Currently, fertility preservation options include pretreatment hormonal stimulation and egg harvesting for females and sperm banking for males.[237] In addition, efforts to minimize impact on fertility, such as reducing the dosage of radiation or eliminating gonadotoxic agents from the treatment regimen, can be used to preserve fertility. Options such as adoption and third-party reproduction (i.e., use of a gestational carrier) are also available for cancer survivors; however, these options can be cost prohibitive. Typical fees average $4,200 for egg donors and $40,000 to $120,000 for a gestational surrogate (including the associated medical and legal fees),[238] and costs of adoption can exceed $40,000.[239] Further, a history of cancer may be seen as an inability to provide a stable home by adoption agencies and/or birth parents and can impact a survivor's eligibility or appeal.[239,240]

FEMALE CANCER SURVIVORS

Infertility in females can either be an acute concern or chronic issue following cancer treatment and can result from the treatment reducing the number of primordial follicles, affecting a woman's hormonal levels, or interfering with ovarian, fallopian tube, uterine, or cervical function.[232] Human females are born with a finite number of primordial follicles; a subset of these will develop into oocytes and be released during ovulation from puberty until menopause. The number of oocytes decreases over the lifespan and are not replenished.[72] Chemotherapy and radiotherapy are particularly toxic for these primordial follicles and can result in ovarian failure (manifested by irregular menses or amenorrhea) during active treatment.[241] Younger women are more likely to resume regular menstrual patterns sometime after ending treatment compared to those who are closer to natural menopause.[242,243] The closer a woman is to natural menopause at the time of cancer treatment, the more likely treatment will induce menopause. Thus, women who have delayed planned childbearing may be particularly impacted by infertility resulting from iatrogenic menopause. In addition, while resuming regular menses following treatment is related to lower rates of infertility, female cancer survivors are at increased risk of eventual premature menopause, which, in addition to the break imposed by treatments and recovery, can further limit a woman's window of fertility.[232] Vascular changes following treatment and anatomical changes following surgery (such as oophorectomies) can also impact fertility,[232] and the risk of congenital malformations, intrauterine growth retardation, and spontaneous miscarriage is increased during pelvic or whole body radiation.[244,245]

Fertility preservation options for female cancer survivors include prophylaxis and traditional fertility intervention. Prophylaxis involves protecting the ova or ovaries during cancer therapy. Invasive methods include oophoropexy, which can be used to shield the ovaries by surgically moving them out of the field of radiation. While this method has been shown to preserve fertility for some patients,[241] there is still a decreased chance of a successful pregnancy.[246] Pharmacologic prophylaxis can also be used during chemotherapy or radiation to suppress function and protect ovarian tissue. Leuprolide acetate and other gonadotropin releasing hormone (GnRH) agonists are regularly used in premenopausal women to reduce recurrence risk among patients with hormone-receptor–positive breast cancer.[247,248] Broad use in other chemotherapy patients to protect ovarian function is less common[249,250]; however, large randomized controlled trials are in progress.[232]

Fertility treatment for women often involves collecting mature oocytes and cryopreserving the ova or embryos.[235] This method is not appropriate for all patients as it requires hormonal stimulation that is contraindicated for some hormone-sensitive diagnoses, necessitates sperm from a donor or partner for fertilization, and cannot be used to preserve fertility in patients that have not yet reached puberty. In addition, hormonal stimulation requires a delay in treatment that may not be feasible for all patients. While previous methods resulted in relatively low pregnancy rates,[234,235,246] current methods have significantly improved the chances of successful implantation and pregnancy.[235,251,252] Recent studies have shown pregnancy rates of 63% and 39% per transfer and implantation, respectively.[253] Other experimental options for female fertility preservation includes cryopreservation of ovarian tissue to be used in future autotransplantation, xenotransplanation, or in vitro maturation.[234]

MALE CANCER SURVIVORS

Infertility among male cancer survivors results from anatomical changes,[232,254] hormonal insufficiency from either the downregulation of endocrine substances from tumors (e.g., testicular germ cell tumors)[255] or androgen suppression as part of treatment,[232,256] or from the damage/depletion of germinal sperm cells.[232] As with females, pretreatment fertility predicts future fertility following cancer treatment. Semen analysis can be used to assess spermatogenesis and provide a fair assessment of fertility.[246] Regarding pediatric cancer survivors, men are approximately half as likely to father a child than their healthy siblings,[257] with the most severe fertility consequences of cancer treatment seen in those treated for hypothalamic-pituitary tumors,[258] who completed testicular radiation,[257] who were treated with combination chemotherapy,[257] and who were older at diagnosis.[257,258] While the testes are particularly sensitive to radiation, they will often be protected during irradiation except in targeted therapy or whole body radiation.[246] While even low levels of radiation can impair gonadal function, this is transient and does not appear to impact fertility after treatment has ended.[259]

For male cancer survivors, the only established method for fertility preservation is semen cryopreservation.[255] While this is a simple procedure, it is underutilized. It is recommended that patients bank sperm prior to cancer treatment, but studies have shown that successful pregnancies can result from intracytoplasmic sperm injection that utilizes sperm banked after the start of treatment.[260] Studies have found that only 24% of male cancer survivors bank semen, and very few of these men actually utilize it.[261] This is particularly unfortunate given high rates of successful live births from banked samples among cancer survivors (36%–57%).[262–264]

PEDIATRIC CANCER SURVIVORS

The options for fertility preservation among pediatric cancer survivors who were pubescent at the time of diagnosis/treatment are essentially the same as those for adults (e.g., oocyte and sperm cryopreservation); however, there are a number of unique considerations for younger children. One issue is the need to obtain both consent and assent prior to medical procedures. In the majority of states, parental consent must be obtained for most medical treatments of children younger than 18 years old (the age of medical consent is as young as 14 years old in some states),[265] but it is also necessary to obtain the child's assent (defined by the American Academy of Pediatrics Committee on Bioethics as developmentally appropriate discussion of illness, treatments, or procedures and a solicitation of willingness and preference for treatment).[266] The possibility should be considered that decisions made by parents while the patient is younger may not reflect the wishes of the patient when he or she is older.[237,267] A more important issue is that there are currently no options for fertility preservation in patients who have not yet entered puberty.[255] There are experimental approaches being investigated among males that have yet to start spermarche. These include the use of a GnRH agonist and cryopreservation of testicular tissue with the intent of obtaining future mature spermatozoa for autotransplantation, xenotransplantation, or in vitro maturation in animal models.[234] More research is clearly needed to develop fertility options for those who receive cancer treatments at a young age.

SUMMARY

Cancer treatments can result in anatomical, hormonal, or gonadotoxic changes that can lead to acute or long-term infertility among survivors. Some chemotherapy and radiotherapy treatments are particularly gonadotoxic and can result in azoospermia or amenorrhea. Current methods of fertility preservation include hormonal stimulation and egg harvesting for women and sperm cryopreservation for men. There is evidence supporting prophylaxsis, such as oophoropexy. Other options, such as adoption or third-party reproduction, can also be utilized by cancer survivors experiencing problems with fertility. Uptake of fertility preservation options remains low among cancer survivors due to lack of information, delays in treatment,[235] and cost. In addition, while there are some experimental techniques, there are currently no widely available fertility preservation options for pediatric cancer survivors that undergo treatment prior to puberty.

CONCLUSION

Advances in cancer care have resulted in increasing numbers of survivors. This increase prompts a need for care focused on long-term survivorship issues in addition to traditional disease-focused treatment.[1-3] Many cancer survivors report concerns about sexuality and fertility that can last for years following treatment and negatively impact quality of life.[5-8] Body image disruption, negative self-attributions, and other psychological concerns contribute to and result from sexual difficulties. Infertility is an equally concerning sequela for male and female survivors who have not completed planned childbearing. Fertility preservation efforts are thwarted by possible delays in cancer treatment, cost, or poor communication between patients/families and providers. Many healthcare providers do not regularly discuss any of these concerns with their patients; these conversations need to be a part of routine cancer care.[14-20] Given both the immediate and long-term consequences in both adult and pediatric populations, it is imperative for providers to address these concerns. Cancer can have a devastating impact on sexual function and fertility, but effective treatments are available and stand to improve quality of life for millions.

REFERENCES

1. De Moor JS, Mariotto AB, Parry C, et al. Cancer survivors in the United States: prevalence across the survivorship trajectory and implications for care. *Cancer Epidemiol Biomarkers Prev.* 2013;22(4):561–570.

2. Centers for Disease Control and Prevention. *A National Action Plan for Cancer Survivorship: Advancing Public Health Strategies.* Atlanta, GA: Author; 2004.

3. Ryerson AB, Eheman CR, Altekruse SF, et al. Annual report to the nation on the status of cancer, 1975–2012, featuring the increasing incidence of liver cancer. *Cancer.* 2016;122(9):1312–1337.

4. Siegel RL, Miller KD, Jemal A. Cancer statistics, 2016. *CA Cancer J Clin.* 2016;66(1):7–30.

5. Soothill K, Morris S, Harman J, Francis B, Thomas C, McIllmurray M. The significant unmet needs of cancer patients: probing psychosocial concerns. *Support Care Cancer.* 2001;9(8):597–605.

6. Bower JE, Ganz PA, Desmond KA, Rowland JH, Meyerowitz BE, Belin TR. Fatigue in breast cancer survivors: occurrence, correlates, and impact on quality of life. *J Clin Oncol.* 2000;18(4):743–753.

7. Polsky D, Doshi JA, Marcus S, et al. Long-term risk for depressive symptoms after a medical diagnosis. *Arch Intern Med.* 2005;165(11):1260–1266.

8. Hewitt M, Rowland JH, Yancik R. Cancer survivors in the United States: age, health, and disability. *J Gerontol Ser A: Biol Sci Med Sci*. 2003;58(1):M82–M91.

9. Burwell SR, Case LD, Kaelin C, Avis NE. Sexual problems in younger women after breast cancer surgery. *J Clin Oncol*. 2006;24(18):2815–2821.

10. Ganz PA, Desmond KA, Leedham B, Rowland JH, Meyerowitz BE, Belin TR. Quality of life in long-term, disease-free survivors of breast cancer: a follow-up study. *J Natl Cancer Inst*. 2002;94(1):39–49.

11. Carter J, Raviv L, Applegarth L, et al. A cross-sectional study of the psychosexual impact of cancer-related infertility in women: third-party reproductive assistance. *J Cancer Survivor*. 2010;4(3):236–246.

12. Bober SL, Varela VS. Sexuality in adult cancer survivors: challenges and intervention. *J Clin Oncol*. 2012;30(30):3712–3719.

13. Van Dijk E, van Dulmen-den Broeder E, Kaspers G, Van Dam E, Braam K, Huisman J. Psychosexual functioning of childhood cancer survivors. *Psychooncology*. 2008;17(5):506–511.

14. Schover LR, Brey K, Lichtin A, Lipshultz LI, Jeha S. Knowledge and experience regarding cancer, infertility, and sperm banking in younger male survivors. *J Clin Oncol*. 2002;20(7):1880–1889.

15. Halley MC, May SG, Rendle KAS, Frosch DL, Kurian AW. Beyond barriers: fundamental "disconnects" underlying the treatment of breast cancer patients' sexual health. *Culture Health Sex*. 2014;16(9):1169–1180.

16. Flynn KE, Reese JB, Jeffery DD, et al. Patient experiences with communication about sex during and after treatment for cancer. *Psychooncology*. 2012;21(6):594–601.

17. Hawkins Y, Ussher J, Gilbert E, Perz J, Sandoval M, Sundquist K. Changes in sexuality and intimacy after the diagnosis and treatment of cancer: the experience of partners in a sexual relationship with a person with cancer. *Cancer Nurs*. 2009;32(4):271–280.

18. Zebrack BJ, Casillas J, Nohr L, Adams H, Zeltzer LK. Fertility issues for young adult survivors of childhood cancer. *Psychooncology*. 2004;13(10):689–699.

19. Lindau ST, Gavrilova N, Anderson D. Sexual morbidity in very long term survivors of vaginal and cervical cancer: a comparison to national norms. *Gynecol Oncol*. 2007;106(2):413–418.

20. Hendren SK, O'Connor BI, Liu M, et al. Prevalence of male and female sexual dysfunction is high following surgery for rectal cancer. *Ann Surg*. 2005;242(2):212–223.

21. Cash TF, Jakatdar TA, Williams EF. The Body Image Quality of Life Inventory: further validation with college men and women. *Body Image*. 2004;1(3):279–287.

22. Cash TF. *Cognitive-Behavioral Perspectives on Body Image*. New York: Guilford Press; 2002.

23. Weaver AD, Byers ES. The relationships among body image, body mass index, exercise, and sexual functioning in heterosexual women. *Psych Women Q*. 2006;30(4):333–339.

24. Wiederman M. Body image and sexual functioning. In: Cash TF, Pruzinsky T, eds. *Body Image: A Handbook of Theory, Research, and Clinical practice*. New York: Guilford Press, 2002:287–294.

25. Pujols Y, Meston CM, Seal BN. The association between sexual satisfaction and body image in women. *J Sex Med*. 2010;7(2 Pt 2):905–916.

26. Fobair P, Stewart SL, Chang S, D'Onofrio C, Banks PJ, Bloom JR. Body image and sexual problems in young women with breast cancer. *Psychooncology*. 2006;15(7):579–594.

27. Mercadante S, Vitrano V, Catania V. Sexual issues in early and late stage cancer: a review. *Support Care Cancer*. 2010;18(6):659–665.

28. Cash TF, Maikkula CL, Yamamiya Y. "Baring the body in the bedroom": body image, sexual self-schemas, and sexual functioning among college women and men. *Electr J Human Sex*. 2004;7:1–9.

29. Koch PB, Mansfield PK, Thurau D, Carey M. "Feeling frumpy": the relationships between body image and sexual response changes in midlife women. *J Sex Res*. 2005;42(3):215–223.

30. Seal BN, Bradford A, Meston CM. The association between body esteem and sexual desire among college women. *Arch Sex Behav*. 2009;38(5):866–872.

31. Sanchez DT, Kiefer AK. Body concerns in and out of the bedroom: implications for sexual pleasure and problems. *Arch Sex Behav*. 2007;36(6):808–820.

32. Ackard DM, Kearney-Cooke A, Peterson CB. Effect of body image and self-image on women's sexual behaviors. *Int J Eat Disord*. 2000;28(4):422–429.

33. Speer JJ, Hillenberg B, Sugrue DP, et al. Study of sexual functioning determinants in breast cancer survivors. *Breast J*. 2005;11(6):440–447.

34. Helms RL, O'Hea EL, Corso M. Body image issues in women with breast cancer. *Psychol Health Med*. 2008;13(3):313–325.

35. Brown H, Randle J. Living with a stoma: a review of the literature. *J Clin Nurs*. 2005;14(1):74–81.

36. Andersen BL, Hacker NF. Psychosexual adjustment after vulvar surgery. *Obstetr Gynecol*. 1983;62(4):457.

37. Romero FR, dos Santos Romero KRP, de Mattos MAE, Garcia CRC, de Carvalho Fernandes R, Perez MDC. Sexual function after partial penectomy for penile cancer. *Urology*. 2005;66(6):1292–1295.

38. Aerts L, Christiaens M, Enzlin P, Neven P, Amant F. Sexual functioning in women after mastectomy versus breast conserving therapy for early-stage breast cancer: a prospective controlled study. *Breast*. 2014;23(5):629–636.

39. Engel J, Kerr J, Schlesinger-Raab A, Sauer H, Hölzel D. Quality of life following breast-conserving therapy or mastectomy: results of a 5-year prospective study. *Breast J*. 2004;10(3):223–231.

40. Kiebert G, De Haes J, Van de Velde C. The impact of breast-conserving treatment and mastectomy on the quality of life of early-stage breast cancer patients: a review. *J Clin Oncol*. 1991;9(6):1059–1070.

41. Moyer A. Psychosocial outcomes of breast-conserving surgery versus mastectomy: a meta-analytic review. *Health Psychol*. 1997;16(3):284.

42. Schover LR, Yetman RJ, Tuason LJ, et al. Partial mastectomy and breast reconstruction: a comparison of their effects on psychosocial adjustment, body image, and sexuality. *Cancer*. 1995;75(1):54–64.

43. Metcalfe KA, Semple J, Quan M-L, et al. Changes in psychosocial functioning 1 year after mastectomy alone, delayed breast reconstruction, or immediate breast reconstruction. *Ann Surg Oncol*. 2012;19(1):233–241.

44. Yurek D, Farrar W, Andersen BL. Breast cancer surgery: comparing surgical groups and determining individual differences in postoperative sexuality and body change stress. *J Consult Clin Psychol*. 2000;68(4):697–709.

45. Rowland JH, Desmond KA, Meyerowitz BE, Belin TR, Wyatt GE, Ganz PA. Role of breast reconstructive surgery in physical and emotional outcomes among breast cancer survivors. *J Natl Cancer Inst*. 2000;92(17):1422–1429.

46. National Cancer Institute. Tackling the conundrum of cachexia in cancer. 2011; https://www.cancer.gov/about-cancer/treatment/research/cachexia. Accessed November 7, 2016.

47. Fearon K. Cancer cachexia: Developing multimodal therapy for a multidimensional problem. *Eur J Cancer*. 2008;44(8):1124–1132.

48. Harrington CB, Hansen JA, Moskowitz M, Todd BL, Feuerstein M. It's not over when it's over: long-term symptoms in cancer survivors: a systematic review. *Int J Psychiatry Med*. 2010;40(2):163–181.

49. Schover LR. Sexuality and fertility after cancer. *ASH Educ Program Book*. 2005;2005(1):523–527.

50. Barnas JL, Pierpaoli S, Ladd P, et al. The prevalence and nature of orgasmic dysfunction after radical prostatectomy. *BJU Int*. 2004;94(4):603–605.

51. American Psychiatric Association. *Diagnostic and Statistical Manual of Mental Disorders*, 5th ed. Washington, DC: Author; 2013.

52. Ganz PA, Desmond KA, Belin TR, Meyerowitz BE, Rowland JH. Predictors of sexual health in women after a breast cancer diagnosis. *J Clin Oncol*. 1999;17(8):2371–2380.

53. Masters W, Johnson VE. *Human Sexual Response*. Boston: Little, Brown; 1966.

54. Kaplan HS. *The New Sex Therapy*. New York: Brunner/Mazel; 1974.

55. Basson R. Human sex-response cycles. *J Sex Marital Ther.* 2001;27(1):33–43.

56. Berner M, Günzler C. Efficacy of psychosocial interventions in men and women with sexual dysfunctions—a systematic review of controlled clinical trials. *J Sex Med.* 2012;9(12):3089–3107.

57. Günzler C, Berner MM. Efficacy of psychosocial interventions in men and women with sexual dysfunctions—a systematic review of controlled clinical trials. *J Sex Med.* 2012;9(12):3108–3125.

58. Hatzichristou D, Rosen RC, Broderick G, et al. Clinical evaluation and management strategy for sexual dysfunction in men and women. *J Sex Med.* 2004;1(1):49–57.

59. Bober SL, Reese JB, Barbera L, et al. How to ask and what to do: a guide for clinical inquiry and intervention regarding female sexual health after cancer. *Curr Opin Support Palliat Care.* 2016;10(1):44–54.

60. Sadovsky R, Basson R, Krychman M, et al. Cancer and sexual problems. *J Sex Med.* 2010;7(1 Pt 2):349–373.

61. Perz J, Ussher JM, Gilbert E. Constructions of sex and intimacy after cancer: Q methodology study of people with cancer, their partners, and health professionals. *BMC Cancer.* 2013;13(1):1–13.

62. Laumann EO, Glasser DB, Neves RCS, Moreira E. A population-based survey of sexual activity, sexual problems and associated help-seeking behavior patterns in mature adults in the United States of America. *Int J Impot Res.* 2009;21(3):171–178.

63. Moreira E, Hartmann U, Glasser D, Gingell C. A population survey of sexual activity, sexual dysfunction and associated helpseeking behavior in middle-aged and older adults in Germany. *Eur J Med Res.* 2005;10(10):434.

64. Simons JS, Carey MP. Prevalence of sexual dysfunctions: results from a decade of research. *Arch Sex Behav.* 2001;30(2):177–219.

65. Shifren JL, Monz BU, Russo PA, Segreti A, Johannes CB. Sexual problems and distress in United States women: prevalence and correlates. *Obstet Gynecol.* 2008;112(5):970–978.

66. Moreira E, Brock G, Glasser DB, et al. Help-seeking behaviour for sexual problems: the Global Study of Sexual Attitudes and Behaviors. *Int J Clin Pract.* 2005;59(1):6–16.

67. Lindau ST, Schumm LP, Laumann EO, Levinson W, O'Muircheartaigh CA, Waite LJ. A study of sexuality and health among older adults in the United States. *N Engl J Med.* 2007;357(8):762–774.

68. Shifren JL, Monz BU, Russo PA, Segreti A, Johannes CB. Sexual problems and distress in United States women: prevalence and correlates. *Obstetr Gynecol.* 2008;112(5):970–978.

69. Biglia N, Moggio G, Peano E, et al. Effects of surgical and adjuvant therapies for breast cancer on sexuality, cognitive functions, and body weight. *J Sex Med.* 2010;7(5):1891–1900.

70. Carpenter K, Andersen B. Psychological and sexual aspects of gynecologic cancer. *Global Library of Women's Medicine.* 2008. doi: 10.3843/GLOWM.10277.

71. Donovan KA, Taliaferro LA, Alvarez EM, Jacobsen PB, Roetzheim RG, Wenham RM. Sexual health in women treated for cervical cancer: characteristics and correlates. *Gynecol Oncol.* 2007;104(2):428–434.

72. Goswami D, Conway GS. Premature ovarian failure. *Hum Reprod Update.* 2005;11(4):391–410.

73. Barni S, Mondin R. Sexual dysfunction in treated breast cancer patients. *Ann Oncol.* 1997;8(2):149–153.

74. Jensen PT, Groenvold M, Klee MC, Thranov I, Petersen MA, Machin D. Early-stage cervical carcinoma, radical hysterectomy, and sexual function. *Cancer.* 2004;100(1):97–106.

75. Saewong S, Choobun T. Effects of radiotherapy on sexual activity in women with cervical cancer. *J Med Assoc Thailand.* 2005;88:S11.

76. Sherwin BB, Gelfand MM. The role of androgen in the maintenance of sexual functioning in oophorectomized women. *Psychosom Med.* 1987;49(4):397–409.

77. McCoy NL, Davidson JM. A longitudinal study of the effects of menopause on sexuality. *Maturitas.* 1985;7(3):203–210.

78. Judd HL, Judd GE, Lucas WE, Yen SS. Endocrine function of the postmenopausal ovary: concentration of androgens and estrogens in ovarian and peripheral vein blood. *J Clin Endocrinol Metab.* 1974;39(6):1020–1024.

79. Zussman L, Zussman S, Sunley R, Bjornson E. Sexual response after hysterectomy-oophorectomy: recent studies and reconsideration of psychogenesis. *Am J Obstet Gynecol.* 1981;140(7):725–729.

80. Amato P, Buster JE. Diagnosis and treatment of hypoactive sexual desire disorder. *Clin Obstet Gynecol.* 2009;52(4):666–674.

81. Davis SR, Braunstein GD. Efficacy and safety of testosterone in the management of hypoactive sexual desire disorder in postmenopausal women. *J Sex Med.* 2012;9(4):1134–1148.

82. Sherwin BB. Randomized clinical trials of combined estrogen-androgen preparations: effects on sexual functioning. *Fertil Steril.* 2002;77:49–54.

83. Shifren JL, Braunstein GD, Simon JA, et al. Transdermal testosterone treatment in women with impaired sexual function after oophorectomy. *N Engl J Med.* 2000;343(10):682–688.

84. Buster JE, Kingsberg SA, Aguirre O, et al. Testosterone patch for low sexual desire in surgically menopausal women: a randomized trial. *Obstet Gynecol.* 2005;105(5, Part 1):944–952.

85. Heiman JR. Treating low sexual desire—new findings for testosterone in women. *N Engl J Med.* 2008;359(19):2047–2049.

86. Kaaks R, Berrino F, Key T, et al. Serum sex steroids in premenopausal women and breast cancer risk within the European Prospective Investigation into Cancer and Nutrition (EPIC). *J Natl Cancer Inst.* 2005;97(10):755–765.

87. Kaaks R, Rinaldi S, Key T, et al. Postmenopausal serum androgens, oestrogens and breast cancer risk: the European prospective investigation into cancer and nutrition. *Endocr Relat Cancer.* 2005;12(4):1071–1082.

88. Zeleniuch-Jacquotte A, Shore R, Koenig K, et al. Postmenopausal levels of oestrogen, androgen, and SHBG and breast cancer: long-term results of a prospective study. *Br J Cancer.* 2004;90(1):153–159.

89. Missmer SA, Eliassen AH, Barbieri RL, Hankinson SE. Endogenous estrogen, androgen, and progesterone concentrations and breast cancer risk among postmenopausal women. *J Natl Cancer Inst.* 2004;96(24):1856–1865.

90. Junko Y, Takara Y, Hiroji O. Aromatization of androstenedione by normal and neoplastic endometrium of the uterus. *J Steroid Biochem.* 1985;22(1):63–66.

91. Yamamoto T, Kitawaki J, Urabe M, et al. Estrogen productivity of endometrium and endometrial cancer tissue; influence of aromatase on proliferation of endometrial cancer cells. *J Steroid Biochem Mol Biol.* 1993;44(4):463–468.

92. Segraves RT, Balon R. Recognizing and reversing sexual side effects of medications. In: Levine SB, ed. *Handbook of Clinical Sexuality for Mental Health Professionals:* New York: Brunner-Routledge; 2003:377–393.

93. Moll JL, Brown CS. The use of monoamine pharmacological agents in the treatment of sexual dysfunction: evidence in the literature. *J Sex Med.* 2011;8:956–970.

94. Puppo G, Puppo V. US Food and Drug Administration approval of Addyi (flibanserin) for treatment of hypoactive sexual desire disorder. *Eur Urol.* 2016;69(2):379–380.

95. Jaspers L, Feys F, Bramer WM, Franco OH, Leusink P, Laan ET. Efficacy and safety of flibanserin for the treatment of hypoactive sexual desire disorder in women: a systematic review and meta-analysis. *JAMA Intern Med.* 2016;176(4):453–462.

96. McCabe MP. Evaluation of a cognitive behavior therapy program for people with sexual dysfunction. *J Sex Marital Ther.* 2001;27(3):259–271.

97. Ravart M, Trudel G, Marchand A, Turgeon L, Aubin S. The efficacy of a cognitive behavioural treatment model for hypoactive sexual desire disorder: an outcome study. *Can J Human Sex.* 1996;5(4):279.

98. Trudel G, Marchand A, Ravart M, Aubin S, Turgeon L, Fortier P. The effect of a cognitive-behavioral group treatment program on hypoactive sexual desire in women. *Sex Relation Ther.* 2001;16(2):145–164.

99. Hawton K, Catalan J, Fagg J. Low sexual desire: sex therapy results and prognostic factors. *Behav Res Ther.* 1991;29(3):217–224.

100. Schover LR, LoPiccolo J. Treatment effectiveness for dysfunctions of sexual desire. *J Sex Marital Ther.* 1982;8(3):179–197.

101. Masters WH, Johnson VE. *Human Sexual Inadequacy.* Boston: Little, Brown; 1970.

102. Bergeron S, Binik YM, Khalifa S, et al. A randomized comparison of group cognitive-behavioral therapy, surface electromyographic biofeedback, and vestibulectomy in the treatment of dyspareunia resulting from vulvar vestibulitis. *Pain.* 2001;91(3):297–306.

103. Ter Kuile MM, Weijenborg PT. A cognitive-behavioral group program for women with vulvar vestibulitis syndrome (VVS): factors associated with treatment success. *J Sex Marital Ther.* 2006;32(3):199–213.

104. Heiman JR. Psychologic treatments for female sexual dysfunction: are they effective and do we need them? *Arch Sex Behav.* 2002;31(5):445–450.

105. Kinsey A, Pomeroy W, Martin C, Gebhard P. *Sexual Behavior in the Human Female.* Philadelphia: W. B. Saunders; 1953.

106. Meston CM. The psychophysiological assessment of female sexual function. *J Sex Educ Ther.* 2000;25(1):6–16.

107. Basson R. The female sexual response: a different model. *J Sex Marital Ther.* 2000;26(1):51–65.

108. Heiman JR. A psychophysiological exploration of sexual arousal patterns in females and males. *Psychophysiology.* 1977;14(3):266–274.

109. Korff J, Geer JH. The relationship between sexual arousal experience and genital response. *Psychophysiology.* 1983;20(2):121–127.

110. Sakheim DK, Barlow DH, Beck JG, Abrahamson DJ. The effect of an increased awareness of erectile cues on sexual arousal. *Behav Res Ther.* 1984;22(2):151–158.

111. Frank JEJE. Diagnosis and treatment of female sexual dysfunction. *Am Fam Physician.* 2008;77(5):635–642.

112. Pieterse Q, Maas C, Ter Kuile M, et al. An observational longitudinal study to evaluate miction, defecation, and sexual function after radical hysterectomy with pelvic lymphadenectomy for early-stage cervical cancer. *Int J Gynecol Cancer.* 2006;16(3):1119–1129.

113. Basson R, Brotto LA, Laan E, Redmond G, Utian WH. Assessment and management of women's sexual dysfunctions: problematic desire and arousal. *J Sex Med.* 2005;2(3):291–300.

114. Basson R. Women's sexual dysfunction: revised and expanded definitions. *CMAJ.* 2005;172(10): 1327–1333.

115. Brotto LA, Erskine Y, Carey M, et al. A brief mindfulness-based cognitive behavioral intervention improves sexual functioning versus wait-list control in women treated for gynecologic cancer. *Gynecol Oncol.* 2012;125(2):320–325.

116. Laumann EO, Nicolosi A, Glasser DB, et al. Sexual problems among women and men aged 40–80 y: prevalence and correlates identified in the Global Study of Sexual Attitudes and Behaviors. *Int J Impot Res.* 2005;17(1):39–57.

117. Laumann EO, Paik A, Rosen RC. Sexual dysfunction in the United States: prevalence and predictors. *JAMA.* 1999;281(6):537–544.

118. Burstein HJ, Temin S, Anderson H, et al. Adjuvant endocrine therapy for women with hormone receptor–positive breast cancer: American Society of Clinical Oncology clinical practice guideline focused update. *J Clin Oncol.* 2014;32(21):2255–2269.

119. Mok K, Juraskova I, Friedlander M. The impact of aromatase inhibitors on sexual functioning: current knowledge and future research directions. *Breast.* 2008;17(5):436–440.

120. Derzko C, Elliott S, Lam W. Management of sexual dysfunction in postmenopausal breast cancer patients taking adjuvant aromatase inhibitor therapy. *Curr Oncol.* 2007;14(Suppl. 1):s20–s40.

121. Mortimer JE, Boucher L, Baty J, Knapp DL, Ryan E, Rowland JH. Effect of Tamoxifen on sexual functioning in patients with breast cancer. *J Clin Oncol.* 1999;17(5):1488–1492.

122. Day R, Ganz PA, Costantino JP, Cronin WM, Wickerham DL, Fisher B. Health-related quality of life and tamoxifen in breast cancer prevention: a report from the National Surgical Adjuvant Breast and Bowel Project P-1 Study. *J Clin Oncol.* 1999;17(9):2659–2669.

123. Berglund G, Nystedt M, Bolund C, Sjödén P-O, Rutquist L-E. Effect of endocrine treatment on sexuality in premenopausal breast cancer patients: a prospective randomized study. *J Clin Oncol.* 2001;19(11):2788–2796.

124. Jensen PT, Groenvold M, Klee MC, Thranov I, Petersen MA, Machin D. Longitudinal study of sexual function and vaginal changes after radiotherapy for cervical cancer. *Int J Radiat Oncol Biol Phys.* 2003;56(4):937–949.

125. Biglia N, Peano E, Sgandurra P, et al. Low-dose vaginal estrogens or vaginal moisturizer in breast cancer survivors with urogenital atrophy: a preliminary study. *Gynecol Endocrinol.* 2010;26(6): 404–412.

126. Al-Baghdadi O, Ewies AAA. Topical estrogen therapy in the management of postmenopausal vaginal atrophy: an up-to-date overview. *Climacteric.* 2009;12(2):91–105.

127. Sinha A, Ewies A. Non-hormonal topical treatment of vulvovaginal atrophy: an up-to-date overview. *Climacteric.* 2013;16(3):305–312.

128. Lee Y-K, Chung HH, Kim JW, Park N-H, Song Y-S, Kang S-B. Vaginal pH-balanced gel for the control of atrophic vaginitis among breast cancer survivors: a randomized controlled trial. *Obstet Gynecol.* 2011;117(4):922–927.

129. Loprinzi CL, Abu-Ghazaleh S, Sloan JA, et al. Phase III randomized double-blind study to evaluate the efficacy of a polycarbophil-based vaginal moisturizer in women with breast cancer. *J Clin Oncol.* 1997;15(3):969–973.

130. Johnston SL, Farrell S, Bouchard C, et al. The detection and management of vaginal atrophy. *J Obstetr Gynaecol Canada.* 2004;26(5):503–515.

131. Basson R, McInnes R, Smith MD, Hodgson G, Nandan K. Efficacy and safety of Sildenafil Citrate in women with sexual dysfunction associated with female sexual arousal disorder. *J Womens Health Gender-Based Med.* 2002;11(4):367–377.

132. Kaplan SA, Reis RB, Kohn IJ, et al. Safety and efficacy of sildenafil in postmenopausal women with sexual dysfunction. *Urology.* 1999;53(3):481–486.

133. Mah K, Binik YM. The nature of human orgasm: a critical review of major trends. *Clin Psychol Rev.* 2001;21(6):823–856.

134. Meston CM. The effects of hysterectomy on sexual arousal in women with a history of benign uterine fibroids. *Arch Sex Behav.* 2004;33(1):31–42.

135. Meston CM, Levin RJ, Sipski ML, Hull EM, Heiman JR. Women's orgasm. *Annu Rev Sex Res.* 2004;15:173–257.

136. Öberg K, Fugl-Meyer AR, Fugl-Meyer KS. On categorization and quantification of women's sexual dysfunctions: an epidemiological approach. *Int J Impot Res.* 2004;16(3):261–269.

137. Hendrickx L, Gijs L, Enzlin P. Prevalence rates of sexual difficulties and associated distress in heterosexual men and women: results from an Internet survey in Flanders. *J Sex Res.* 2014;51(1):1–12.

138. Bancroft J, Loftus J, Long JS. Distress about sex: a national survey of women in heterosexual relationships. *Arch Sex Behav.* 2003;32(3):193–208.

139. Christensen BS, Gronbaek M, Osler M, Pedersen BV, Graugaard C, Frisch M. Sexual dysfunctions and difficulties in Denmark: prevalence and associated sociodemographic factors. *Arch Sex Behav.* 2011;40(1):121–132.

140. Fugl-Meyer AR, Fugl-Meyer K. Sexual disabilities, problems, and satisfaction in 18–74-year-old Swedes. *Scand J Sex*. 1999;2:79–105.

141. Shifren JL, Monz BU, Russo PA, Segreti A, Johannes CB. Sexual problems and distress in United States women: prevalence and correlates. *Obstet Gynecol*. 2008;112(5):970–978.

142. Donovan KA, Thompson LM, Hoffe SE. Sexual function in colorectal cancer survivors. *Cancer Control*. 2010;17(1):44–51.

143. Zippe CD, Raina R, Shah AD, et al. Female sexual dysfunction after radical cystectomy: a new outcome measure. *Urology*. 2004;63(6):1153–1157.

144. Humphreys C, Tallman B, Altmaier E, Barnette V. Sexual functioning in patients undergoing bone marrow transplantation: a longitudinal study. *Bone Marrow Transplant*. 2007;39(8):491–496.

145. Syrjala KL, Kurland BF, Abrams JR, Sanders JE, Heiman JR. Sexual function changes during the 5 years after high-dose treatment and hematopoietic cell transplantation for malignancy, with case-matched controls at 5 years. *Blood*. 2008;111(3):989–996.

146. Fooladi E, Davis SR. An update on the pharmacological management of female sexual dysfunction. *Exp Opin Pharmacother*. 2012;13(15):2131–2142.

147. Basson R. Pharmacotherapy for women's sexual dysfunction. *Exp Opin Pharmacother*. 2009;10(10):1631–1648.

148. Laan E, Rellini AH, Barnes T. Standard operating procedures for female orgasmic disorder: consensus of the International Society for Sexual Medicine. *J Sex Med*. 2013;10(1):74–82.

149. Andersen BL. Primary orgasmic dysfunction: diagnostic considerations and review of treatment. *Psychol Bull*. 1983;93(1):105–136.

150. Heiman JR, Meston CM. Empirically validated treatment for sexual dysfunction. *Annu Rev Sex Res*. 1997;8:148–194.

151. Hurlbert DF, Apt C. The coital alignment technique and directed masturbation: a comparative study on female orgasm. *J Sex Marital Ther*. 1995;21(1):21–29.

152. Lebow JL, Chambers AL, Christensen A, Johnson SM. Research on the treatment of couple distress. *J Marital Family Ther*. 2012;38(1):145–168.

153. Stephenson KR, Rellini AH, Meston CM. Relationship satisfaction as a predictor of treatment response during cognitive behavioral sex therapy. *Arch Sex Behav*. 2013;42(1):143–152.

154. Roughan PA, Kunst L. Do pelvic floor exercises really improve orgasmic potential? *J Sex Marital Ther*. 1981;7(3):223–229.

155. Chambless DL, Sultan FE, Stern TE, O'Neill C, Garrison S, Jackson A. Effect of pubococcygeal exercise on coital orgasm in women. *J Consult Clin Psychol*. 1984;52(1):114–118.

156. da Silva Lara LA, Montenegro ML, Franco MM, Abreu DCC, de Sá Rosa e Silva ACJ, Ferreira CHJ. Is the sexual satisfaction of postmenopausal women enhanced by physical exercise and pelvic floor muscle training? *J Sex Med*. 2012;9(1):218–223.

157. Messé M, Geer J. Voluntary vaginal musculature contractions as an enhancer of sexual arousal. *Arch Sex Behav*. 1985;14(1):13–28.

158. Lowenstein L, Gruenwald I, Gartman I, et al. Can stronger pelvic muscle floor improve sexual function? *Int Urogynecol J*. 2010;21:553–556.

159. Zahariou AG, Karamouti MV, Papaioannou PD. Pelvic floor muscle training improves sexual function of women with stress urinary incontinence. *Int Urogynecol J*. 2008;19(3):401–406.

160. Beji NK, Yalcin O, Erkan HA. The effect of pelvic floor training on sexual function of treated patients. *Int Urogynecol J*. 2003;14(4):234–238.

161. Pauls RN, Marinkovic SP, Silva WA, Rooney CM, Kleeman SD, Karram MM. Effects of sacral neuromodulation on female sexual function. *Int Urogynecol J*. 2007;18(4):391–395.

162. Zabihi N, Mourtzinos A, Maher MG, Raz S, Rodriguez LV. The effects of bilateral caudal epidural S2–4 neuromodulation on female sexual function. *Int Urogynecol J*. 2008;19(5):697–700.

163. Rivalta M, Sighinolfi MC, De Stefani S, et al. Biofeedback, electrical stimulation, pelvic floor muscle exercises, and vaginal cones: a combined rehabilitative approach for sexual dysfunction associated with urinary incontinence. *J Sex Med*. 2009;6(6):1674–1677.

164. Billups KL, Berman L, Berman J, Metz ME, Glennon ME, Goldstein I. A new non-pharmacological vacuum therapy for female sexual dysfunction. *J Sex Marital Ther*. 2001;27(5):435–441.

165. Schroder M, Mell LK, Hurteau JA, et al. Clitoral therapy device for treatment of sexual dysfunction in irradiated cervical cancer patients. *Int J Radiat Oncol Biol Phys*. 2005;61(4):1078–1086.

166. Wilson SK, Delk JR, Billups KL. Treating symptoms of female sexual arousal with the Eros-Clitoral Therapy Device. *J Gend Specif Med*. 2001;4(2):54–58.

167. Bergmark K, Åvall-Lundqvist E, Dickman PW, Henningsohn L, Steineck G. Vaginal changes and sexuality in women with a history of cervical cancer. *N Engl J Med*. 1999;340(18):1383–1389.

169. Spinelli S, Chiodi S, Costantini S, et al. Female genital tract graft-versus-host disease following allogeneic bone marrow transplantation. *Haematologica*. 2003;88(10):1163–1168.

169. Zantomio D, Grigg AP, MacGregor L, Panek-Hudson Y, Szer J, Ayton R. Female genital tract graft-versus-host disease: incidence, risk factors and recommendations for management. *Bone Marrow Transplant*. 2006;38(8):567–572.

170. Brotto LA, Heiman JR. Mindfulness in sex therapy: applications for women with sexual difficulties following gynecologic cancer. *Sex Relation Ther*. 2007;22(1):3–11.

171. Carter J, Goldfrank D, Schover LR. Simple strategies for vaginal health promotion in cancer survivors. *J Sex Med*. 2011;8(2):549–559.

172. Miles T, Johnson N. Vaginal dilator therapy for women receiving pelvic radiotherapy. *Cochrane Database Sys Rev*. 2014;2.

173. Goetsch MF, Lim JY, Caughey AB. A practical solution for dyspareunia in breast cancer survivors: a randomized controlled trial. *J Clin Oncol*. 2015;33(30):3394–3400.

174. Meuleman EJ, van Lankveld JJ. Male sexual desire disorder. In: Mirone V, ed. *Clinical Uro-andrology*. Berlin: Springer; 2015:133–146.

175. Morales A, Buvat J, Gooren LJ, et al. Endocrine aspects of sexual dysfunction in men. *J Sex Med*. 2004;1(1):69–81.

176. van Lankveld JJ, Grotjohann Y. Psychiatric comorbidity in heterosexual couples with sexual dysfunction assessed with the Composite International Diagnostic Interview. *Arch Sex Behav*. 2000;29(5):479–498.

177. Beck JG, Bozman AW. Gender differences in sexual desire: the effects of anger and anxiety. *Arch Sex Behav*. 1995;24(6):595–612.

178. Baldwin DS. Depression and sexual dysfunction. *Br Med Bull*. 2001;57:81–99.

179. Chung E, Brock G. Sexual rehabilitation and cancer survivorship: a state of art review of current literature and management strategies in male sexual dysfunction among prostate cancer survivors. *J Sex Med*. 2013;10(Suppl. 1):102–111.

180. Isidori AM, Giannetta E, Gianfrilli D, et al. Effects of testosterone on sexual function in men: results of a meta-analysis. *Clin Endocrinol*. 2005;63(4):381–394.

181. Travison TG, Morley JE, Araujo AB, O'Donnell AB, McKinlay JB. The relationship between libido and testosterone levels in aging men. *Int J Clin Endocrinol Metab*. 2006;91(7):2509–2513.

182. Fowler FJ, McNaughton Collins M, Walker Corkery E, Elliott DB, Barry MJ. The impact of androgen deprivation on quality of life after radical prostatectomy for prostate carcinoma. *Cancer*. 2002;95(2):287–295.

183. DiBlasio CJ, Malcolm JB, Derweesh IH, et al. Patterns of sexual and erectile dysfunction and response to treatment in patients receiving androgen deprivation therapy for prostate cancer. *BJU Int*. 2008;102(1):39–43.

184. Potosky AL, Knopf K, Clegg LX, et al. Quality-of-life outcomes after primary androgen deprivation therapy: results from the prostate cancer outcomes study. *J Clin Oncol.* 2001;19(17):3750–3757.

185. Basaria S, Lieb J, Tang AM, et al. Long-term effects of androgen deprivation therapy in prostate cancer patients. *Clin Endocrinol.* 2002;56(6):779–786.

186. Incrocci L, Hop WC, Wijnmaalen A, Slob AK. Treatment outcome, body image, and sexual functioning after orchiectomy and radiotherapy for Stage I–II testicular seminoma. *Int J Radiat Oncol Biol Phys.* 2002;53(5):1165–1173.

187. Wang C, Nieschlag E, Swerdloff RS, et al. ISA, ISSAM, EAU, EAA and ASA recommendations: investigation, treatment and monitoring of late-onset hypogonadism in males. *Aging Male.* 2009;12(1):5–12.

188. Morales A, Black AM, Emerson LE. Testosterone administration to men with testosterone deficiency syndrome after external beam radiotherapy for localized prostate cancer: preliminary observations. *BJU Int.* 2009;103(1):62–64.

189. Pastuszak A, Pearlman A, Godoy G, Miles BJ, Lipshultz L, Khera M. Testosterone replacement therapy in the setting of prostate cancer treated with radiation. *Int J Impot Res.* 2013;25(1):24–28.

190. Morgentaler A, Lipshultz LI, Bennett R, Sweeney M, Avila D, Khera M. Testosterone therapy in men with untreated prostate cancer. *J Urol.* 2011;185(4):1256–1261.

191. Canada AL, Neese LE, Sui D, Schover LR. Pilot intervention to enhance sexual rehabilitation for couples after treatment for localized prostate carcinoma. *Cancer.* 2005;104(12):2689–2700.

192. Booth AM. Physiology of male sexual function. *Ann Intern Med.* 1980;92(2 Pt. 2):329–331.

193. Laumann EO, Paik A, Rosen RC. Sexual dysfunction in the United States: prevalence and predictors. *JAMA.* 1999;281(6):537–544.

194. Johannes CB, Araujo AB, Feldman HA, Derby CA, Kleinman KP, McKinlay JB. Incidence of erectile dysfunction in men 40 to 69 years old: longitudinal results from the Massachusetts Male Aging Study. *J Urol.* 2000;163(2):460–463.

195. Braun M, Wassmer G, Klotz T, Reifenrath B, Mathers M, Engelmann U. Epidemiology of erectile dysfunction: results of the Cologne Male Survey. *Int J Impot Res.* 2000;12(6):305–311.

196. Roumeguere T, Wespes E, Carpentier Y, Hoffmann P, Schulman C. Erectile dysfunction is associated with a high prevalence of hyperlipidemia and coronary heart disease risk. *Eur Urol.* 2003;44(3):355–359.

197. Wiechno P, Demkow T, Kubiak K, Sadowska M, Kamińska J. The quality of life and hormonal disturbances in testicular cancer survivors in Cisplatin era. *Eur Urol.* 2007;52(5):1448–1455.

198. Jonker-Pool G, Van de Wiel HB, Hoekstra HJ, et al. Sexual functioning after treatment for testicular cancer: review and meta-analysis of 36 empirical studies between 1975–2000. *Arch Sex Behav.* 2001;30(1):55–74.

199. Krouse R, Grant M, Ferrell B, Dean G, Nelson R, Chu D. Quality of life outcomes in 599 cancer and non-cancer patients with colostomies. *J Surg Res.* 2007;138(1):79–87.

200. Tal R, Alphs HH, Krebs P, Nelson CJ, Mulhall JP. Erectile function recovery rate after radical prostatectomy: a meta-analysis. *J Sex Med.* 2009;6(9):2538–2546.

201. Geary ES, Dendinger TE, Freiha FS, Stamey TA. Nerve sparing radical prostatectomy: a different view. *J Urol.* 1995;154(1):145–149.

202. Tsujimura A, Matsumiya K, Miyagawa Y, et al. Relation between erectile dysfunction and urinary incontinence after nerve-sparing and non-nerve-sparing radical prostatectomy. *Urol Int.* 2004;73(1):31–35.

203. Tal R, Valenzuela R, Aviv N, et al. Persistent erectile dysfunction following radical prostatectomy: the association between nerve-sparing status and the prevalence and chronology of venous leak. *J Sex Med.* 2009;6(10):2813–2819.

204. Mulhall JP, Secin FP, Guillonneau B. Artery sparing radical prostatectomy: myth or reality? *J Urol.* 2008;179(3):827–831.

205. Schwartz EJ, Wong P, Graydon RJ. Sildenafil preserves intracorporeal smooth muscle after radical retropubic prostatectomy. *J Urol.* 2004;171(2):771–774.

206. Potosky AL, Davis WW, Hoffman RM, et al. Five-year outcomes after prostatectomy or radiotherapy for prostate cancer: the Prostate Cancer Outcomes Study. *J Natl Cancer Inst.* 2004;96(18):1358–1367.

207. Sanda MG, Dunn RL, Michalski J, et al. Quality of life and satisfaction with outcome among prostate-cancer survivors. *N Engl J Med.* 2008;358(12):1250–1261.

208. van der Wielen GJ, van Putten WL, Incrocci L. Sexual function after three-dimensional conformal radiotherapy for prostate cancer: results from a dose-escalation trial. *Int J Radiat Oncol Biol Phys.* 2007;68(2):479–484.

209. Mantz C, Song P, Farhangi E, et al. Potency probability following conformal megavoltage radiotherapy using conventional doses for localized prostate cancer. *Int J Radiat Oncol Biol Phys.* 1997;37(3):551–557.

210. Litwin MS, Flanders SC, Pasta DJ, Stoddard ML, Lubeck DP, Henning JM. Sexual function and bother after radical prostatectomy or radiation for prostate cancer: multivariate quality-of-life analysis from CaPSURE. *Urology.* 1999;54(3):503–508.

211. Zelefsky MJ, Eid JF. Elucidating the etiology of erectile dysfunction after definitive therapy for prostatic cancer. *Int J Radiat Oncol Biol Phys.* 1998;40(1):129–133.

212. DiBiase SJ, Wallner K, Tralins K, Sutlief S. Brachytherapy radiation doses to the neurovascular bundles. *Int J Radiat Oncol Biol Phys.* 2000;46(5):1301–1307.

213. Merrick GS, Wallner K, Butler WM, Galbreath RW, Lief JH, Benson ML. A comparison of radiation dose to the bulb of the penis in men with and without prostate brachytherapy-induced erectile dysfunction. *Int J Radiat Oncol Biol Phys.* 2001;50(3):597–604.

214. Miles C, Candy B, Jones L, Williams R, Tookman A, King M. Interventions for sexual dysfunction following treatments for cancer. *Cochrane Database Sys Rev.* 2007;4.

215. McMahon CG. High dose sildenafil citrate as a salvage therapy for severe erectile dysfunction. *Int J Impot Res.* 2002;14(6):533–538.

216. Shindel AW. 2009 update on phosphodiesterase type 5 inhibitor therapy part 1: recent studies on routine dosing for penile rehabilitation, lower urinary tract symptoms, and other indications (CME). *J Sex Med.* 2009;6(7):1794–1808; quiz 1793, 1809–1710.

217. Stember DS, Mulhall JP. The concept of erectile function preservation (penile rehabilitation) in the patient after brachytherapy for prostate cancer. *Brachytherapy.* 2012;11(2):87–96.

218. Wang R. Penile rehabilitation after radical prostatectomy: where do we stand and where are we going? *J Sex Med.* 2007;4(4):1085–1097.

219. Stephenson RA, Mori M, Hsieh Y-C, et al. Treatment of erectile dysfunction following therapy for clinically localized prostate cancer: patient reported use and outcomes from the Surveillance, Epidemiology, and End Results Prostate Cancer Outcomes Study. *J Urol.* 2005;174(2):646–650.

220. Schover LR, Fouladi RT, Warneke CL, et al. The use of treatments for erectile dysfunction among survivors of prostate carcinoma. *Cancer.* 2002;95(11):2397–2407.

221. Melnik T, Soares B, Nasello AG. Psychosocial interventions for erectile dysfunction. *Cochrane Database Sys Rev.* 2007;5.

222. Koeman M, Van Driel M, Weijmar Schultz W, Mensink H. Orgasm after radical prostatectomy. *Br J Urol.* 1996;77(6):861–864.

223. Lee J, Hersey K, Lee CT, Fleshner N. Climacturia following radical prostatectomy: prevalence and risk factors. *J Urol.* 2006;176(6):2562–2565.

224. Abouassaly R, Lane BR, Lakin MM, Klein EA, Gill IS. Ejaculatory urine incontinence after radical prostatectomy. *Urology.* 2006;68(6):1248–1252.

225. Choi JM, Nelson CJ, Stasi J, Mulhall JP. Orgasm associated incontinence (climacturia) following radical pelvic surgery: rates of occurrence and predictors. *J Urol.* 2007;177(6):2223–2226.

226. Nilsson AE, Carlsson S, Johansson E, et al. Orgasm-associated urinary incontinence and sexual life after radical prostatectomy. *J Sex Med.* 2011;8(9):2632–2639.

227. Zebrack BJ, Foley S, Wittmann D, Leonard M. Sexual functioning in young adult survivors of childhood cancer. *Psychooncology.* 2010;19(8):814–822.

228. Bober SL, Zhou ES, Chen B, Manley PE, Kenney LB, Recklitis CJ. Sexual function in childhood cancer survivors: a report from Project REACH. *J Sex Med.* 2013;10(8):2084–2093.

229. Ritenour CW, Seidel KD, Leisenring W, et al. Erectile dysfunction in male survivors of childhood cancer—a report from the Childhood Cancer Survivor Study. *J Sex Med.* 2016;13(6):945–954.

230. Ford JS, Kawashima T, Whitton J, et al. Psychosexual functioning among adult female survivors of childhood cancer: a report from the Childhood Cancer Survivor Study. *J Clin Oncol.* 2014;32(28):3126–3136.

231. Zegers-Hochschild F, Adamson GD, de Mouzon J, et al. The International Committee for Monitoring Assisted Reproductive Technology (ICMART) and the World Health Organization (WHO) revised glossary on ART terminology, 2009. *Hum Reprod.* 2009;24(11): 2683–2687.

232. Lee SJ, Schover LR, Partridge AH, et al. American Society of Clinical Oncology recommendations on fertility preservation in cancer patients. *J Clin Oncol.* 2006;24(18):2917–2931.

233. Green D, Galvin H, Horne B. The psycho-social impact of infertility on young male cancer survivors: a qualitative investigation. *Psychooncology.* 2003;12(2):141–152.

234. Nieman CL, Kazer R, Brannigan RE, et al. Cancer survivors and infertility: a review of a new problem and novel answers. *J Support Oncol.* 2006;4(4):171–178.

235. Sonmezer M, Oktay K. Fertility preservation in female patients. *Hum Reprod Update.* 2004;10(3):251–266.

236. National Cancer Institute. A to Z list of cancer drugs. 2017; https://www.cancer.gov/about-cancer/treatment/drugs. Accessed March 29, 2017.

237. Jeruss JS, Woodruff TK. Preservation of fertility in patients with cancer. *N Engl J Med.* 2009;360(9):902–911.

238. Chambers GM, Adamson GD, Eijkemans MJ. Acceptable cost for the patient and society. *Fertil Steril.* 2013;100(2):319–327.

239. Gateway CWI. *Costs of Adopting.* Washington, DC: U.S. Department of Health and Human Services, Children's Bureau; 2011.

240. Rosen A. Third-party reproduction and adoption in cancer patients. *J Natl Cancer Inst Monogr.* 2005;(34):91–93.

241. Meirow D, Nugent D. The effects of radiotherapy and chemotherapy on female reproduction. *Hum Reprod Update.* 2001;7(6):535–543.

242. Bath LE, Critchley HO, Chambers SE, Anderson RA, Kelnar CJ, Wallace WHB. Ovarian and uterine characteristics after total body irradiation in childhood and adolescence: response to sex steroid replacement. *BJOG.* 1999;106(12):1265–1272.

243. Green DM, Kawashima T, Stovall M, et al. Fertility of female survivors of childhood cancer: a report from the Childhood Cancer Survivor Study. *J Clin Oncol.* 2009;27(16):2677–2685.

244. Critchley H, Wallace WHB, Shalet SM, Mamtora H, Higginson J, Anderson D. Abdominal irradiation in childhood; the potential for pregnancy. *BJOG.* 1992;99(5):392–394.

245. Wallace W, Thomson A. Preservation of fertility in children treated for cancer. *Arch Dis Child.* 2003;88(6):493–496.

246. Wallace WHB, Anderson RA, Irvine DS. Fertility preservation for young patients with cancer: who is at risk and what can be offered? *Lancet Oncol.* 2005;6(4):209–218.

247. Pagani O, Regan MM, Walley BA, et al. Adjuvant exemestane with ovarian suppression in premenopausal breast cancer. *N Engl J Med.* 2014;371(2):107–118.

248. Francis PA, Regan MM, Fleming GF, et al. Adjuvant ovarian suppression in premenopausal breast cancer. *N Engl J Med*. 2015;372(5):436–446.

249. Blumenfeld Z, Avivi I, Linn S, Epelbaum R, Ben-Shahar M, Haim N. Endocrinology: prevention of irreversible chemotherapy-induced ovarian damage in young women with lymphoma by a gonadotrophin-releasing hormone agonist in parallel to chemotherapy. *Hum Reprod*. 1996;11(8):1620–1626.

250. Blumenfeld Z. Ovarian rescue/protection from chemotherapeutic agents. *J Soc Gynecol Investig*. 2001;8(1 Suppl.):S60–S64.

251. Kuwayama M. Highly efficient vitrification for cryopreservation of human oocytes and embryos: the Cryotop method. *Theriogenology*. 2007;67(1):73–80.

252. Kuwayama M, Vajta G, Kato O, Leibo SP. Highly efficient vitrification method for cryopreservation of human oocytes. *Reprod Biomed Online*. 2005;11(3):300–308.

253. Kasai M, Mukaida T. Cryopreservation of animal and human embryos by vitrification. *Reprod Biomed Online*. 2004;9(2):164–170.

254. Simon B, Lee SJ, Partridge AH, Runowicz CD. Preserving fertility after cancer. *CA Cancer J Clin*. 2005;55(4):211–228.

255. Dohle GR. Male infertility in cancer patients: review of the literature. *Int J Urol*. 2010;17(4):327–331.

256. Dohle G, Smit M, Weber R. Androgens and male fertility. *World J Urol*. 2003;21(5):341–345.

257. Green DM, Kawashima T, Stovall M, et al. Fertility of male survivors of childhood cancer: a report from the Childhood Cancer Survivor Study. *J Clin Oncol*. 2010;28(2):332–339.

258. Relander T, Cavallin-Ståhl E, Garwicz S, Olsson AM, Willén M. Gonadal and sexual function in men treated for childhood cancer. *Med Pediatr Oncol*. 2000;35(1):52–63.

259. Centola GM, Keller JW, Henzler M, Rubin P. Effect of low-dose testicular irradiation on sperm count and fertility in patients with testicular seminoma. *J Androl*. 1994;15(6):608–613.

260. Tournaye H, Goossens E, Verheyen G, et al. Preserving the reproductive potential of men and boys with cancer: current concepts and future prospects. *Hum Reprod Update*. 2004;10(6):525–532.

261. Schover LR, Brey K, Lichtin A, Lipshultz LI, Jeha S. Knowledge and experience regarding cancer, infertility, and sperm banking in younger male survivors. *J Clin Oncol*. 2002;20(7):1880–1889.

262. Hourvitz A, Goldschlag DE, Davis OK, Gosden LV, Palermo GD, Rosenwaks Z. Intracytoplasmic sperm injection (ICSI) using cryopreserved sperm from men with malignant neoplasm yields high pregnancy rates. *Fertil Steril*. 2008;90(3):557–563.

263. Van Casteren N, van Santbrink E, Van Inzen W, Romijn J, Dohle G. Use rate and assisted reproduction technologies outcome of cryopreserved semen from 629 cancer patients. *Fertil Steril*. 2008;90(6):2245–2250.

264. Hallak J, Hendin BN, Thomas AJ, Agarwal A. Investigation of fertilizing capacity of cryopreserved spermatozoa from patients with cancer. *J Urol*. 1998;159(4):1217–1220.

265. National District Attorneys Association. Minor consent to medical treatment laws. 2013; http://www.ndaa.org/pdf/Minor%20Consent%20to%20Medical%20Treatment%20(2).pdf. Accessed March 31, 2017.

266. Bioethics Co. Informed consent, parental permission, and assent in pediatric practice. *Pediatrics*. 1995;95(2):314–317.

267. Kohrman A, Clayton EW, Frader JE, et al. Informed consent, parental permission, and assent in pediatric practice. *Pediatrics*. 1995;95(2):314–317.

CHAPTER 10

LYMPHEDEMA AND BODY IMAGE DISTURBANCE

Sarah M. DeSnyder, Simona F. Shaitelman, and Mark V. Schaverien

It always pains me to look at myself in the mirror. I am reminded of all my body has gone through in the last year. As if it isn't enough losing my breasts to surgery, I now have to deal with lymphedema on my left arm. And unlike the other treatments that are now over, there is no end in sight with the lymphedema. I am told one of the reasons I am high risk is because of the surgery to clear my lymph nodes to stop the cancer from spreading. But I feel that this suffering is unbearable in its own way! There is stabbing pain that starts in my arm and radiates to my hands. I have tried wearing a special sleeve and keeping it elevated whenever I can, but I can't find relief. The pain only makes me think about all I can't do. Forget wearing my favorite dress, my arm does not fit through the sleeve anymore; forget doing handicrafts like I used to, the stiffness and swelling even affects my fingers. I feel as if my problem arm is as heavy as a ton of bricks. It is so unsightly, I sometimes joke that I have an alien arm, and that it is not really part of me. And although I try to keep a brave front, deep down I feel so unhappy about how my body look and feels.

> *—56-year-old female survivor of breast cancer*

I used to be an avid hiker and loved my time outdoors. However, I was diagnosed with sarcoma on my thigh and had to undergo surgery and radiation therapy. Just as I was ready to move on, I developed a swelling in the treated leg that was diagnosed as lymphedema. I was sent to a physical therapist that specializes in lymphedema. My leg was placed in wrap, and with several weeks of massage treatment it got better. Even now, walking makes my leg feel weak and I prop the leg up whenever I get the chance. But what bugs me the most is that I am not able to be as active and engage in outdoor activities as I used to. I am also constantly worried that I might reinjure the site or get an insect bite if I am outdoors that will lead to an infection. There are days when I feel let down by my body and get really upset. But I am not going to let this bring me now. I just need to tell myself, even if the symptoms never completely go away, it can be managed.

> *—28-year-old male survivor of sarcoma*

INTRODUCTION

Lymphedema is a common condition, estimated to occur in approximately 15.5% of cancer survivors. While primary lymphedema can occur as a result of inherited traits, the focus of this chapter is on secondary lymphedema resulting from cancer treatment. Secondary lymphedema has been estimated to affect 3 million to 5 million people in the United States and over 150 million people worldwide, and lymphedema is a significant health economic burden to both patients and society.[1–4]

In the Western world, secondary lymphedema occurs predominantly as a side effect of cancer treatment, including administration of some chemotherapeutics, surgery to the regional lymph node basins, and adjuvant radiation therapy. Depending on the site of the primary tumor, it may affect the upper extremity, one or both of the lower extremities, the trunk, or the head and neck region. Although the majority of cases will occur within 24 months of surgery, lymphedema may occur decades after surgery; and once at risk for lymphedema patients remain at lifelong risk.[5,6] The incidence of lymphedema is highest in patients following treatment for breast cancer, affecting over 20% of the 2.5 million breast cancer survivors in the United States and millions more worldwide.[7,8] Lymphedema also affects a large proportion of survivors with other malignancies, including melanoma (16%), gynecological cancer (20%), genitourinary cancer (10%), head/neck cancer (4%), and sarcoma (30%).[9]

Studies within the field of psychosocial oncology have shed light on the profound effect of lymphedema secondary to treatment of cancer on quality of life, body image, activities of daily living, and financial stress.[10,11] It has been said that the burden of living with lymphedema can be greater than the cancer itself.[12] In addition to the edema, lymphedema may result in chronic skin changes, fibrosis, loss of sensation, deformity of the afflicted region of the body, and pain.[13] Even after patients have been cured of their cancer, lymphedema and the compression garments worn to control their swelling serve as a lifelong reminder of the cancer. Not only do patients have an edematous limb that may be uncomfortable and restrict movement and function, they have to undergo a time-consuming daily routine of skin care, manual or pneumatic lymphatic drainage, and application of wrapping and/or compression garments. In addition, the excess limb volume and functional restrictions are social stigmata drawing unwanted attention to the lymphedematous limb. Lower extremity lymphedema may be particularly debilitating as conservative and surgical treatments are less effective, gait can be profoundly affected, and long-term orthopedic sequelae can occur in the hip and knees. Lymphedema of the head and neck following cancer treatment is an unrecognized condition that confers additional morbidity to already compromised patients, in particular to swallowing, breathing, and speech.[14,15] The highly visible nature of the condition results in profound negative psychosocial sequelae such as reduced self-esteem and poor socialization.[16]

Lymphedema is a dreaded complication of cancer care which is a constant reminder to cancer survivors of their cancer and its treatments. Not surprisingly, lymphedema may profoundly impact body image. In this chapter, we define lymphedema, explain the stages of lymphedema, describe risk factors for lymphedema, illustrate treatments for lymphedema, and discuss available literature that describes the impact of lymphedema on body image.

WHAT IS LYMPHEDEMA?

The lymphatic system is composed of lymphatic vessels as well as lymph nodes. Lymphatic fluid is moved throughout the body within both deep and superficial lymphatic vessels. Lymphatic fluid passes through lymph nodes where harmful substances such as viruses, bacteria, and waste products are filtered out of the lymph fluid and destroyed by leukocytes. The lymph fluid is then returned to the circulation via the thoracic duct.

Normal lymphatic function occurs when there is passive uptake of interstitial fluid into and intrinsic contraction of the lymphatic vessels. Lymphedema results when a disequilibrium occurs among the microvascular filtration capillaries, the lymphatic venules, and the lymphatic drainage system. Damage to the lymphatic vessels and/or lymph nodes results in disruption of this continuous flow of lymph with resulting hypertension of the lymphatic vessels and malfunction of the valves through which passive uptake of lymph occurs. Eventually, failure of the lymphatic vessels occurs resulting in stasis of the lymph fluid with subsequent build-up of this fluid (swelling) and finally fibrosis of the surrounding connective tissue.

STAGES OF LYMPHEDEMA

Four stages of lymphedema have been used to describe its severity (Table 10.1, Figure 10.1).[17] These descriptions are based on the degree of swelling as well as the degree of changes in the surrounding connective tissue. It is important to note that although most patients, particularly those with breast cancer, will achieve control of their lymphedema thus making it a chronic ailment, failure to achieve such control may result in progression of their lymphedema, repeated potentially limb threatening infections, impaired limb function, and even development of angiosarcoma, a rare but deadly malignancy.

RISK FACTORS FOR LYMPHEDEMA

In this section, we focus on risk factors for lymphedema. While the vast majority of lymphedema literature focus on breast cancer patients, the risk factors and precautions are applicable to lymphedema resulting from the treatments of other cancers as well. Certainly treatments for breast cancer, most notably surgery and radiation, place cancer patients at risk for lymphedema. However, there are other factors that may pose significant risk for the development of lymphedema. It is important that patients understand that their risk of lymphedema is sustained for the duration of their lives.[5,6]

TABLE 10.1: Stages of Lymphedema

Stage of Lymphedema	Description	Treatment
0 (or 1a)	No clinical evidence of swelling.	Compression sleeve +/– specialized exercises
	May have symptoms of heaviness or fatigue of the extremity.	
	Limb volume changes up to 5% above baseline may be detected.	
1	Swelling and/or pitting of the skin reversible with elevation,	Compression sleeve +/– specialized exercises
	decreased physical activity, or self-directed manual therapy.	+/– complete decongestive therapy
2	Swelling no longer spontaneously reversible.	Complete decongestive therapy
	Swelling may be decreased by elevation, decreased physical activity.	
	or self-directed manual therapy, but some swelling will persist.	
	Inflammation of the connective tissue will cause firmness of the skin.	
3	Known as lymphostatic elephantitis.	Complete decongestive therapy
	Inflammatory changes result in thickening of the skin and fibrosis of the subcutaneous tissue.	

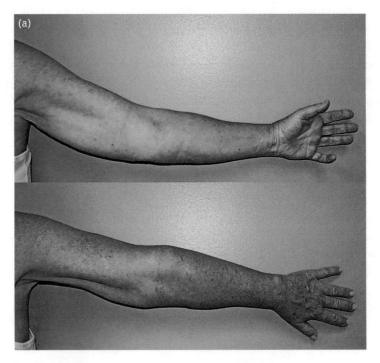

(a)

FIGURE 10.1.a: Lymphedema Stage 1.

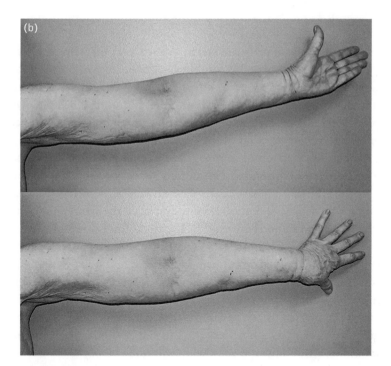

FIGURE 10.1b: Lymphedema - Stage 2

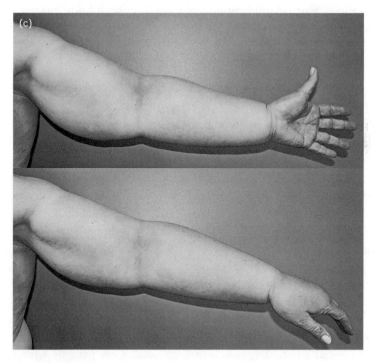

FIGURE 10.1.c: Lymphedema - Stage 3

TREATMENTS FOR CANCER

The lymphatic system can be directly affected by both surgery that removes lymph nodes or causes injury to lymph vessels, as well as resulting scar tissue formation. Surgical treatments for cancer have evolved and continue to do so employing less invasive techniques while providing equivalent local-regional control with lower morbidity, including lymphedema. As an example, historically, evaluation of the draining lymph nodes of both melanoma and breast cancer required removal of all of the lymph nodes within the at-risk lymph nodal basin. However, the introduction of sentinel lymph node biopsy as a method to sample these lymph nodes has revolutionized lymph node evaluation.[18,19] Importantly, multiple randomized controlled trials in breast cancer patients have all shown no difference in long-term outcomes for those who did not have removal of all the lymph nodes in the setting of a negative sentinel lymph node biopsy.[20,21] The trend toward less invasive axillary surgery has continued to evolve for breast cancer patients to include lesser axillary surgery for those planned for breast-conserving surgery with whole breast irradiation who have limited axillary disease on sentinel lymph node biopsy.[22] It has also been suggested that breast cancer patients who are node positive at diagnosis who have resolution of axillary disease with neoadjuvant chemotherapy as noted at the time of surgery with lymph node sampling may not need removal of all lymph nodes.[23–26] This safe minimization of lymph node surgery is critical as those who undergo sentinel lymph node biopsy alone have been shown to have fewer complications including wound infections, axillary seromas, paresthesias, shoulder pain, weakness, axillary web syndrome, and lymphedema.[27] It is known that these complications, particularly lymphedema, result in both body image and emotional disturbances including anxiety and depression.[28]

RADIATION

Radiation is a critical component of cancer treatment for many patients. Patients may have changes in their body as a result of radiation that may alter both physical appearance and function, including redness, flaking, and swelling of the treated area. Although these changes will mostly resolve after treatment is completed, some long-lasting side effects may occur such as skin pigment changes, changes in skin texture, restrictions in range of motion, and, for those with head and neck cancer, dysphagia. In addition to these physical and functional changes, radiation is known to increase the risk of lymphedema.

While the vast majority of studies have focused on lymph node surgery as the primary cause of lymphedema, information regarding radiation as a cause of lymphedema is limited. When radiation is delivered to the lymph nodes, it typically targets the lymph nodes not removed by the surgeon that are still at risk of harboring occult micrometastatic disease. Advances in treatment planning techniques over the past two decades have enabled more specific targeting of only those particular lymph nodes that are at risk, while minimizing irradiation of normal adjacent organs. Studies focusing on patients with breast cancer have demonstrated survival benefit with regional nodal irradiation for those with locally advanced disease and even some women with early-stage but high-risk disease.[29–31] The exact incidence of lymphedema associated with regional nodal radiation in the literature is variable, but in general, regional nodal radiation may nearly double the risk of lymphedema in breast cancer patients, and this risk is likely highest among patients who also undergo an axillary lymph node dissection.[30]

RISK-REDUCING BEHAVIORS

Women with breast cancer who are at risk for lymphedema have long been counseled to avoid blood pressure measurements, blood draws, injections, intravenous line placement, and trauma in an attempt to avoid developing cellulitis and lymphedema to the at-risk arm.[32–34] This extensive list of "do nots" has been advised despite data demonstrating the benefit of avoiding these procedures.[33] Certainly, this list of "dos" and "do nots" is a source of profound anxiety for at-risk patients. In addition, patients who develop lymphedema may blame themselves for this side effect. However, recent data has demonstrated that significant factors associated with development of lymphedema include elevated body mass index, axillary lymph node dissection, regional nodal irradiation, and cellulitis.[35] This study, which analyzed data on over 600 breast cancer patients at risk for lymphedema who underwent over 3,000 measurements of limb volume over a median follow-up of 24 months, demonstrated that ipsilateral blood draws, injections, blood pressure readings, and air travel of both short and long duration were not associated with arm volume increases. Importantly, this collection of data adds to existing evidence that elevated body mass index is a risk factor for the development of lymphedema following breast cancer treatments.[36,37] It is critical that patients at risk for lymphedema with an elevated body mass index are counseled about the importance of losing weight and that all patients are counseled about the importance of maintaining a healthy, active lifestyle in an effort to maintain a normal body mass index. While it is important for patients with obesity to be counseled about their associated risk of lymphedema, it is also important to recognize that obesity is a risk factor for body image disturbance. In particular, patients with a history of large fluctuations in body weight may be predisposed to worse body image related to breast cancer and development of lymphedema.[38]

EDUCATING PATIENTS ABOUT THE RISK OF LYMPHEDEMA

Guidelines published by the American Cancer Society and the American Society of Clinical Oncology focus on the need to counsel patients at risk for lymphedema about risk-reducing behaviors as well as the importance of weight loss for those at-risk patients who are either overweight or obese.[39] Three phases of lymphedema education have been recommended and are summarized in Table 10.2.[39–41] Orem's Self-Care Theory states that patients must be knowledgeable about the potential sequelae of their treatments so they can develop health promotion behaviors.[42] It is critical that patients have adequate information about the potential to develop lymphedema to ensure that they are our partners in their care. Ensuring patients are knowledgeable about their risk for lymphedema and the signs and symptoms

TABLE 10.2: Lymphedema Education

Phase of care	Goals of education
Pretreatment	Aimed at awareness
	Set the stage for posttreatment education
Postoperative education	Focus on prevention and symptoms awareness
	Discussion of risk factors and risk-reduction strategies
	Discussion of evidence-based precautions
	Discussion of psychosocial aspects of lymphedema
Continuing education	Continue to reinforce postoperative education

that may occur prior to swelling provides patients the best opportunity for early detection and intervention, thus maximizing the potential to achieve the best outcomes from lymphedema treatment, thereby decreasing body image sequelae. Importantly, patients' perceived lack of information about lymphedema may increase their distress level.[43] This educational construct is similar to how body image concerns are best addressed where preemptive discussions and early recognition of body image concerns can facilitate ease of treatment.

At the University of Texas MD Anderson Cancer Center, we provide patients an education packet at the time of their preoperative appointment. Key content areas include a description of what lymphedema is, precautions for risk reduction, and what signs and symptoms should prompt medical attention. Recently, a pilot study was undertaken in our Nellie B. Connally Breast Center to improve lymphedema education. Patients undergoing axillary surgery underwent a baseline assessment of their lymphedema knowledge followed by a nurse-guided education session which included the viewing of a lymphedema education video.[44] Patients were administered the same assessment after the session as well as at their postoperative appointment. At their postoperative assessment, patients demonstrated retention of 87% of their lymphedema knowledge. In addition, all patients indicated they derived benefit from the session and 73% indicated that they went on to seek additional knowledge about lymphedema after the session. To improve and standardize lymphedema education for our patients, a brief video which could become a part of routine work flow in our center was produced to educate patients about lymphedema. Patients planned for axillary surgery view this video at their preoperative assessment and may also access the video at any time through their patient portal.

TREATMENT OF LYMPHEDEMA

Lymphedema is a chronic condition. Patients diagnosed with lymphedema must undergo complex, time-consuming, and expensive treatments to achieve good control of their symptoms. While patients with stage 0 and state 1 lymphedema may be treated with a compression sleeve and specialized exercises, some patients with stage 1 lymphedema may be advised to undergo complete decongestive therapy. For those with stage 2 and

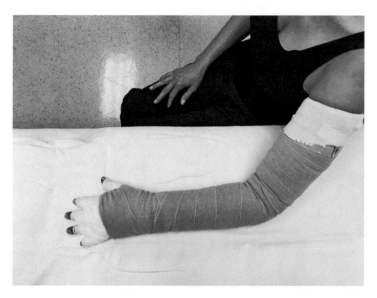

FIGURE 10.2: Compression bandaging.

state 3 lymphedema, standard of care treatment is complete decongestive therapy by a lymphedema-certified physical therapist. This involves two to four weeks of manual lymphatic drainage, compression bandaging, and instruction regarding a home care program geared toward autonomous management.[45] Manual lymphatic drainage employs light massage techniques to stimulate superficial lymphatic vessels and lymph nodes to improve efficiency of fluid movement from the arm into the body as well as to strengthen collaterals in the chest to promote increased receipt of lymphatic fluid. Compression bandaging, as shown in Figure 10.2, is performed to provide graduated tissue support following manual lymphatic drainage with a goal of preventing lymphatic fluid from refluxing back into the tissues, stopping the formation of additional lymphatic fluid, and softening the tissue fibrosis and/or skin thickening. Gentle exercise is an important component of complete decongestive therapy. It is important to note that exercises must always be performed with compression bandages intact. These gentle exercises act to squeeze the lymphatics between the bandages and the muscles to encourage fluid movement from the arm into the trunk as well as to soften the tissue fibrosis and/or skin thickening. In addition, the teaching of self-care is a critical component of complete decongestive therapy. Patients are taught how to don and doff compression bandages and garments, how to safely perform exercises, how to preserve skin integrity, and how to monitor for and respond appropriately to infection.

Compression garments, such as that depicted in Figure 10.3, can also be worn to prevent further swelling of the lymphedematous limb. There are specialized compression sleeves or stockings that provide support in different compression classes to match patient need. Most patients do not have an issue with wearing compression garments; however, it is worth noting that wearing a compression garment may be uncomfortable or distressing to some. The act of putting it on can be time-consuming. Some patients balk at the idea of wearing a compression garment for the entire day every day and, for some, a night compression sleeve. Further, ready-made garments are available; however, their fit may be less precise and thus

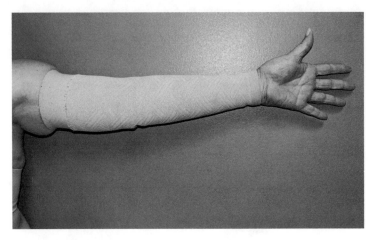

FIGURE 10.3: Compression garment.

may be less comfortable, especially if a person has longer/shorter limbs. The appearance of the garment may also be a concern as they are usually visible when worn with clothes that do not cover the entire limb, as in the case of short-sleeved tops or shorts/skirts. It is also noteworthy that the most common color for compression garments is beige and thus may not match the skin tone of darker-complected individuals. These factors can affect compliance of wearing the compression garments.

EFFECT OF LYMPHEDEMA ON BODY IMAGE

Lymphedema has complex, multidimensional effects on social factors in patients with cancer, including body image, sexuality, social relationships, and leisure and recreational activities.[46–48] Body image encompasses the relationship between patient perceptions, cognitions, emotions, and behaviors regarding physical appearance and is increasingly being recognized as an important predictor of health-related quality of life.[49–51] Body image dissatisfaction is a central psychological and interpersonal issue for patients with cancer, as the physical changes patients undergo during and as a result of cancer treatment can result in profound changes to physical appearance and functioning.[52,53] In addition, personal investment in body image relates to body integrity, where self-worth is dependent on physical integrity of the body.[54] This may have relevance to the psychosocial impairment and depression experienced by patients with lymphedema, where the visible deformity of the extremity debilitates perceived body integrity. Oliveri and colleagues surveyed 245 breast cancer survivors, 31% of whom reported arm/hand swelling since the time of their surgery. Of those who reported lymphedema, 32% stated that their swelling interfered with perceptions about their general appearance and 36% reported that their clothing choice was impacted by the swelling.[46] Speck and colleagues evaluated breast cancer survivors both at risk of and afflicted with lymphedema after one year of strength training.[47] Importantly, they found that this twice-weekly intervention positively impacted self-perceptions of appearance as well as health, physical strength, sexuality, relationships, and social functioning. This highlights the need for preemptive interventions targeting body image for those both at risk of and afflicted with lymphedema.

Adverse psychological effects of body image changes include debilitating levels of social anxiety and clinical depression as well as deterioration in relationships with partners and impaired sexuality. Body image dissatisfaction has demonstrated independent association with depression in various populations.[55,56] It is known that physical symptoms caused by lymphedema can negatively impact body image.[57–60] Ridner and colleagues collected expressive writings from 52 breast cancer patients afflicted with lymphedema.[57] Analysis of these writings revealed perceptions of marginalization from healthcare providers as well as perceptions of loss including body image disturbances, decreased functionality, uncertainty, and relationship alterations. Within the subtheme of body image, two-thirds of those with lymphedema indicated persistent maladaptive thoughts about the appearance of the afflicted extremity. Many described their arm negatively and indicated they felt damaged. In addition, they described altering their clothing choice to hide their afflicted arm and even not attending social functions when they were unable to hide their afflicted arm. Another study of breast cancer survivors reported that lymphedema was particularly distressing because it was unexpected and they had not imagined how lymphedema and the resulting symptoms would impact their daily lives.[59] Yang and colleagues surveyed 191 breast cancer survivors specifically examining the impact of their disease on sexuality.[60] They found that poor body image and objectively identified lymphedema were both predictive of sexual dissatisfaction. Importantly, pain severity has also been linked along with body image dissatisfaction to depressive symptoms in patients with lymphedema.[56] This link provides a clear opportunity to intervene as improving pain resulting from lymphedema has a direct positive impact on depression.

It is critical to acknowledge that the body image changes associated with lymphedema may be lifelong, resulting in a deleterious psychological impact on patients and their families long after they are cured from their cancer.[57,61–65] It is not surprising that the visibility of lymphedema results in body image disturbance experienced by patients and that the edema and chronic skin changes result in concerns regarding appearance.[59] As such, limb excess volume is significantly associated with lymphedema-related appearance, with patients who have a high-volume differential reporting greater appearance disturbance.

Certainly, negative perceptions of appearance and body image also have negative effects on self-confidence and sexual relationships.[57,60,66–69] Breast cancer survivors with lymphedema may no longer perceive themselves as attractive or desirable and may be concerned about sexual performance as well as their partner's perception of them.[70] A study which interviewed 17 women with lymphedema about the impact of their lymphedema on body image concerns described that although women noted their sexual concerns were impacted by their breast cancer treatments, their sexual concerns were also impacted by the severity and location of their lymphedema.[71]

Negative self-identity is related to body image disturbance, and visible features of lymphedema may be perceived as a conspicuous sign of disability.[61,63,70] As such, negative self-perception and criticisms from others may also lead to negative body image.[58,66,72] Winch and colleagues described their interviews with women afflicted with lymphedema.[71]

These women cited instances when they had been treated as disabled by others due to their compression garment. Many stated that their swollen extremity could be misunderstood as obesity and generally made them feel ugly. Not surprisingly, affected individuals may attempt to conceal their extremity due to social embarrassment as well as avoid social activities and situations where the limb would be exposed.[58,66,73] Social isolation to avoid scrutiny from others is common in an attempt to avoid the discomfort of being asked why their limb is "large" or "burned."[61,62,74] Not uncommonly, an affected individual with a swollen limb secondary to lymphedema may have feelings of insecurity secondary to body image distortion, alter their daily activities, and change their choice of clothing to better conceal their perceived deformity.[58,66,72,75,76] Additionally, barriers to work activities and recreation exist and have been reported by afflicted patients as resulting in perceived marginalization.[47,48,77–80]

IMPACT OF LYMPHEDEMA ON HEALTH-RELATED QUALITY OF LIFE

It is well recognized that lymphedema and associated symptoms, including swelling, heaviness, tightness, firmness, pain, numbness, stiffness, and impaired limb mobility, have a negative impact on physical and functional well-being, resulting in diminished overall health-related quality of life.[10,11] The Iowa Women's Health Study, a large population-based cohort study of health-related quality of life in 1,287 women with a diagnosis of breast cancer, found that quality of life was lower in patients with lymphedema, with a proportional relationship between the number of arm symptoms and reduced quality of life.[75] Another study demonstrated that symptoms secondary to lymphedema and coping strategies were both associated with physical and functional well-being and that limb volume change correlated with negative physical, functional, and social well-being.[56] A systematic review of all published qualitative studies on the psychosocial impact of lymphedema between 2004 and 2011 consistently found negative psychological impact (negative self-identity, emotional disturbance, psychological distress) and negative social impact (marginalization, financial burden, perceived diminished sexuality, social isolation, perceived social abandonment, public insensitivity, nonsupportive work environment) reported as a result of lymphedema.[52]

ASSESSMENT AND INTERVENTION APPROACHES FOR PATIENTS WITH LYMPHEDEMA

Multidisciplinary collaboration between oncologists, surgeons, psychologists, psychiatrists, nurses, physician assistants, physical therapists, occupational therapists, speech and language pathologists, social workers, and other allied healthcare professionals play a vital role in assessment and delivery of psychosocial interventions to address body image issues in patients with lymphedema. Research findings from psycho-oncology in the field of lymphedema secondary to cancer treatment support the central importance of body image in overall adjustment through the cancer and survivorship journey. The complex relationship between body image, including thoughts, beliefs, and emotions, and mood disturbance in the setting of cancer treatment and its sequelae are not only a result of appearance changes but can also be associated with physical changes including pain, sensation, and function. The certified lymphedema physical therapist has a central and vital role in treating patients with lymphedema as well as with the lifelong management of compression garments to control the edema, reduce limb volume, reduce symptoms secondary to the edema, and prevent progression to chronic lymphedema with associated skin changes.[81]

In the head and neck, treatment of lymphedema can improve function including speech, swallowing, and breathing, as well as physical appearance.[14,15,82] More recently, surgical approaches have been employed to treat lymphedema. These procedures have included lymphovenous bypass which redirects lymphatic fluid into the venous circulation, lymph node transfer which moves healthy lymph nodes to replace removed or damaged lymph nodes, and even debulking procedures which excise damaged tissue. The role of surgical intervention in reducing limb volume, alleviating symptoms, and reducing the risk of progression to the chronic disease state is increasingly being recognized.[83–86] The severity of lymphedema, measured either by subjective symptom burden or objective limb volume change, and the patient's coping strategy and support structure have been demonstrated to be associated with quality of life. There is evidence that emotional support is significantly associated with increased functional well-being in patients with lymphedema, which may be a result of increased ability to manage the daily stresses related to experiencing the condition, as well as perhaps reducing the perceived social nonacceptance.[83] Teo and colleagues surveyed breast cancer patients with lymphedema who underwent microsurgical intervention including either lymphaticovenular bypass or lymph node transfer. They found that denial was a predictor of poorer social well-being and that venting and self-blame predicted poorer emotional well-being. The finding that these maladaptive coping strategies reduce quality of life in patients with lymphedema is important in that it highlights the need to preemptively discuss coping strategies for affected individuals. Understanding the coping strategy employed by individuals affected, including participation or avoidance behaviors, may give the healthcare provider an insight into quality of life and, when necessary, help patients to be directed to appropriate psychosocial services. This is of particular importance in cancer survivors where many support mechanisms and opportunities for intervention may no longer be in place when the condition enters a chronic and more symptomatic stage. For this reason, routine assessment of body image concerns is essential in patients with lymphedema as a potentially critical area to facilitate early intervention.

White's heuristic model of important body image dimensions describes how a people's body image concerns impact their assumptions of others' responses to their appearance changes and their assumptions about others' behaviors resulting in compensatory behavior.[87] Interventions to educate patients, thus aiding them in developing adaptive coping skills as well as helping them to reduce maladaptive coping skills, may be useful. Psychosocial counseling can facilitate patients in accepting their circumstance, helping them to identify sources of social support, and assuaging maladaptive strategies including disengagement, denial, venting, and self-blame. It is critical to recognize that pain intensity and body image dissatisfaction are important factors in understanding depressive symptoms in patients with lymphedema. Screening for symptoms of pain and body image concerns in patients with lymphedema may help to determine those in distress as well as those at risk for depressive symptoms.[56] Intervention to reduce pain secondary to edema and counseling interventions targeting body image dissatisfaction may be beneficial in reducing symptoms of depression. Cognitive-behavioral therapy for body image, which is intended to modify these maladaptive body image beliefs and negative body integrity perceptions, may decrease patient distress. Therapeutic strategies including cognitive restructuring and mindfulness/acceptance techniques may be useful to address these negative thoughts and feelings and to replace them with more neutral or positive ones. These strategies may also mitigate the associated behavioral avoidance and social isolation as a result of having lymphedema.[13]

CONCLUSION

Lymphedema is a dreaded side effect of cancer treatments. Patients who develop lymphedema are at risk for body image disturbances. It is critical for healthcare providers to recognize and treat lymphedema at its earliest stages not only to control lymphedema but to mitigate the detrimental downstream effects of lymphedema including body image disturbance, social anxiety, and depression, all of which affect health-related quality of life. For those who experience diminished health-related quality of life due to lymphedema, healthcare providers must intervene with psychosocial support.

REFERENCES

1. Lawenda BD, Mondry TE, Johnstone PA. Lymphedema: a primer on the identification and management of a chronic condition in oncologic treatment. *CA Cancer J Clin*. 2009;59(1):8–24.

2. Basta MN, Fox JP, Kanchwala SK, et al. Complicated breast cancer-related lymphedema: evaluating health care resource utilization and associated costs of management. *Am J Surg*. 2016;211(1):133–141.

3. Shih YC, Xu Y, Cormier JN, et al. Incidence, treatment costs, and complications of lymphedema after breast cancer among women of working age: a 2-year follow-up study. *J Clin Oncol*. 2009;27(12):2007–2014.

4. Brayton KM, Hirsch AT, PJ OB, Cheville A, Karaca-Mandic P, Rockson SG. Lymphedema prevalence and treatment benefits in cancer: impact of a therapeutic intervention on health outcomes and costs. *PLoS One*. 2014;9(12):e114597.

5. Armer JM, Stewart BR. Post-breast cancer lymphedema: incidence increases from 12 to 30 to 60 months. *Lymphology*. 2010;43(3):118–127.

6. Brennan MJ, Weitz J. Lymphedema 30 years after radical mastectomy. *Am J Phys Med Rehabil*. 1992;71(1):12–14.

7. DiSipio T, Rye S, Newman B, Hayes S. Incidence of unilateral arm lymphoedema after breast cancer: a systematic review and meta-analysis. *Lancet Oncol*. 2013;14(6):500–515.

8. Voss RK, Cromwell KD, Chiang YJ, et al. The long-term risk of upper-extremity lymphedema is two-fold higher in breast cancer patients than in melanoma patients. *J Surg Oncol*. 2015;112(8):834–840.

9. Cormier JN, Askew RL, Mungovan KS, Xing Y, Ross MI, Armer JM. Lymphedema beyond breast cancer: a systematic review and meta-analysis of cancer-related secondary lymphedema. *Cancer*. 2010;116(22):5138–5149.

10. Velanovich V, Szymanski W. Quality of life of breast cancer patients with lymphedema. *Am J Surg*. 1999;177(3):184–187; discussion 188.

11. Heiney SP, McWayne J, Cunningham JE, et al. Quality of life and lymphedema following breast cancer. *Lymphology*. 2007;40(4):177–184.

12. Carter BJ. Women's experiences of lymphedema. *Oncol Nurs Forum*. 1997;24(5):875–882.

13. Passik SD, Newman ML, Brennan M, Tunkel R. Predictors of psychological distress, sexual dysfunction and physical functioning among women with upper extremity lymphedema related to breast can. *Psychooncology*. 1995;4(4):255–263.

14. Deng J, Murphy BA, Dietrich MS, Sinard RJ, Mannion K, Ridner SH. Differences of symptoms in head and neck cancer patients with and without lymphedema. *Support Care Cancer*. 2016;24(3):1305–1316.

15. Deng J, Ridner S, Rothman R, et al. Perceived symptom experience in head and neck cancer patients with lymphedema. *J Palliat Med*. 2016;19(12):1267–1274.

16. McGarvey AC, Osmotherly PG, Hoffman GR, Chiarelli PE. Lymphoedema following treatment for head and neck cancer: impact on patients, and beliefs of health professionals. *Eur J Cancer Care*. 2014;23(3):317–327.

17. International Society of Lymphology. The diagnosis and treatment of peripheral lymphedema: 2013 Consensus Document of the International Society of Lymphology. *Lymphology*. 2013;46:1–11.

18. Morton DL, Wanek L, Nizze JA, Elashoff RM, Wong JH. Improved long-term survival after lymphadenectomy of melanoma metastatic to regional nodes. Analysis of prognostic factors in 1134 patients from the John Wayne Cancer Clinic. *Ann Surg*. 1991;214(4):491–499; discussion 499–501.

19. Giuliano AE, Kirgan DM, Guenther JM, Morton DL. Lymphatic mapping and sentinel lymphadenectomy for breast cancer. *Ann Surg*. 1994;220(3):391–398; discussion 398–401.

20. Ashikaga T, Krag DN, Land SR, et al. Morbidity results from the NSABP B-32 trial comparing sentinel lymph node dissection versus axillary dissection. *J Surg Oncol*. 2010;102(2):111–118.

21. Veronesi U, Viale G, Paganelli G, et al. Sentinel lymph node biopsy in breast cancer: Ten-year results of a randomized controlled study. *Ann Surg*. 2010;251(4):595–600.

22. Giuliano AE, Hunt KK, Ballman KV, et al. Axillary dissection vs no axillary dissection in women with invasive breast cancer and sentinel node metastasis: a randomized clinical trial. *JAMA*. 2011;305(6):569–575.

23. Boughey JC, Suman VJ, Mittendorf EA, et al. Sentinel lymph node surgery after neoadjuvant chemotherapy in patients with node-positive breast cancer: the ACOSOG Z1071 (Alliance) clinical trial. *JAMA*. 2013;310(14):1455–1461.

24. Boileau JF, Poirier B, Basik M, et al. Sentinel node biopsy after neoadjuvant chemotherapy in biopsy-proven node-positive breast cancer: the SN FNAC study. *J Clin Oncol*. 2015;33(3):258–264.

25. Kuehn T, Bauerfeind I, Fehm T, et al. Sentinel-lymph-node biopsy in patients with breast cancer before and after neoadjuvant chemotherapy (SENTINA): a prospective, multicentre cohort study. *Lancet Oncol*. 2013;14(7):609–618.

26. Caudle AS, Yang WT, Krishnamurthy S, et al. Improved axillary evaluation following neoadjuvant therapy for patients with node-positive breast cancer using selective evaluation of clipped nodes: implementation of targeted axillary dissection. *J Clin Oncol*. 2016;34(10):1072–1078.

27. Lucci A, McCall LM, Beitsch PD, et al. Surgical complications associated with sentinel lymph node dissection (SLND) plus axillary lymph node dissection compared with SLND alone in the American College of Surgeons Oncology Group Trial Z0011. *J Clin Oncol*. 2007;25(24):3657–3663.

28. Recchia TL, Prim AC, Luz CM. Upper Limb functionality and quality of life in women with five-year survival after breast cancer surgery. *Revista brasil ginecol obstetr*. 2017;39(3):115–122.

29. Recht A, Comen EA, Fine RE, et al. Postmastectomy radiotherapy: an American Society of Clinical Oncology, American Society for Radiation Oncology, and Society of Surgical Oncology focused guideline update. *Ann Surg Oncol.* 2017;24(1):38–51.

30. Whelan TJ, Olivotto IA, Levine MN. Regional nodal irradiation in early-stage breast cancer. *New Engl J Med.* 2015;373(19):1878–1879.

31. Poortmans PM, Collette S, Kirkove C, et al. Internal mammary and medial supraclavicular irradiation in breast cancer. *New Engl J Med.* 2015;373(4):317–327.

32. American Cancer Society. *Lymphedema: What Every Woman with Breast Cancer Should Know.* New York: American Cancer Society; 2013.

33. NLN Medical Advisory Committee. Position Statement of the National Lymphedema Network: Lymphedema Risk Reduction Practices. National Lymphedema Network, 2012. https://www.lymphnet.org/pdfDocs/nlnriskreduction.pdf

34. McLaughlin SA, Bagaria S, Gibson T, et al. Trends in risk reduction practices for the prevention of lymphedema in the first 12 months after breast cancer surgery. *J Am Coll Surg.* 2013;216(3):380–389; quiz 511–383.

35. Ferguson CM, Swaroop MN, Horick N, et al. Impact of ipsilateral blood draws, injections, blood pressure measurements, and air travel on the risk of lymphedema for patients treated for breast cancer. *J Clin Oncol.* 2016;34(7):691–698.

36. McLaughlin SA, Wright MJ, Morris KT, et al. Prevalence of lymphedema in women with breast cancer 5 years after sentinel lymph node biopsy or axillary dissection: Objective measurements. *J Clin Oncol.* 2008;26(32):5213–5219.

37. Ozaslan C, Kuru B. Lymphedema after treatment of breast cancer. *Am J Surg.* 2004;187(1):69–72.

38. Fazzino TL, Hunter RC, Sporn N, Christifano DN, Befort CA. Weight fluctuation during adulthood and weight gain since breast cancer diagnosis predict multiple dimensions of body image among rural breast cancer survivors. *Psychooncology.* 2017;26(3):392–399.

39. Runowicz CD, Passik SD, Hann D, et al. American Cancer Society Lymphedema Workshop. Workgroup II: Patient education—pre- and posttreatment. *Cancer.* 1998;83(12 Suppl. American):2880–2881.

40. Runowicz CD. Lymphedema: patient and provider education: current status and future trends. *Cancer.* 1998;83(12 Suppl. American):2874–2876.

41. Thiadens SR. Current status of education and treatment resources for lymphedema. *Cancer.* 1998;83(12 Suppl. Am.):2864–2868.

42. Denyes MJ, Orem DE, Bekel G. Self-care: a foundational science. *Nurs Sci Q.* 2001;14(1):48–54.

43. Ridner SH. Pretreatment lymphedema education and identified educational resources in breast cancer patients. *Patient Educ Counsel.* 2006;61(1):72–79.

44. Simmons HM. Preoperative lymphedema education for breast cancer patients. *Nurs Health.* 2015;3(3):69–83.

45. Moseley AL, Carati CJ, Piller NB. A systematic review of common conservative therapies for arm lymphoedema secondary to breast cancer treatment. *Ann Oncol.* 2007;18(4):639–646.

46. Oliveri JM, Day JM, Alfano CM, et al. Arm/hand swelling and perceived functioning among breast cancer survivors 12 years post-diagnosis: CALGB 79804. *J Cancer Survivor Res Pract.* 2008;2(4):233–242.

47. Speck RM, Gross CR, Hormes JM, et al. Changes in the Body Image and Relationship Scale following a one-year strength training trial for breast cancer survivors with or at risk for lymphedema. *Breast Cancer Res Treat.* 2010;121(2):421–430.

48. Miedema B, Hamilton R, Tatemichi S, et al. Predicting recreational difficulties and decreased leisure activities in women 6–12 months post breast cancer surgery. *J Cancer Survivor Res Pract.* 2008;2(4):262–268.

49. Hopwood P, Maguire GP. Body image problems in cancer patients. *Br J Psychiatr Suppl.* 1988(2):47–50.

50. Fingeret MC, Nipomnick SW, Crosby MA, Reece GP. Developing a theoretical framework to illustrate associations among patient satisfaction, body image and quality of life for women undergoing breast reconstruction. *Cancer Treat Rev.* 2013;39(6):673–681.

51. Fingeret MC, Teo I, Epner DE. Managing body image difficulties of adult cancer patients: lessons from available research. *Cancer.* 2014;120(5):633–641.

52. Fu MR, Ridner SH, Hu SH, Stewart BR, Cormier JN, Armer JM. Psychosocial impact of lymphedema: a systematic review of literature from 2004 to 2011. *Psychooncology.* 2013;22(7):1466–1484.

53. Jager G, Doller W, Roth R. Quality-of-life and body image impairments in patients with lymphedema. *Lymphology.* 2006;39(4):193–200.

54. Petronis VM, Carver CS, Antoni MH, Weiss S. Investment in body image and psychosocial well-being among women treated for early stage breast cancer: partial replication and extension. *Psychol Health.* 2003;18(1):1–13.

55. Himelein MJ, Thatcher SS. Depression and body image among women with polycystic ovary syndrome. *J Health Psychol.* 2006;11(4):613–625.

56. Teo I, Novy DM, Chang DW, Cox MG, Fingeret MC. Examining pain, body image, and depressive symptoms in patients with lymphedema secondary to breast cancer. *Psychooncology.* 2015;24(11):1377–1383.

57. Ridner SH, Bonner CM, Deng J, Sinclair VG. Voices from the shadows: living with lymphedema. *Cancer Nurs.* 2012;35(1):E18–E26.

58. Ridner SH, Sinclair V, Deng J, Bonner CM, Kidd N, Dietrich MS. Breast cancer survivors with lymphedema: glimpses of their daily lives. *Clin J Oncol Nurs.* 2012;16(6):609–614.

59. Rosedale M, Fu MR. Confronting the unexpected: temporal, situational, and attributive dimensions of distressing symptom experience for breast cancer survivors. *Oncol Nurs Forum.* 2010;37(1):E28–E33.

60. Yang EJ, Kim SW, Heo CY, Lim JY. Longitudinal changes in sexual problems related to cancer treatment in Korean breast cancer survivors: a prospective cohort study. *Support Care Cancer.* 2011;19(7):909–918.

61. Fu MR, Rosedale M. Breast cancer survivors' experiences of lymphedema-related symptoms. *J Pain Symptom Manage.* 2009;38(6):849–859.

62. Towers A, Carnevale FA, Baker ME. The psychosocial effects of cancer-related lymphedema. *J Palliat Care.* 2008;24(3):134–143.

63. Maxeiner A, Saga E, Downer C, Arthur L. Comparing the psychosocial issues experienced by individuals with primary vs. secondary lymphedema. *Rehabil Oncol.* 2009;27:9–15.

64. Greenslade MV, House CJ. Living with lymphedema: a qualitative study of women's perspectives on prevention and management following breast cancer-related treatment. *Can Oncol Nurs J = Rev can nurs oncol.* 2006;16(3):165–179.

65. Honner A. The information needs of patients with therapy-related lymphoedema. *Cancer Nurs Pract.* 2009;8:21–26.

66. Vassard D, Olsen MH, Zinckernagel L, Vibe-Petersen J, Dalton SO, Johansen C. Psychological consequences of lymphoedema associated with breast cancer: a prospective cohort study. *Eur J Cancer.* 2010;46(18):3211–3218.

67. Ridner SH. Quality of life and a symptom cluster associated with breast cancer treatment-related lymphedema. *Support Care Cancer.* 2005;13(11):904–911.

68. Arndt V, Stegmaier C, Ziegler H, Brenner H. A population-based study of the impact of specific symptoms on quality of life in women with breast cancer 1 year after diagnosis. *Cancer.* 2006;107(10):2496–2503.

69. Hormes JM, Lytle LA, Gross CR, Ahmed RL, Troxel AB, Schmitz KH. The Body Image and Relationships Scale: development and validation of a measure of body image in female breast cancer survivors. *J Clin Oncol.* 2008;26(8):1269–1274.

70. Radina E, Watson W, Faubert K. Lymphoedema and sexual relationships in mid/later life. *J Lympho.* 2008;3(2):21–30.

71. Winch CJ, Sherman KA, Koelmeyer LA, Smith KM, Mackie H, Boyages J. Sexual concerns of women diagnosed with breast cancer-related lymphedema. *Support Care Cancer*. 2015;23(12):3481–3491.

72. O'Toole J, Jammallo LS, Skolny MN, et al. Lymphedema following treatment for breast cancer: a new approach to an old problem. *Crit Rev Oncol Hematol*. 2013;88(2):437–446.

73. Lee SH, Min YS, Park HY, Jung TD. Health-related quality of life in breast cancer patients with lymphedema who survived more than one year after surgery. *J Breast Cancer*. 2012;15(4):449–453.

74. Bogan LK, Powell JM, Dudgeon BJ. Experiences of living with non-cancer-related lymphedema: implications for clinical practice. *Qual Health Res*. 2007;17(2):213–224.

75. Ahmed RL, Prizment A, Lazovich D, Schmitz KH, Folsom AR. Lymphedema and quality of life in breast cancer survivors: the Iowa Women's Health Study. *J Clin Oncol*. 2008;26(35):5689–5696.

76. Pinto M, Gimigliano F, Tatangelo F, et al. Upper limb function and quality of life in breast cancer related lymphedema: a cross-sectional study. *Eur J Phys Rehabil Med*. 2013;49(5):665–673.

77. Lam R, Wallace A, Burbidge B, Franks P, Moffatt C. Experiences of patients with lymphoedema. *J Lympho*. 2006;1(1):16–21.

78. Fu MR. Women at work with breast cancer-related lymphoedema. *J Lympho*. 2008;3(1):20–25.

79. Passik SD, McDonald MV. Psychosocial aspects of upper extremity lymphedema in women treated for breast carcinoma. *Cancer*. 1998;83(12 Suppl. Am.):2817–2820.

80. Beaulac SM, McNair LA, Scott TE, LaMorte WW, Kavanah MT. Lymphedema and quality of life in survivors of early-stage breast cancer. *Arch Surg*. 2002;137(11):1253–1257.

81. Lasinski BB, McKillip Thrift K, Squire D, et al. A systematic review of the evidence for complete decongestive therapy in the treatment of lymphedema from 2004 to 2011. *PM R*. 2012;4(8):580–601.

82. Smith BG, Hutcheson KA, Little LG, et al. Lymphedema outcomes in patients with head and neck cancer. *Otolaryngol Head Neck Surg*. 2015;152(2):284–291.

83. Teo I, Fingeret MC, Liu J, Chang DW. Coping and quality of life of patients following microsurgical treatment for breast cancer-related lymphedema. *J Health Psychol*. 2016;21(12):2983–2993.

84. Silva AK, Chang DW. Vascularized lymph node transfer and lymphovenous bypass: novel treatment strategies for symptomatic lymphedema. *J Surg Oncol*. 2016;113(8):932–939.

85. Shaitelman SF, Cromwell KD, Rasmussen JC, et al. Recent progress in the treatment and prevention of cancer-related lymphedema. *CA Cancer J Clin*. 2015;65(1):55–81.

86. Brorson H. Liposuction in lymphedema treatment. *J Reconstr Microsurg*. 2016;32(1):56–65.

87. White CA. Body image dimensions and cancer: a heuristic cognitive behavioural model. *Psychooncology*. 2000;9(3):183–192.

CHAPTER 11

SPEECH AND SWALLOWING IMPAIRMENT

Jan S. Lewin, Michelle Cororve Fingeret, and Kate A. Hutcheson

Jerry is a 72-year-old man who has recently been diagnosed with laryngeal cancer. He is scheduled to undergo a total laryngectomy for definitive treatment of his cancer. During pretreatment education and evaluation sessions with the speech pathologist, he presents with significant anxiety regarding his ability to cope with the loss of his voice. He is referred for preoperative body image counseling with a psychologist so that he will feel better prepared and supported in managing his social and emotional concerns surrounding future body image changes. He attends several counseling sessions ahead of his surgery designed to normalize and validate his specific body image concerns, help him set realistic and flexible expectations regarding his treatment outcome, and discuss practical strategies for coping with communication challenges during acute postoperative recovery. Following surgery, Jerry engages in intensive functional rehabilitation and remains in body image counseling to facilitate his psychosocial adjustment to use of an electrolarynx. Jerry is encouraged and supported as he explores his emotional reaction to the loss of his natural voice and the manner in which his daily life and functioning has been impacted. Body image counseling also helps Jerry challenge assumptions he is making about how others perceive him and confront his fears of going out in public.

Shondra is a 60-year old woman with a history of oral tongue cancer. She was initially treated with a partial glossectomy (removal of a portion of the tongue) and radiation. She subsequently developed recurrent cancer in the floor of her mouth and underwent a mandibulectomy (removal of a portion of her mandible) and further glossectomy with reconstruction. Shondra is currently a 12-year cancer survivor and has been cancer free for five years. Due to her glossectomy, Shondra's speech is difficult to understand. She finds that her husband often needs to help translate what she is saying to others. Shondra becomes frustrated by the reactions of others when she attempts to communicate and sometimes will emotionally shut down and avoid social interactions altogether. Shondra's treatment has also significantly impaired her ability to swallow, and she relies on the use of a feeding tube. She has felt highly self-conscious about eating around others and is reluctant to participate in social or family gatherings. For the past four years she has been attending a support group, led by a psychologist and speech pathologist, that is part of the National Foundation of Swallowing Disorders. This support group meets once per month for two hours, and she attends this group with her husband. Through this group, Shondra finds great comfort and is inspired by others who, like her, are coping with the effects of dysphagia. She has also felt empowered to begin making her own meals from natural foods which she blends to the right consistency for her feeding tube. Shondra has felt increasingly comfortable with eating in public through her feeding tube and often provides tips to the group about traveling with her feeding supplies as she and her husband have begun to travel around the world.

INTRODUCTION

Speech and swallowing dysfunction are frequent consequences of head and neck cancer and its treatment. The diagnosis of cancer of the head and neck imparts a tremendous impact on the individual's physical, psychological, and social functioning and carries significant patient burden that affects the ability to communicate, impedes the return to personal and work routines, disrupts quality of life, and ultimately impacts the emotional and psychological well-being associated with survivorship. As demonstrated by two case examples presented at the outset of this chapter, newly diagnosed patients as well as long-term survivors can experience difficulties coping with changes to speech and swallowing as a result of cancer treatment and can benefit greatly from interventions to facilitate their psychosocial adjustment.

Unlike tumors that affect other parts of the body that are concealed or hidden from view, tumors that affect the head and neck are most often visibly obvious. Thus, the treatment and its consequences will almost certainly be associated with concerns regarding physical appearance and body image, self- concept, self-esteem, and self-worth.[1-5] Body image, as discussed throughout this book, is recognized to extend beyond one's view of physical appearance, to include perceptions, thoughts, and feelings about the entire body and its functioning. Body image associated with functional loss in cancer patients is covered broadly in Chapter 8. In this chapter, we focus specifically on the manner in which body image is affected by functional impairments in speech and swallowing. Patients with head and neck cancer, specifically, experience functional disabilities associated with the tumor itself as well as treatment-related morbidity, both of which may have long-term disabling outcomes years after the patient has recovered from the cancer treatment. The problems associated with the loss of normal function are often predictable and almost always affect the ability to speak and swallow. Thus, pretreatment evaluation and counseling and posttreatment intervention must be timely and precise to optimize patient outcomes, lessen long-term disabilities, and facilitate successful recovery.

TREATMENT IMPACT

Over the past two decades, the focus of treatment, whether surgical or nonsurgical, has transitioned from strictly cure and survival to organ preservation with an associated emphasis on functional preservation and quality of life. Speech and swallowing dysfunction after surgical resection varies depending on the extent of the surgery, the type of reconstruction, and the surgeon's preference in surgical technique. When radiation therapy accompanies surgery, or is given in combination with chemotherapy as an adjuvant modality, the effects are generally intensified and worsen the functional deficits. As medical and surgical treatments evolve and improve, more patients with head and neck tumors are being cured or surviving with stable disease. The advantage of endoscopic surgeries using laser and robotic technology to treat cancers of the head and neck, over nonsurgical alternatives that use intensity-modulated radiation therapy protocols with photon or proton beams, or adaptive radiation protocols to preserve function, continues to be investigated.

What we do know is that patients' goals have not changed significantly; their posttreatment expectations continue to be able to (a) eat by mouth, (b) speak using their natural laryngeal voice, and (c) appear unchanged from their pre-cancer appearance.[6] Despite the advances in organ-sparing treatment protocols, the functional sequelae for speech and swallowing are often severe and vary depending on the modality or combination of treatment modalities selected to cure the cancer. Impaired swallowing, dysphagia, is a dose-limiting toxicity of chemoradiation therapy for head and neck cancers. Even more important, dysphagia is also the primary functional concern of patients treated with nonsurgical therapy, drives perception of quality of life after chemoradiation therapy, and significantly predicts pneumonia in long-term survivorship.[7-9]

As the treatment for head and neck cancer has intensified, so too have the treatment-associated complications. Despite a reduction in the occurrence of total organ ablation, in favor of organ preservation, experience has shown that organ preservation does not ensure preservation of function. Unfortunately, data now shows that for some patients who have been treated with radiation therapy, the long-term late effects generally result in severe dysfunction, primarily dysphagia, years after the cancer treatment has ended, that, in most cases, is refractory to current standard methods of behavioral dysphagia therapy.[10] These long-term effects can induce significant body image distress. Likewise, high rates of aspiration[10,11] are often silent (without patient awareness or reaction) that result in aspiration pneumonia and chronic gastrostomy tube dependence in the posttreatment period. Given the current advances in speech and swallowing rehabilitation, in some cases, complete resection produces better functional outcomes and superior quality of life than treatments that spare but cripple the organ. Clearly, patient outcomes will vary both in terms of the cancer treatment response as well as the response to rehabilitation or restoration. Thus, anatomical preservation does not ensure functional preservation nor is the potential for recovery a guarantee for functional success. At the present time, the exact predictors of functional outcomes still remain unclear.

MULTIDISCIPLINARY TEAM

In all cases, speech and swallowing success ultimately depends on a strong, collegial collaboration between the speech pathologist and the other members of the multidisciplinary team (i.e., medical oncology, radiation oncology, head and neck surgery, plastic and reconstructive surgery, nutrition, social work, psychiatry and psychology, dental oncology, physical and occupational therapy) to ensure cancer cure, functional restoration, and optimal psychosocial adjustment. This point cannot be overemphasized. Pretreatment evaluation and planning for functional rehabilitation should begin immediately after diagnosis and involve the entire oncologic care and rehabilitative team. In particular, the need for speech and swallowing therapy is often unexpected for both the patient and family who frequently find it surprising as the ability to speak and swallow after treatment is commonly anticipated to spontaneously recover without the need for intervention. Both data and experience have shown that recovery and rehabilitation are optimized when there is ongoing dialogue and similar sharing of information provided to the patient by all members of the interdisciplinary team.[12]

Mental health professionals, who can at times be overlooked as essential members of the multidisciplinary team, play a vital role in helping patients with managing their expectations for treatment outcome and ameliorating the psychological and social impact of changes to speech and swallowing during treatment and into cancer survivorship. As demonstrated at the outset of this chapter, healthcare professionals with body image expertise can help patients develop practical strategies for coping with communication challenges, reduce preoccupation and distress related to functional impairment, and address social isolation and behavioral avoidance due to changes in speech and swallowing. However, in order for mental health professionals to adequately treat these patients, they must have a strong collegial relationship with the speech pathologist and other members of the treatment team as well as a basic understanding of processes involved in speech and swallowing, functional assessment techniques, and functional rehabilitation related to head and neck cancer.

PROCESSES INVOLVED IN NORMAL SPEECH AND SWALLOWING

The ability to speak and swallow depend on highly complex processes that incorporate a series of precisely coordinated biomechanical events and physiologic interactions of oral, pharyngeal, and laryngeal anatomy. Figures 11.1 and 11.2 show normal anatomy seen radiographically and through a flexible fiberoptic endoscope. Structural contacts and oropharyngeal cavity shapes are the key determinants of speech intelligibility, vocal resonance, and swallowing competency. Therefore, any surgical or nonsurgical insult to these structures or their movements, such as those that result from head and neck cancer, will affect these processes. In general, speech production is affected primarily by cancers that involve the oral tongue or other structures of the oral cavity and voice production by tumors that affect the larynx. Although swallowing can be affected by any cancer within the aerodigestive

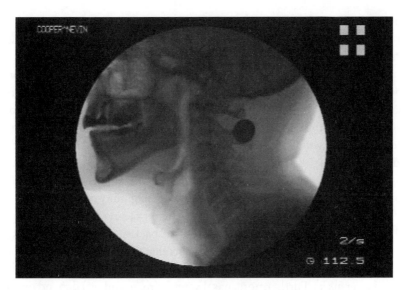

FIGURE 11.1: Normal aerodigestive tract visualized radiographically on modified barium swallow examination.

tract, in most instances, the greatest impact on swallowing occurs form tumors that affect the base of the tongue or pharynx.

Speech production and intelligibility depend on precise and timely contact by the articulators of the oral cavity, mainly the lips, tongue, and soft palate, that rapidly change the configuration of the vocal tract. Although articulation is the main contributor to speech intelligibility, speech understandability is also influenced by voice quality and resonance. Thus, tumors of the head and neck can alter the ability to produce sound as well as interfere with the quality of the voice, that is, the perceptual features that distinguish the way one person sounds from that of another. The voice changes as a function of tumor or posttreatment effect. For example, the voice may sound breathy and weak when one of the vocal folds is paralyzed

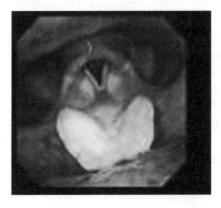

FIGURE 11.2: Normal laryngeal anatomy visualized transnasally through a flexible fiberoptic endoscope. (See Color Insert)

and cannot approximate the unimpaired side resulting in air loss and wastage. Alternatively, surgery or radiation therapy often disrupts the ability of the vocal folds to vibrate and therefore results in complaints of a hoarse or raspy sounding voice. Additionally, patients with maxillary and other palatal defects that impair normal velopharyngeal motion or oronasal seal experience changes in vocal resonance associated with excessive nasal airflow referred to as hypernasal speech. In contrast, hyponasality results from obstruction to the normal passage of airflow through the nasal cavity. Hyponasal speech production often sounds similar to the sound associated with an upper respiratory infection or "cold." Hence, any cancer that affects structures such as the larynx, specifically vocal fold function, or fills the recesses of the naso-, oro-, or laryngopharynx will result in changes in the quality of the voice (loudness, pitch, resonance) and therefore, indirectly, affect the intelligibility of speech.

Speech intelligibility primarily depends on articulatory contacts. Sound production may be bilabial (m, p, and b) or velar and articulated in the back of the mouth against the velum, (k and g). The valving of airflow through the larynx that involves the opening or closing of the vocal folds provides the voiced versus voiceless distinction between sounds (b versus p, d versus t, and g versus k). Furthermore, nasal sounds (m, n, and ng) depend on the valving action from the velum that lowers the soft palate to allow sound to resonate within the nasal cavity. And finally, in the case of vowel production, the shape and height of the tongue are the key determinants of vowel distinction. Therefore, any tumor that affects these structures and movements will also ultimately affect speech intelligibility.

STAGES AND MECHANICS OF SWALLOWING

The act of swallowing includes four phases: the oral preparatory, oral, pharyngeal, and esophageal phases or stages. The oropharyngeal swallow consists of the first three stages only and is primarily the focus of most speech pathologists. The oropharyngeal region and oropharyngeal phase of swallowing is most often affected by head and neck cancer. In general, the oropharyngeal swallow begins at the lips and ends as the food bolus enters the cervical esophageal inlet at the level of the cricopharyngeus muscle and involves both voluntary and involuntary control mechanisms. Normal swallowing, regardless of the type of food or liquid being swallowed, should take no longer than one to two seconds in normal individuals. Although oropharyngeal swallowing disorders directly affect the esophageal component of the swallow, diagnosis of abnormalities associated with the esophageal stage of swallowing remain the responsibility of the diagnostic radiologist or gastroenterologist. While interdisciplinary collaboration is important for accurate, comprehensive diagnosis and treatment of swallowing impairments, the speech pathologist mainly evaluates and treats oropharyngeal swallowing disorders that are responsive to functional interventions such as changes in posture and exercises that strengthen and increase the range of motion of muscles involved in the act of swallowing.

Key anatomy and physiologic requirements define each of the stages of swallowing. The tongue is the fundamental organ for normal speech and swallowing. Oral tongue control and strength are important to ensure efficient mastication and posterior propulsion of foods and liquids to the pharynx during the oral phase of the swallow but are also necessary contributors to the pharyngeal phase of swallowing. Any treatment that alters, particularly, the posterior aspect of the tongue will likely cause a delay in the timely triggering of the pharyngeal swallow and result in other problems associated with the efficient propulsion and transit through the oropharynx. Because the extent and location of tongue resections are critically related to swallowing outcomes, surgeries that suture the tongue to the floor of the mouth or buccal mucosa are rarely performed because of the severe limitation to the mobility and range of motion of the remaining tongue that results in severe speech and swallowing deficits.

FUNCTIONAL ASSESSMENT

Standardized functional assessments remain a critical component of comprehensive patient care and outcomes research. The importance of pretreatment functional assessment of speech, voice, and swallowing in patients with head and neck cancer cannot be overemphasized.[12,13] Pretreatment evaluation allows collection of baseline data that is critical because it documents pretreatment function, helps establish a proactive plan of intervention, and establishes a foundation for later posttreatment comparison. Clinical experience and published reports show that the results of these studies are often strong predictors of treatment outcomes and help identify patients who are better suited for surgery versus organ-preserving procedures. For example, aspiration, vocal fold paresis, feeding tube dependence, and tracheostomy prior to treatment have been reported as adverse prognostic indicators of posttreatment functional recovery.[14] In addition, when appropriately analyzed and interpreted, the results of these procedures not only establish the etiology of dysfunction but also are key determinants of the specific intervention or combined interventions, behavioral strategies, exercises, or surgery that will best treat the problem, thereby avoiding the use of rehabilitative techniques, surgical or otherwise, that are not indicated or suitable for remediating the dysfunction. Finally, the results of pretreatment evaluation (which must be shared with the patient and all members of the multidisciplinary team) offer realistic posttreatment functional expectations that frequently facilitate patient understanding, acceptance, and compliance with both cancer and rehabilitative treatment recommendations. Baseline examination allows clinicians to assess outcomes and draw conclusions that cannot be determined without appropriate pretreatment functional examination. These reasons, among others, establish the foundation for baseline functional evaluation as best practice for all patients with or treated for head and neck cancer.

A complete functional examination includes clinician-driven examinations that rely on clinical appraisal along with those that include instrumental and imaging studies and clinician-rated scales. In addition, a comprehensive functional examination must also recognize patient perception and therefore include patient-reported outcomes such as quality of life questionnaires and symptom performance inventories. The most common studies for pretreatment assessment of baseline function are summarized next.

METHODS OF EVALUATION (FUNCTIONAL ASSESSMENT)

CLINICAL/BEDSIDE

The clinical or bedside examination is useful because it is based on observation of swallowing in a more natural, relaxed environment similar to actual patient routine. However, it is important to remember that clinical observation lacks the sensitivity of instrumental examination and should never be used in place of more objective examinations. The bedside swallowing examination often precedes the instrumental examination, such as the modified barium swallow (MBS) and flexible endoscopic evaluation of swallowing (FEES) study. It allows a basic screening to identify patients who have functional competency and who do not require instrumental examination. The bedside examination also helps determine the timing or readiness to begin oral intake. Not all patients require instrumental examination as these tests can be expensive and impractical. More important, they are generally associated with a resource burden that may be avoided when clinical examinations show no further need for examination. Figure 11.3 illustrates a basic clinical/beside evaluation.

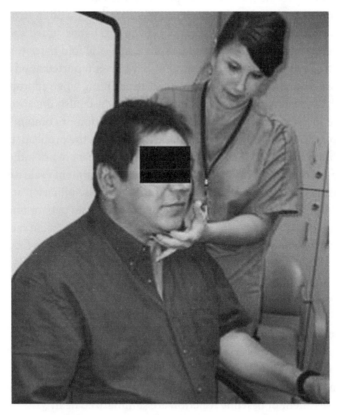

FIGURE 11.3: A clinician performing a clinical/beside evaluation.

Although clinical examinations provide important information that is critical to the patient's functional status, the bedside observation of swallowing function cannot reliably determine or rule out silent aspiration nor can it diagnose pharyngeal swallowing disorders. Diagnoses of swallowing disorders should never be made based on inference from clinical examination. In these cases, an instrumental examination (MBS or FEES) should be performed to reliably evaluate oropharyngeal physiology. The goal of the clinical bedside examination is to integrate overt and subtle observations to make recommendations regarding the need for further, more objective swallowing assessment.

PATIENT-REPORTED OUTCOMES

A variety of assessments are available to examine both speech and swallowing that include both quality-of-life and symptom scales. Measures of patient report rely on patient perception of functional abilities. Data, however, have shown that patients' report of their functional competency is frequently unreliable and more often does not accurately reflect physiologic performance and actual abilities.[15] Patients, particularly in long-term survivorship, frequently report normal swallowing despite abnormal findings of silent aspiration shown on MBS studies.[16,17] Conversely, patients also report abnormal swallowing function associated with radiation-induced xerostomia or acute treatment toxicities such as pain despite functional MBS findings.

A variety of assessments are available to measure voice perception that provide patient-rated assessment of and handicap related to such vocal characteristics as breathiness, strain, and asthenia.[18–20] Unfortunately, although there are multiple tools for assessing voice and swallowing function, there are relatively few assessments specifically designed for evaluation of speech intelligibility.[21]

The importance of patient experience and opinion are critical components of functional recovery and performance and should not be disregarded. However, only instrumental examination, such as the MBS study or FEES in the case of swallowing, or laryngeal videostroboscopy in cases of vocal dysfunction, can provide information regarding physiology and disorder that ultimately identifies the etiology of dysfunction. Because anecdotal experience and research findings clearly recognize the discrepancy between patients' perceptions of their handicap versus instrumental findings of dysfunction, comprehensive examination should always include both measures to ensure accurate interpretation of functional status.

MODIFIED BARIUM SWALLOW

Perhaps the most widely used and likely still the gold standard of instrumental swallowing evaluations is the MBS study, also referred to as the videofluoroscopic assessment of swallowing. MBS radiographically evaluates all phases of oropharyngeal swallowing from the time the food enters the mouth until it passes into the cervical esophagus. The MBS is performed jointly by a speech pathologist and a radiologist. Swallowing is evaluated as

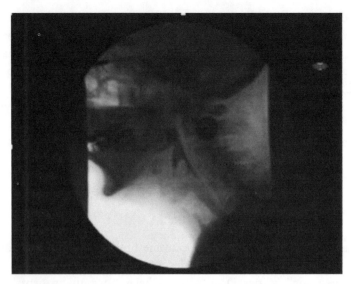

FIGURE 11.4: Swallowing seen radiographically on a modified barium swallow study.

the patient ingests radio-opaque liquids, pastes, and solid foods, because swallowing physiology varies according to the consistency and amount of food presented. This anatomic and physiologic evaluation of swallowing is in contrast to the traditional barium esophagram, or barium swallow, in which the primary purpose is to evaluate the structural integrity of the esophagus and to identify the presence of aspiration.

Furthermore, the MBS study provides critical information that allows for the differential diagnosis of the swallowing disorder and helps to identify the causes of the aspiration. On the basis of the physiologic findings, appropriate compensatory strategies can be selected to remediate the swallowing problem and their effectiveness evaluated in real time while the patient is undergoing the study. Swallowing is illustrated during a MBS study shown in Figure 11.4.

FLEXIBLE ENDOSCOPIC EVALUATION OF SWALLOWING

FEES provides an excellent alternative to the MBS study because it can be easily performed as a clinical procedure or at bedside for patients who cannot tolerate or are not candidates for videofluoroscopic assessment of oropharyngeal swallowing. FEES uses a flexible endoscope placed transnasally to examine the pharyngeal swallow while providing direct visualization of laryngeal anatomy. FEES has been shown equally effective to the MBS study in detecting aspiration and does not expose the patient to radiation.[22]

FEES may be preferred for patients who have malignancies of the larynx as it provides the best view of glottic competency, including airway protection and vocal fold mobility. An additional advantage of FEES is that it can be paired with sensory testing to better

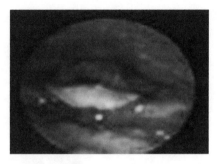

FIGURE 11.5: FEES shows stasis of the food bolus in the vallecular recesses. (See Color Insert)

determine the etiology of the dysphagia as it relates to laryngeal sensitivity, unlike the MBS in which this is difficult to do and must be assumed based on the occurrence of silent aspiration.[23] Moreover, FEES can provide the patient with immediate biofeedback and visualization that are often beneficial during therapy sessions.

Unfortunately, the disadvantage of FEES is its inability to visualize the oral preparatory and the oral phases of swallowing during examination. Thus, all oral phase disorders and some pharyngeal disorders of swallowing must be inferred, limiting the usefulness of FEES in patients with tumors of the oral cavity and oropharynx. Similar to the MBS study, FEES provides excellent feedback regarding the effectiveness of swallowing compensations and strategies. Figure 11.5 illustrates swallowing during FEES.

LARYNGEAL VIDEOSTROBOSCOPY

Laryngeal videostroboscopic evaluation of vocal functioning is routinely performed in a clinic setting using either a rigid or flexible fiberoptic endoscope. Videostroboscopy allows direct observation of the apparent motion of the vocal folds and provides valuable information regarding vocal fold vibration as well as an immediate and magnified image of the presence or absence of pathology that often is not detectable using standard methods of indirect laryngoscopy. Videostroboscopy assesses patterns of vocal fold motion and vibration, including true vocal fold approximation, the symmetry and regularity of motion, and the presence of mucosal wave as an indicator of vibratory integrity. Videostroboscopy, therefore, is a useful tool because it provides a permanent record for documentation and comparison of laryngeal functioning. Videostroboscopy is an essential component of the physical examination of head and neck cancer patients with hypopharyngeal or laryngeal disease and should be performed as a baseline evaluation and for routine surveillance of laryngeal functioning after cancer treatment. Figures 11.6 and 11.7 show videostroboscopic examination of vocal function and a typical glottic image seen via oral endoscopy using a rigid endoscope.

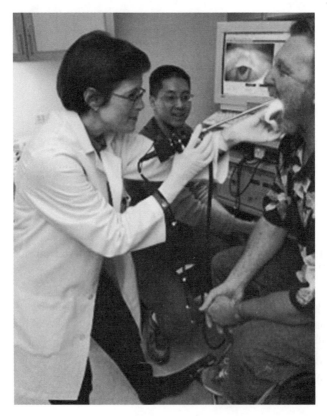

FIGURE 11.6: Examination of vocal functioning performed using a rigid endoscope placed transorally.

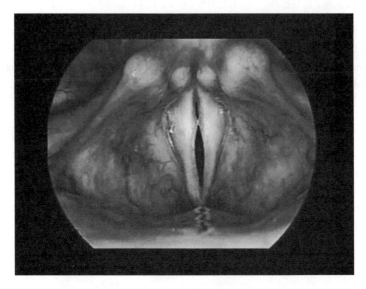

FIGURE 11.7: Resulting glottic image from Figure 11.6. (See Color Insert)

FUNCTIONAL OUTCOMES
AFTER SURGERY

In general, functional outcomes after head and neck surgery vary widely and are primarily related to the surgeon's experience and technique but are also impacted by patient characteristics that include patient preference, family/caregiver support, access to rehabilitation, and financial considerations. In most cases, the primary impact to postsurgical speech and swallowing outcomes occurs based on (a) the site of the disease, (b) the surgical approach, (c) the type of closure, and (d) management of neck disease.

Clearly, the location of the disease and its relationship to speech and swallowing will be important to postoperative function. The size of the tumor and the amount of extension to other adjacent structures are also critical predictors of the ability to speak and swallow after surgery. In contemporary practice, the use of open partial procedures, such as supraglottic laryngectomy and hemi-laryngectomy, are rare because of the increased morbidity and complications, increased length of hospital stay, and increased damage to structures adjacent to the primary tumor associated with these procedures when compared with contemporary transoral methods. The advantages of muscle physiology preservation, better medical recovery, less hospitalization, and faster functional return have resulted in a transition away from ablative surgeries with open surgical procedures in favor of organ preservation that depend on minimally invasive transoral resections to treat many cancers of the head and neck.

It is not surprising that in most cases bigger resections portend worse swallowing function. Experience has shown that patients swallow better after primary surgical closures of smaller resections than they do when large flap reconstructions are required. Furthermore, additional risk of postoperative morbidity occurs when adjuvant neck dissections are performed. Resection of neck disease may result in neck fibrosis, lymphedema, and reduced range of motion, among other complications that reduce postsurgical speech and swallowing function and ultimately quality of life.

Reconstruction of oropharyngeal defects continues to evolve and remains a critical predictor of speech and swallowing outcomes. Reconstructive procedures must use sufficient tissue to fill the defect but prevent pooling of secretions, preserve remaining lingual mobility, and restore as much as possible the shape and volume of the remaining lingual and pharyngeal structure to maintain residual function and avoid tissue bulk. Early studies showed that partial tongue resections which remove 50% or less of the mobile tongue that are then closed primarily have the best functional outcomes.[24] However, preservation of swallowing function after major tongue resections can also be achieved and have been documented.[25–27] In fact, the assumption that total resection of the tongue (total glossectomy) will relegate the patient gastrostomy tube dependent because of the inability to swallow orally have summarily been shown false.[28]

Data and experience have taught us that the degree of swallowing impairment depends also on the quality of the reconstruction in addition to the extent of tongue resection. Unfortunately, at the present time, there is no surgical reconstructive alternative that can reliably restore the intricate interplay between swallowing sensation and physiologic function. Despite current data that demonstrates the ability of innervated cutaneous flap reconstructions to recover lingual sensation, the ability of these procedures to restore function remains controversial.[29] Hence, for the present, it would appear that biologic success does not always ensure functional success.

Mandibular continuity is important after surgery particularly during mastication to maintain balance and symmetry during the oral preparation of the food bolus and in concert with the lips, teeth, and buccal cavity to help prevent anterior loss of food from the mouth. Even though the mandible supports periodontal structures and is the foundation for the tongue and muscles of the floor of mouth, swallowing deficits in the absence of marked deformities after mandibular resection are generally relatively minor. Mandibular preservation has not been shown predictive of improved swallowing outcomes in surgically treated patients with head and neck cancer.[30] Together, the extent of mandibular resection along with the involvement of the floor of mouth and tongue will generally determine the degree of swallowing impairment. As long as the tongue is mobile and mandibular contour is preserved, most patients will be able to form a food bolus and propel it through the oral cavity during the oral stage of the swallow.

In some instances, oral prostheses including palatal augmentation devices and obturators are extremely beneficial to speech and swallowing in patients who have undergone palatal resection. These devices help restore the articulatory contacts, prevent nasal air escape, and avoid nasal regurgitation of food through the nasopharyngeal port after maxillectomy compromises the oronasal seal or when soft palate resection results in velopharyngeal insufficiency. Generally, obturation is difficult in patients who have undergone partial velar resection and are left with a mobile soft palate remnant. In these cases, complete velar resection may provide better functional rehabilitation because of the ability to adequately obturate the entire defect and avoid the problems associated with a poorly fitting obturator that cannot maintain a consistent seal because of the continuous movement from the remaining leftover palate.[31] Figure 11.8 illustrates common palatal augmentation devices and obturators.

Probably one of the most important contributors to the ability to safely swallow without aspiration is that furnished by the suprahyoid musculature because of the attachments they provide from the floor of the mouth to the mandible, and hyoid bone, and then indirectly

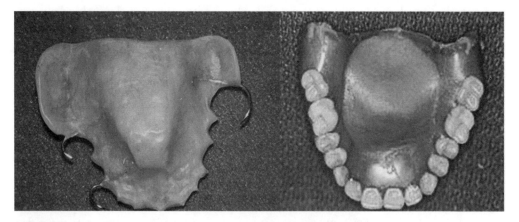

FIGURE 11.8: Palatal augmentation devices commonly used to obturate palatal defects.

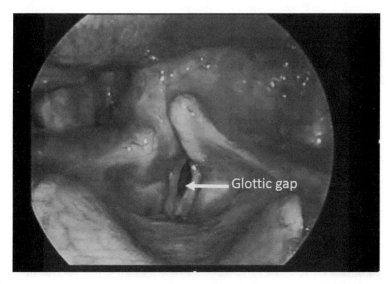

FIGURE 11.9: Left true vocal fold paralysis and a glottic gap during phonation. (See Color Insert)

to the larynx. When the suprahyoid musculature is impaired, either surgically or because of the effects of irradiation, the risk for aspiration increases because of the disruption to the vertical elevation and anterior movement of the larynx that directs the food and liquid away from the entrance to the larynx thereby protecting the airway from aspiration during swallowing. In addition to airway protection, these movements are essential to open the upper esophageal sphincter (cricopharyngeus) so that spillage into the airway is avoided and food is directed into the esophagus. Although unrestricted hyolaryngeal excursion plays a significant role in airway protection, the ability of the true vocal folds to completely approximate is also important to prevent aspiration of food and liquid from entering the airway. Despite the importance of true vocal fold closure, glottic closure is not essential to airway protection and functional swallowing. For example, patients with unilateral true vocal fold paralysis often compensate for glottic incompetency by using other mechanisms of airway closure to safely swallow without aspiration. Thus, airway protection is not solely dependent on the ability of the true vocal folds to close. Safe swallowing despite left true vocal fold paralysis and glottic incompetency is shown in Figures 11.9, 11.10 and 11.11.

Alternatively, vocal fold closure is the key determinant of voice production and vocal quality. Disease that impedes or alters vocal fold closure and vibration will result in dysphonia. The glottic site of the cancer and the depth of tissue invasion are key determinates in treatment selection. Cancers that deeply invade the vocal cord or ones that involve the anterior commissure are often better treated with nonsurgical alternatives that avoid large defects and impede vocal fold approximation that result in glottic incompetency, poor vocal quality, and risk of aspiration. Unfortunately, there are few alternatives to augment or correct large, fibrotic defects of the glottis that result in poor quality of life for patients who are cured of their disease and for whom the prognosis for long-term survival is good. In these cases, nonsurgical alternatives frequently offer better long-term functional outcomes.

Surgical treatment for advanced cancers of the larynx in particular is generally associated with problems of both voice and swallowing. Contemporary treatment for advanced

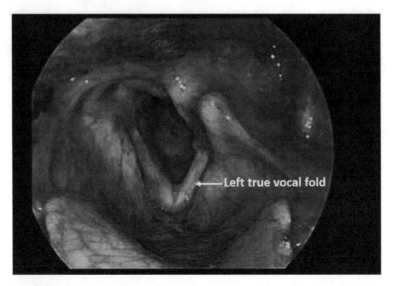

FIGURE 11.10: Shows the lateral positioning and foreshortening associated with left true vocal fold paralysis. (See Color Insert)

cancer of the larynx includes larynx-preserving resection that is often accompanied by adjuvant regimens of radiation therapy alone or in combination with chemotherapy. Although ablatives surgeries such as total laryngectomy and pharyngolaryngectomy are less frequently performed because of the widespread popularity of nonsurgical organ preservation, they remain viable alternatives for the treatment of advanced cancer of the larynx that is not treatable with conservation alternatives and as salvage procedures for patients with persistent or recurrent laryngeal cancer when larynx preservation strategies fail. Both data

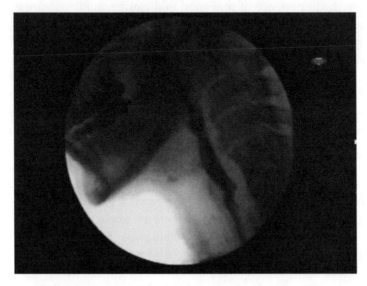

FIGURE 11.11: Illustrates safe swallowing without aspiration despite the vocal fold paralysis as seen on the modified barium swallow examination. Note that there is no aspiration into the trachea.

and experience have shown that, in some cases, speech and swallowing function after total organ resection remain far superior to those surgeries that spare but cripple the organ.

FUNCTIONAL OUTCOMES AFTER RADIATION THERAPY

Regardless of the clinical intent of radiation therapy as a definitive treatment modality, whether given in combination with chemotherapy for organ preservation, as an adjuvant treatment following surgery, or for palliation of patients with incurable disease, it produces tissue changes that affect speech and swallowing function immediately after treatment and frequently continue to impact function long after treatment has finished, well into the survivorship years.

In general, radiation therapy has a greater impact on swallowing than it does on speech production. Acute effects of radiation therapy also frequently result in painful symptoms that exacerbate swallowing problems and limit the patient's ability to maintain oral intake through the duration of treatment. The addition of chemotherapy is believed to exacerbate these effects. Both experience and data have shown that the cumulative adverse impact of radiation therapy on function can rival or exceed the sequelae from surgery.

Radiation-associated dysphagia (RAD) may develop during radiation as an acute toxicity of treatment but is generally associated with the occurrence of oropharyngeal fibrosis, neuropathy, and sensory alteration resulting from chronic tissue changes. Most patients who develop acute RAD will experience at least partial recovery of swallowing function as edema and mucositis resolve, but it is not uncommon for dysphagia to persist or occur months or years after the completion radiation or chemoradiation therapy. In most cases swallowing function is acceptable but swallowing is never normal. That is, patients who have been irradiated for head and neck cancer usually experience the ability to eat by mouth again that is best characterized as a "new normal" while a smaller minority, approximately 13%, suffer clinically significant levels of chronic dysphagia as a consequential late effect of the acute toxicities of aggressive cancer therapy.[32] The degree of swallowing recovery has been shown to be associated with the level of tumor burden and baseline function, treatment intensity (radiation particle, dose-volume distribution, systemic therapy), and supportive care. Despite a better understanding of the relationship between radiation therapy and the swallowing effects of treatment, the long-term outcomes remain unclear, and investigations of the ability of dose-limiting treatments to reduce normal tissue damage and preserve function, such as intensity modulated radiation therapy versus intensity modulated proton therapy versus adapted radiation protocols, continue.[33,34]

Although our current ability to identify those patients who are likely in danger of developing long-term dysphagia after radiation therapy continues to be investigated, several risk factors have been reported. The site of the primary tumor and the T-stage will impact the type and severity of dysphagia after radiation treatment. Of all patients with cancers of the head and neck, patients with hypopharyngeal tumors are at risk for the greatest degree of swallowing impairment.[35] Furthermore, patients who have difficulty swallowing before treatment are also at higher risk for chronic dysphagia and permanent feeding tube dependency.[36] Among patients with primary tumors of the oropharynx, data estimates that 7% to 31% will develop chronic aspiration,[35,37] 11% will develop aspiration pneumonia,[30] and 4% will remain chronically feeding tube dependent in survivorship after chemoradiation.[36] Among patients with cancers of the larynx or hypopharynx, it is estimated that 22% to 30% will develop chronic aspiration and/or pneumonia,[38,39] and 5% will be chronically feeding tube dependent.[40] Likewise, prolonged intervals of nothing per oral (NPO) for longer than two weeks during radiation therapy (RT) or chemoradiation therapy (CRT) are associated with poorer swallowing outcomes.[41] Therefore, it is important that patients continue to swallow, even if it is their own saliva, throughout the course of RT or CRT as much as possible, and even brief intervals of NPO should be avoided.[42]

Normal tissue effects that produce RAD appear to occur both in the acute posttreatment phase and throughout the course of survivorship. These effects also seem to be cumulative. In the early months after RT or CRT, the dysphagia-aspiration-related structures (e.g., the pharyngeal muscles and larynx) in the radiation field become edematous and then stiffen over time as fibrosis sets in as a chronic sequela of treatment. It is thought that acute and persistent RAD in the first one to two years reflects varying degrees of muscle edema, fibrosis, and disuse atrophy.[42] More recently, neuropathic injury has been recognized as a significant contributor to the late onset of radiation-associated dysphagia. Tongue base retraction, hyoid movement, laryngeal lift, and pharyngeal contraction have been shown abnormal in 50% to 75% of patients who have been previously irradiated.[36,43] The resulting effect to normal swallowing is impaired supraglottic closure and abnormal pharyngeal contraction in patients who experience RAD. Figures 11.12 and 11.13 show severe fibrosis years after the completion of radiation therapy.

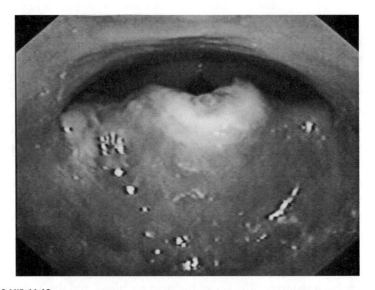

FIGURES 11.12 AND 11.13: Severe fibrosis that distorts normal anatomy years after the completion of radiation therapy. Note the anatomical abnormalities seen in both figures. Distorted and enlarged epiglottis and valleculae that trap debris in Figure 11.12. Thickened, fibrotic epiglottis that is continuous with pharyngeal mucosa is seen on Figure 11.13. (See Color Insert)

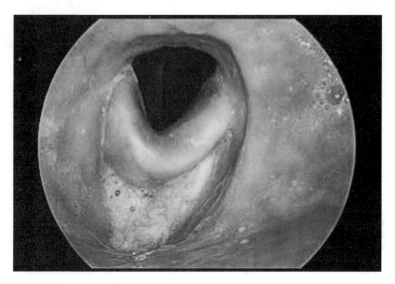

FIGURES 11.12 AND 11.13: Continued

COMMON COMPLICATIONS OF TREATMENT

Xerostomia (dry mouth) and mucositis (inflammation and ulceration of the body's mucous membrane) are common complications resulting from radiation-induced damage to the salivary glands and mucosal tissue of the upper aerodigestive tract. Xerostomia is one of the most disconcerting complaints by patients who have been treated with radiation as there is no good, effective, long-lasting management to relieve dry mouth. Acute mucositis is also associated with long-term dysphagia and has also been reported to be a significant dose-limiting toxicity of chemotherapy and radiation treatment regimens. Patients experience thick, tenacious secretions that are difficult to swallow or expectorate and often result in gagging, regurgitation, and, in some cases, aspiration.[44] The unfortunate consequences to swallowing are reduced lingual speed, slow oral transit of food, aberrant tongue movements, and slowed swallow initiation.[45] Other complication, including trismus ("lock jaw"), dys- or ageusia (changes in or loss of taste), and dysosmia (changes in smell), are additional complications that disrupt speech and swallowing often beginning acutely and worsening throughout treatment.

An often underrecognized but markedly debilitating complication of head and neck cancer treatment that is unequivocally associated with poor body image, symptom burden, functional deterioration, and poor quality of life is head and neck lymphedema (HNL; see also Chapter 10). Unfortunately, despite the positive outcomes that can be achieved with proper therapy, HNL continues to be undertreated and poorly managed. HNL has been estimated to occur in up to 75% of treated head and neck patients. HNL is characterized by tissue swelling resulting from the blockage of normal drainage pathways in the lymphatic system. Surgery that removes lymph nodes along with the tumor itself are key causes of HNL, but the strongest impact is generally associated with radiation effects that impair

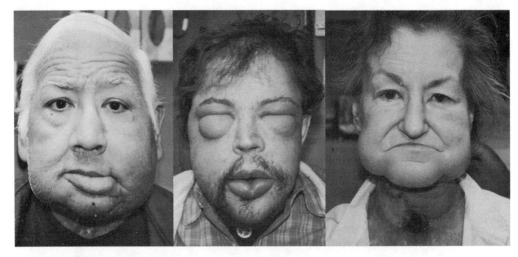

FIGURE 11.14: Typical presentations of head and neck lymphedema in patients treated for head and neck cancer. (See Color Insert)

vessel contractility, or "lymphangiomotoricity," that mainly cause vessel obstruction. If left untreated, HNL along with permanent fibrosis can result in persistent cosmetic, functional, and psychosocial changes that remain uncomfortable and irreversible, the consequences of which impede speech, respiration, voice, and swallowing.[46,47] Figure 11.14 represents typical presentations of patients with HNL after treatment of their head and neck cancer.

A recent analysis of the data from more than 1,200 head and neck cancer survivors with HNL showed that 68% of patients with functional complaints reported swallowing problems. Swallowing dysfunction is plainly apparent in the radiographic views shown in Figure 11.15. More important, the same investigators showed that 60% of patients experience a dramatic reduction in HNL regardless of complete or partial adherence to therapy that can be self-administered by the patient through a home program of exercise. Additionally, significant restrictions in posture and gait can also occur because of severe myofascial fibrosis. Figures 11.16 and 11.17 illustrate the debilitating effect and dramatic improvement after therapy in affected patients.

FUNCTIONAL REHABILITATION

Impairment in voice production associated primarily with the treatment for cancer of the larynx, including both surgical and nonsurgical management, can range from breathy, hoarse, weak vocal production to complete aphonia. Depending on the etiology, speech therapy alone or in combination with surgery designed to improve and optimize voice production may be beneficial, particularly in cases of unilateral vocal fold paralysis. Speech and swallowing assessment along with laryngeal videostroboscopy are critical elements that guide the proper selection of surgical versus nonsurgical treatment. In appropriately selected cases, injection medialization laryngoplasty (thyroplasty) offers temporary correction for

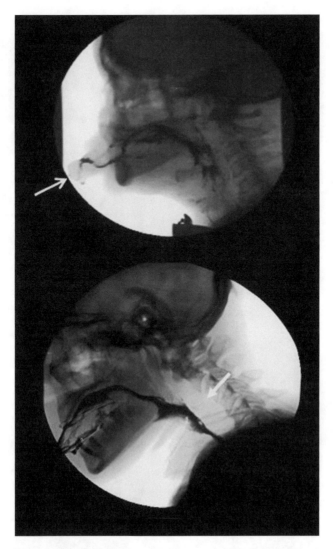

FIGURE 11.15: Note the significant problems resulting from lymphedema in the lips that results in loss of food and drooling from the mouth and the restriction of food through the pharynx because of prevertebral lymphedema that narrows the pharyngeal lumen.

relief of acute aspiration along with restoration of phonatory production related to glottic incompetence. Alternatively, for patients with long-standing vocal fold paralysis and glottic insufficiency, permanent medialization thyroplasty offers the opportunity for return of near-normal vocal function and improved glottic airway protection.[48,49]

Probably the most significant voice disorder requiring specialized expertise is the rehabilitation of voice after total laryngectomy. Although a thorough discussion of alaryngeal rehabilitation goes beyond the scope of this chapter, the major focus of functional rehabilitation after total laryngectomy comprises three primary approaches used to restore oral communication after total resection of the larynx: (a) use of the artificial larynx, more commonly referred to as the electrolarynx; (b) traditional methods of esophageal speech

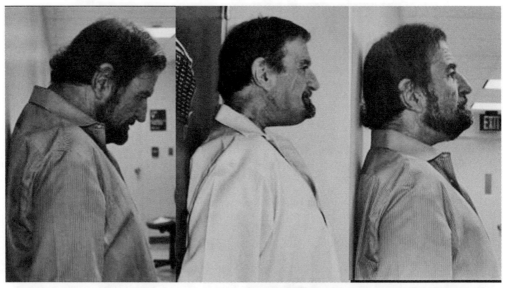
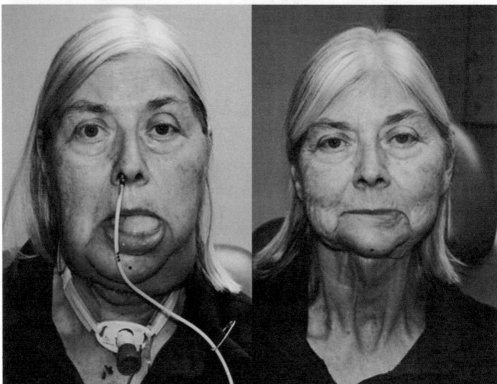

FIGURES 11.16 AND 11.17: Dramatic changes are seen in patients treated for severe head and neck lymphedema and myofascial dysfunction. (See Color Insert)

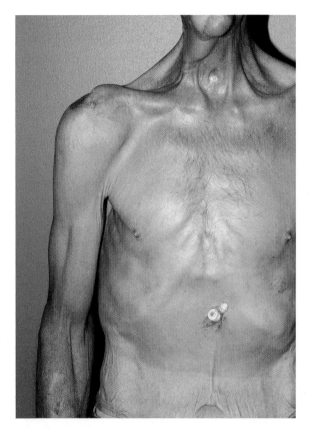

FIGURE 7.1. Patient with cachexia, required a G-tube to facilitate nutrition.

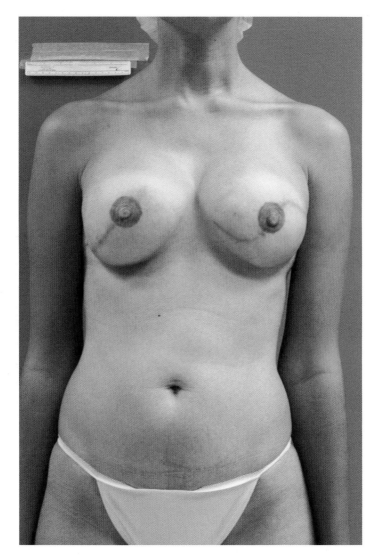

FIGURE 7.2. Patient with bilateral total mastectomy and implant-based breast reconstruction.

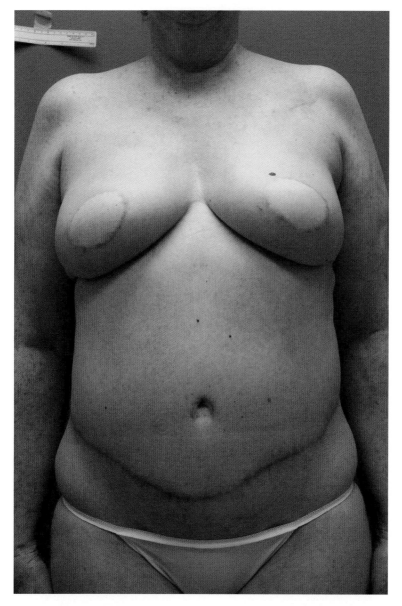

FIGURE 7.3. Patient with bilateral skin sparing mastectomy with autologous flap breast reconstruction using transverse rectus abdominis myocutaneous (TRAM) flap.

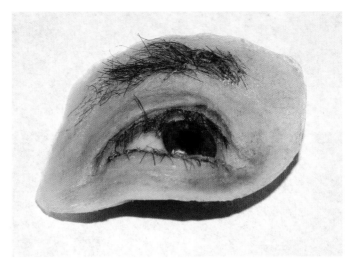

FIGURE 7.4. Example of eye prosthesis created for a patient.

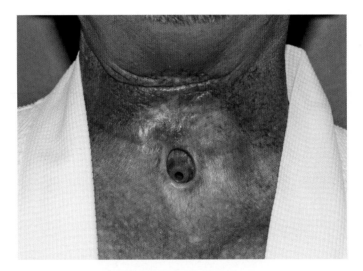

FIGURE 7.5. Patient with stoma after radiation and laryngectomy.

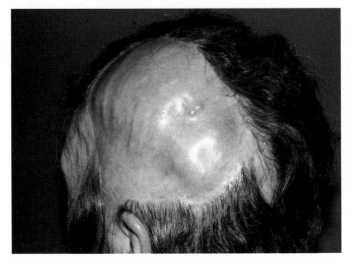

FIGURE 7.6. Patient with alopecia after scalp cancer and free flap.

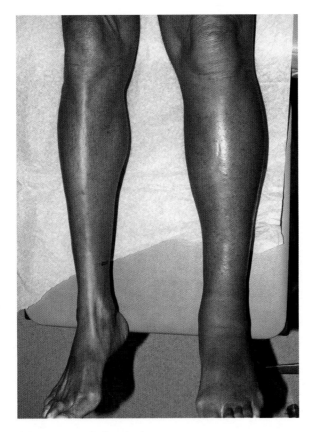

FIGURE 7.7. Patient with lower extremity lymphedema.

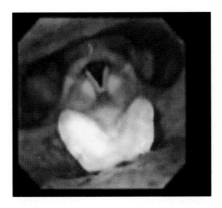

FIGURE 11.2. Normal laryngeal anatomy visualized transnasally through a flexible fiberoptic endoscope.

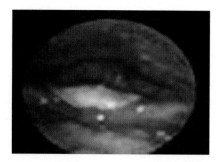

FIGURE 11.5. FEES shows stasis of the food bolus in the vallecular recesses.

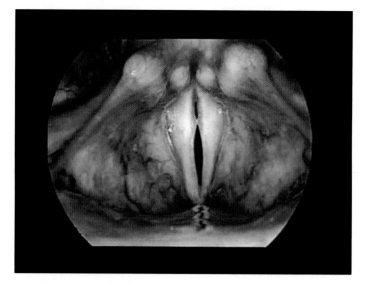

FIGURE 11.7. Resulting glottic image from Figure 11.6.

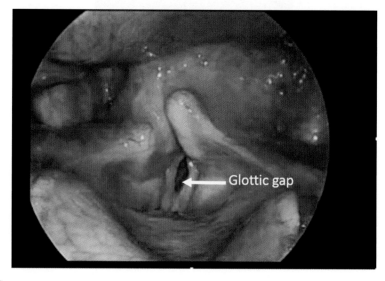

FIGURE 11.9. Left true vocal fold paralysis and a glottic gap during phonation.

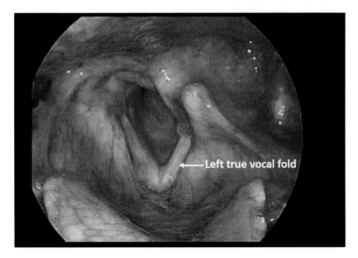

FIGURE 11.10. Shows the lateral positioning and foreshortening associated with left true vocal fold paralysis.

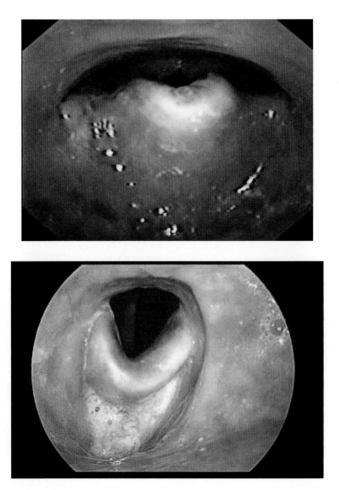

FIGURES 11.12 AND 11.13. Severe fibrosis that distorts normal anatomy years after the completion of radiation therapy. Note the anatomical abnormalities seen in both figures. Distorted and enlarged epiglottis and valleculae that trap debris in Figure 11.12. Thickened, fibrotic epiglottis that is continuous with pharyngeal mucosa is seen on Figure 11.13.

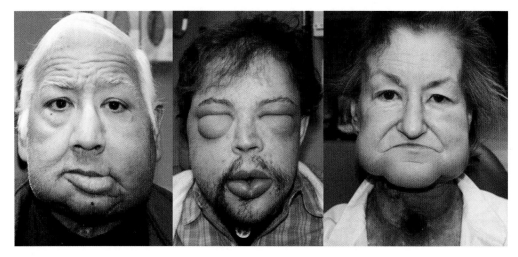

FIGURE 11.14. Typical presentations of head and neck lymphedema in patients treated for head and neck cancer.

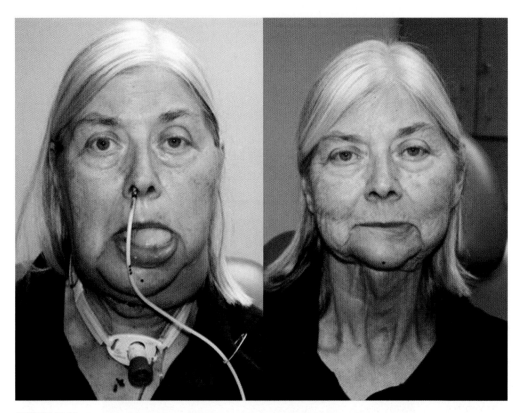

FIGURES 11.17. Dramatic changes are seen in patients treated for severe head and neck lymphedema and myofascial dysfunction.

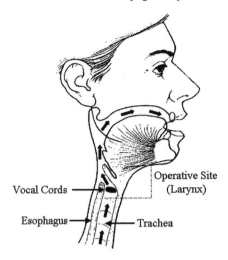

Before Laryngectomy

Vocal Cords

Operative Site
(Larynx)

Esophagus

Trachea

FIGURE 11.18: Normal aerodigestive anatomy before total laryngectomy. Voice is produced by the vocal cords.

production; and (c) tracheoesophageal voice restoration. The selection of the optimal alternative depends on appropriate patient selection, patient motivation, and clinician expertise with the selected alaryngeal speech alternative. Although not every patient is a candidate for all methods of alaryngeal speech production, the decision should be patient driven. Unilateral decisions of choice made by the physician, family, or speech pathologist should be discouraged as they are never the best course of action for the patient. It is important to remember that patients who have undergone total laryngectomy suffer from a loss of sound production as a result of the loss of vocal fold vibration. Unless the structures of the oral cavity are impaired, speech production is usually quite intelligible once sound production has been restored, regardless of the method of alaryngeal speech alternative. Hence, total laryngectomy results in loss of sound, not speech. The goal of rehabilitation is, therefore, to restore the patient's speech as closely as possible to that of his or her premorbid state, keeping in mind that no person undergoing total laryngectomy should be without some method of functional speech production. Figure 11.18 illustrates a schematic of the vocal cords before total laryngectomy. The three methods of alaryngeal speech production are illustrated in Figures 11.19, 11.20, and 11.21.

SWALLOWING REHABILITATION
AFTER RADIATION THERAPY

Preventive swallowing therapy is considered the best practice for patients treated with curative RT or CRT for head and neck cancer. Because of the acute toxicities associated with treatment including mucositis, salivary dysfunction, and dysgeusia, eating often becomes

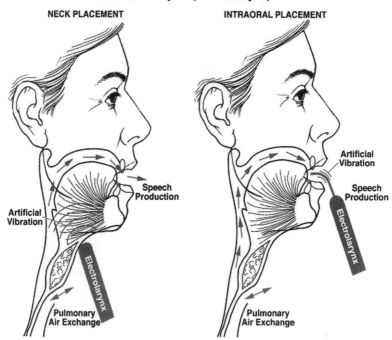

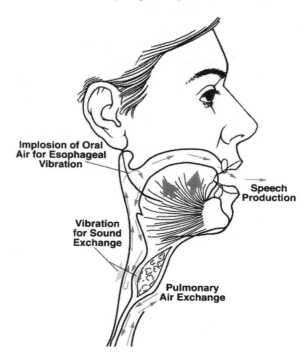

FIGURES 11.19, 11.20, 11.21: Alaryngeal speech production after total laryngectomy using three different speech methods.

Tracheoesophageal (TE) Speech

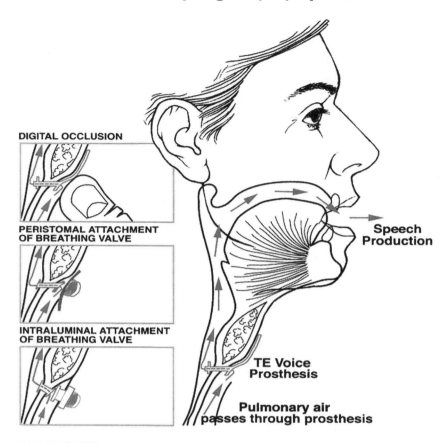

DIGITAL OCCLUSION

PERISTOMAL ATTACHMENT OF BREATHING VALVE

INTRALUMINAL ATTACHMENT OF BREATHING VALVE

Speech Production

TE Voice Prosthesis

Pulmonary air passes through prosthesis

FIGURES 11.19, 11.20, 11.21: Continued

unpleasant and thus is avoided. For this reason, at least half of patients require a feeding tube to maintain nutrition through treatment, and the majority stop eating solid foods because of the effort and pain that usually accompanies swallowing.[50–52] The loss of the normal resistive load on the pharyngeal musculature that occurs when patients stop eating solid foods is the central premise of proactive swallowing therapy—the "use it or lose it" model. It is this model of early, aggressive swallowing therapy that is critical to mitigate the muscular wasting and remodeling that occurs after even brief intervals of disuse. Preventive or proactive swallowing therapy thus avoids periods of NPO and endorses adherence to swallowing exercise. The benefits of swallowing behaviors (eat and exercise) have been reported by numerous investigators in randomized trials and observational studies. The benefit of preventive swallowing therapy include reduced loss of functional swallow ability,[53] superior swallowing-related quality of life,[54] better tongue base and epiglottic movement,[55] larger post chemoradiation muscle mass of the genioglossus, mylohyoid, and hyoglossus muscles based on magnetic resonance imaging,[56] shorter duration of gastrostomy,[50,51] and greater return to normal diet.[57]

Multidisciplinary management of other acute chemoradiation toxicities besides dysphagia, including pain, mucositis, odynophagia, dysgeusia, and weight loss, among others, is critical to facilitate safe oral intake throughout treatment. Prophylactic neuropathic pain management has also been associated with lower pain scores, decreased percutaneous endoscopic gastrostomy (PEG) utilization, and decreased aspiration after chemoradiation. The authors suggested that optimization of pain management allowed patients to keep eating and adhere to exercises that ultimately resulted in a physiologic advantage in preservation of swallowing function.[58]

Chronic RAD is a challenging clinical problem and one that is difficult to treat. Intensive swallowing therapy attempts to optimize functional abilities and patient perception of their swallowing dysfunction despite the unlikely reversal of chronic and late RAD. Most patients with persistent posttreatment dysphagia can learn with therapy to better compensate for the problem. These techniques help patients minimize or clear aspiration, improve swallowing efficiency, and optimize diet. One of the most important goals of swallowing therapy is to maximize quality of life while simultaneously minimizing the risk of life-threatening aspiration pneumonia. There is no single best approach to dysphagia therapy for chronic posttreatment swallowing dysfunction. Dysphagia therapy should be individualized and incorporate targeted treatment based on the results of instrumental testing (e.g., MBS study or FEES). In the absence of sufficient comparative data, best practice dictates that swallowing therapy begin with a comprehensive examination that incorporates both patient-reported outcomes and the results of instrumental testing along with adherence to established exercise principles based on swallowing physiology.

PSYCHOSOCIAL EVALUATION AND TREATMENT

While this chapter has primarily involved delineating principles and practices for functional assessment and rehabilitation of speech and swallowing impairment for patients with head and neck cancer, the comprehensive management of these patients includes attention to psychosocial issues that inevitably arise with body image changes that affect function. Research conducted with patients surgically treated for head and neck cancer indicated that patients with speech and eating concerns experience body image difficulties at least equivalent to or even more so than that of head and neck cancer patients with concerns tied to physical appearance.[59] In this study, patients with eating and speech concerns were significantly more likely to be avoidant of social activities and to report interest in psychosocial interventions to address body image concerns compared to patients with only appearance-related concerns. These findings suggest the importance of providing care that extends beyond functional rehabilitation and specifically addresses coping with body image issues.

Fundamental elements of conducting a clinical assessment of body image concerns for cancer patients is covered elsewhere in this book (see Chapter 3). Considerations for assessment of body image in patients with speech and swallowing impairment include evaluating the nature and extent of functional as well as any appearance-related concerns the patient may be experiencing. Key areas of assessment involve evaluating the degree to which a patient has realistic/unrealistic expectations regarding treatment outcome; preoccupation with concerns about upcoming or recent changes to appearance and function; distress associated with changes to appearance and function, avoidance of viewing oneself in the mirror due to appearance concerns; avoidance of social situations due to concerns about appearance, speech, or eating; and romantic relationship distress due to changes in appearance and function.

With regard to body image treatment, a range of intervention approaches are covered in Chapters 4 and 15. It can be useful to consider body image interventions which surround three main time points of a patient's cancer treatment trajectory: (a) interventions designed to facilitate treatment decisions that will affect a patient's body image, (b) interventions that help patients cope with recent body image changes, and (c) interventions that help promote body image acceptance during survivorship. Within the context of individual therapy, there are a number of treatment strategies that may be used to facilitate body image coping. Normalizing and validating body image concerns, whether they are appearance-related and/or involve changes to speech and swallowing, is a fundamental treatment strategy and critical for reducing shame and embarrassment for having such concerns.[60] Speech and swallowing difficulties can range in severity, and it is crucial for patients with relatively mild difficulties to have a safe place to explore difficulties they may be having with adjustment. In many cases, these patients will feel guilty for struggling with milder forms of dysphagia or speech articulation especially when they encounter other patients in their treatment setting with more severe functional deficits. Problem-solving and social skills training can be particularly useful to facilitate coping with recent body image changes. Cognitive restructuring, behavioral activation, gradual exposure/desensitization to mirror viewing, and mindfulness are also recognized as useful treatment strategies to facilitate coping with body image changes.[60]

Support groups, such as those available through the National Foundation of Swallowing Disorders, provide an opportunity for patients to obtain peer support from individuals facing similar issues. Although evidence for the effectiveness of support group interventions is less clear than desirable, there is broad consensus that such groups can increase a patient's self-confidence in coping with side effects of an illness and its treatment, provide needed emotional support, and improve knowledge and coping skills.[61] Support groups can be entirely peer-led; alternatively they can be led or co-led by healthcare professionals. In our experience, we have found that such groups when led by professionals provide opportunities to bring in a range of expert speakers to deliver presentations on medical topics of interest to the group. For example, our dysphagia support group, co-led by a psychologist and speech pathologist, has addressed topics such as management of lymphedema, thyroid functioning in patients with head and neck cancer, treatment-related side effects associated with damage to hearing and vestibular systems, telephone access and alternative communication strategies, dental oncology, radiation oncology, and PEG tubes. Participants have shared the following feedback regarding their participation in this group:

> *"I like to gain knowledge from experts in the field. I also take comfort from interacting with survivors like me, and I enjoy sharing any bits of information with new survivors. I am a 14-year cancer survivor."*

"I've liked knowing that I'm not alone in this. That there are others that understand what I'm going through. The program topics have been very helpful to me in moving forward in my 'new' life. Finding my new normal."

"Having the opportunity to interact with other couples and families that are experiencing a similar situation really has helped me feel less alone and isolated. I have gotten a great deal of emotional support from just sitting in group. My husband has benefitted from getting to see other caregivers and by having the opportunity to open up in a safe environment with people who understand what we are going through."

CONCLUSION

The severity of functional deficits and associated body image disturbance alongside the complexity of speech and swallowing rehabilitation for patients with head and neck cancer has significantly increased—patients are younger, the demand for success is greater, the complications are more severe, the treatments, both surgical and nonsurgical, more intense, and the effects of treatment are more debilitating. Achieving successful speech and swallowing after treatment for head and neck cancer demands strong expertise from a dedicated multidisciplinary team of specialists who understand the unique problems associated with the treatment of the patient with head and neck cancer and who share goals for survival, functional success, and optimal psychosocial outcomes for patients who battle malignancies of the head and neck.

ACKNOWLEDGMENT

Dr. Hutcheson receives grant support from the MD Anderson Institutional Research Grant Program and the National Cancer Institute (R03 CA188162). Dr. Hutcheson also receives grant support from the National Institute of Dental and Craniofacial Research (1R56DE025248-01). Dr. Jan Lewin and Dr. Katherine Hutcheson have received research grants from National Institutes of Health Center Core Grant (5P30CA016672).

These listed funders/supporters played no role in the study design, collection, and analysis, interpretation of data, manuscript writing, or decision to submit the report for publication.

Dr. Lewin had full access to all of the data in the study and takes responsibility for the integrity of the data and the accuracy of the data analysis.

The authors are grateful for the editorial assistance of Ms. Janet Hampton and project administration and support by Ms. Martha P. Barrow, data analyst. The authors also acknowledge the Section of Speech Pathology & Audiology at MD Anderson Cancer Center for patient care and data collection efforts. They also thank our head and neck cancer patients who made this chapter possible.

REFERENCES

1. Chen SC, Yu PJ, Hong MY, et al. Communication dysfunction, body image, and symptom severity in post-operative head and neck cancer patients: factors associated with the amount of speaking after treatment. *Support Care Cancer.* 2015;23(8):2375–2382.

2. Liu HE. Changes of satisfaction with appearance and working status for head and neck tumour patients. *J Clin Nurs.* 2008;17(14):1930–1938.

3. Batioglu-Karaaltin A, Binbay Z, Yigit O, Donmez Z. Evaluation of life quality, self-confidence and sexual functions in patients with total and partial laryngectomy. *Auris Nasus Larynx.* 2017;44(2):188–194.

4. Yilmaz M, Yener M, Yollu U, et al. Depression, self-esteem and sexual function in laryngeal cancer patients. *Clin Otolaryngol.* 2015;40(4):349–354.

5. Fingeret MC, Yuan Y, Urbauer D, Weston J, Nipomnick S, Weber R. The nature and extent of body image concerns among surgically treated patients with head and neck cancer. *Psychooncology.* 2012;21(8):836–844.

6. List MA, Stracks J, Colangelo L, et al. How do head and neck cancer patients prioritize treatment outcomes before initiating treatment? *J Clin Oncol.* 2000;18(4):877–884.

7. Wilson JA, Carding PN, Patterson JM. Dysphagia after nonsurgical head and neck cancer treatment: patients' perspectives. *Otolaryngol Head Neck Surg.* 2011;145(5):767–771.

8. Hunter KU, Schipper M, Feng FY, et al. Toxicities affecting quality of life after chemo-IMRT of oropharyngeal cancer: prospective study of patient-reported, observer-rated, and objective outcomes. *Int J Radiat Oncol Biol Phys.* 2013;85(4):935–940.

9. Hunter KU, Lee OE, Lyden TH, et al. Aspiration pneumonia after chemo-intensity-modulated radiation therapy of oropharyngeal carcinoma and its clinical and dysphagia-related predictors. *Head Neck.* 2014;36(1):120–125.

10. Hutcheson KA, Lewin JS, Barringer DA, et al. Late dysphagia after radiotherapy-based treatment of head and neck cancer. *Cancer.* 2012;118(23):5793–5799.

11. Eisbruch A. Dysphagia and aspiration after chemoradiotherapy for head-and-neck cancer: Which anatomic structures are affected and can they be spared by IMRT? *Int J Radiat Oncol Biol Phys.* 2004;60(5):1425–1439.

12. Starmer HM, Liu Z, Akst LM, Gourin C. Attendance in voice therapy: Can an interdisciplinary care model have an impact? *Ann Otol Rhinol Laryngol.* 2014;123(2):117–123.

13. Starmer HM, Gourin CG. Is speech language pathologist evaluation necessary in the nonoperative treatment of head and neck cancer? *Laryngoscope.* 2013;123(7):1571–1572.

14. Hutcheson KA, Lewin JS. Functional outcomes after chemoradiotherapy of laryngeal and pharyngeal cancers. *Curr Oncol Rep.* 2012;14(2):158–165.

15. Hunter KU, Lee OE, Lyden TH, et al. Aspiration pneumonia after chemo-intensity-modulated radiation therapy of oropharyngeal carcinoma and its clinical and dysphagia-related predictors. *Head Neck.* 2014;36(1):120–125.

16. Gillespie MB, Brodsky MB, Day TA, Sharma AK, Lee FS, Martin-Harris B. Laryngeal penetration and aspiration during swallowing after the treatment of advanced oropharyngeal cancer. *Arch Otolaryngol Head Neck Surg.* 2005;131(7):615–619.

17. Rogus-Pulia NM, Pierce MC, Mittal BB, Zecker SG, Logemann JA. Changes in swallowing physiology and patient perception of swallowing function following chemoradiation for head and neck cancer. *Dysphagia.* 2014;29(2):223–233.

18. Jacobson BH, Johnson A, Grywalski C, Silbergleit A, Jacobson G, Benninger MS, Newman CW. The Voice Handicap Index (VHI): development and validation. *Am J Speech Lang Pathol.* 1997;6:66–70.

19. Rosen CA, Lee AS, Osborne J, Zullo T, Murry T. Development and validation of the voice handicap index-10. *Larngoscope*. 2004;114(9):1549–1556.

20. Hogikyan, G. Sethuraman. Validation of an instrument to measure voice-related quality of life (V-RQOL). *J Voice*. 1999;13(4):557–569.

21. Rinkel RN, Leeuw IM, van Reij EJ, Aaronson NK, Leemans CR. Speech handicap index in patients with oral and pharyngeal cancer: better understanding of patients' complaints. *Head Neck*. 2008;30:868–874.

22. Colodny N. Interjudge and intrajudge reliabilities in fiberoptic endoscopic evaluation of swallowing (fees) using the penetration-aspiration scale: a replication study. *Dysphagia*. 2002;17(4):308–315.

23. Aviv JE, Kim T, Sacco RL, et al. FEESST: a new bedside endoscopic test of the motor and sensory components of swallowing. *Ann Otol Rhinol Laryngol*. 1998;107(5 Pt 1):378–387.

24. McConnel FM, Pauloski BR, Logemann JA, et al. Functional results of primary closure vs flaps in oropharyngeal reconstruction: a prospective study of speech and swallowing. *Arch Otolaryngol Head Neck Surg*. 1998;124(6):625–630.

25. Kimata Y, Uchiyama K, Ebihara S, et al. Postoperative complications and functional results after total glossectomy with microvascular reconstruction. *Plast Reconstr Surg*. 2000;106(5):1028–1035.

26. Chien CY, Su CY, Hwang CF, Chuang HC, Jeng SF, Chen YC. Ablation of advanced tongue or base of tongue cancer and reconstruction with free flap: functional outcomes. *Eur J Surg Oncol*. 2006;32(3):353–357.

27. van Lierop AC, Basson O, Fagan JJ. Is total glossectomy for advanced carcinoma of the tongue justified? *S Afr J Surg*. 2008;46(1):22–25.

28. Dziegielewski PT, Ho ML, Rieger J, et al. Total glossectomy with laryngeal preservation and free flap reconstruction: objective functional outcomes and systematic review of the literature. *Laryngoscope*. 2013;123(1):140–145.

29. Baas M, Duraku LS, Corten EM, Mureau MA. A systematic review on the sensory reinnervation of free flaps for tongue reconstruction: Does improved sensibility imply functional benefits? *J Plast Reconstr Aesthetic Surg*. 2015;68(8):1025–1035.

30. Allison GR, Rappaport I, Salibian AH, et al. Adaptive mechanisms of speech and swallowing after combined jaw and tongue reconstruction in long-term survivors. *Am J Surg*. 1987;154(4):419–422.

31. Curtis TA, Beumer J. Speech, palatopharyngeal function, and restoration of soft palate defects. In: Beumer J, Curtis TA, Firtell DN, eds. *Maxillofacial Rehabilitation: Prosthodontic and Surgical Considerations*. St. Louis, MO: Mosby; 1979.

32. MD Anderson Head and Neck Cancer Symptom Working Group. Beyond mean pharyngeal constrictor dose for beam path toxicity in non-target swallowing muscles: dose-volume correlates of chronic radiation-associated dysphagia (RAD) after oropharyngeal intensity modulated radiotherapy. *Radiother Oncol*. 2016;118(2):304–314.

33. Feng FY, Kim HM, Lyden TH, et al. Intensity-modulated radiotherapy of head and neck cancer aiming to reduce dysphagia: early dose-effect relationships for the swallowing structures. *Int J Radiat Oncol Biol Phys*. 2007;68(5):1289–1298.

34. Eisbruch A. Dysphagia and aspiration after chemoradiotherapy for head-and-neck cancer: Which anatomic structures are affected and can they be spared by IMRT? *Int J Radiat Oncol Biol Phys*. 2004;60(5):1425–1439.

35. Logemann JA, Rademaker AW, Pauloski BR, et al. Site of disease and treatment protocol as correlates of swallowing function in patients with head and neck cancer treated with chemoradiation. *Head Neck*. 2006;28(1):64–73.

36. Hutcheson KA, Barringer DA, Rosenthal DI, May AH, Roberts DB, Lewin JS. Swallowing outcomes after radiotherapy for laryngeal carcinoma. *Arch Otolaryngol Head Neck Surg*. 2008;134(2):178–183.

37. Starmer HM, Tippett D, Webster K, et al. Swallowing outcomes in patients with oropharyngeal cancer undergoing organ-preservation treatment. *Head Neck*. 2014;36(10):1392–1397.

38. Eisbruch A, Kim HM, Feng FY, et al. Chemo-IMRT of oropharyngeal cancer aiming to reduce dysphagia: swallowing organs late complication probabilities and dosimetric correlates. *Int J Radiat Oncol Biol Phys.* 2011;1:81(3):e93–e99.

39. Hutcheson KA, Lewin JS, Holsinger FC, et al. Long-term functional and survival outcomes after induction chemotherapy and risk-based definitive therapy for locally advanced squamous cell carcinoma of the head and neck. *Head Neck.* 2014;36(4):474–480.

40. Hutcheson KA. Rehabilitation of heavily treated head and neck cancer patients. In: Bernier J, ed. *Head and Neck Cancer: Multimodality Management.* Cham: Springer International; 2016:783–798.

41. Gillespie MB, Brodsky MA, Day TA, Lee F, Martin-Harris B. Swallowing-related quality of life after head and neck cancer treatment. *Laryngoscope.* 2004;114(8):1362–1367.

42. Rosenthal DI, Lewin JS, Eisbruch A. Prevention and treatment of dysphagia and aspiration after chemoradiation for head and neck cancer. *J Clin Oncol.* 2006;24(17):2636–2643.

43. Eisbruch A, Lyden T, Bradford CR, et al. Objective assessment of swallowing dysfunction and aspiration after radiation concurrent with chemotherapy for head-and-neck cancer. *Int J Radiat Oncol Biol Phys.* 2002;53(1):23–28.

44. Rosenthal DI, Trotti A. Strategies for managing radiation-induced mucositis in head and neck cancer. *Semin Radiat Oncol.* 2009;19(1):29–34.

45. Lewin JS. Speech and swallowing following treatment for oral cancer. In: Werning JW, ed. *Oral Cancer.* New York: Thieme Medical; 2007:304–308.

46. Smith BG, Lewin JS. Lymphedema management in head and neck cancer. *Curr Opin Otolaryngol Head Neck Surg.* 2010;18(3):153–158.

47. Smith BG, Hutcheson KA, Little LG, et al. Lymphedema outcomes in patients with head and neck cancer. *Otolaryngol Head Neck Surg.* 2015;152(2):284–291.

48. Kupferman ME. Addressing an unmet need in oncology patients: rehabilitation of upper aerodigestive tract function. *Laryngoscope.* 2011;22(10):2299–2303.

49. Kubik M, Rosen C. Laryngeal framework surgery in the irradiated neck: a retrospective matched cohort study. *Ann Otol Rhinol Laryngol.* 2016;125(10):823–828.

50. Bhayani MK, Hutcheson KA, Barringer DA, et al. Gastrostomy tube placement in patients with oropharyngeal carcinoma treated with radiotherapy or chemoradiotherapy: factors affecting placement and dependence. *Head Neck.* 2013;35(11):1634–1640.

51. Bhayani MK, Hutcheson KA, Barringer DA, Roberts DB, Lewin JS, Lai SY. Gastrostomy tube placement in patients with hypopharyngeal cancer treated with radiotherapy or chemoradiotherapy: Factors affecting placement and dependence. *Head Neck.* 2013;35(11):1641–1646.

52. Setton J, Lee NY, Riaz N, et al. A multi-institution pooled analysis of gastrostomy tube dependence in patients with oropharyngeal cancer treated with definitive intensity-modulated radiotherapy. *Cancer.* 2015;121(2):294–301.

53. Hutcheson KA, Bhayani MK, Beadle BM, et al. Eat and exercise during radiotherapy or chemoradiotherapy for pharyngeal cancers: use it or lose it. *JAMA Otolaryngol Head Neck Surg.* 2013;139(11):1127–1134.

54. Kulbersh BD, Rosenthal EL, McGrew BM, et al. Pretreatment, preoperative swallowing exercises may improve dysphagia quality of life. *Laryngoscope.* 2006;116(6):883–886.

55. Carroll WR, Locher JL, Canon CL, Bohannon IA, McColloch NL, Magnuson JS. Pretreatment swallowing exercises improve swallow function after chemoradiation. *Laryngoscope.* 2008;118(1):39–43.

56. Carnaby-Mann G, Crary MA, Schmalfuss I, Amdur R. "Pharyngocise": randomized controlled trial of preventative exercises to maintain muscle structure and swallowing function during head-and-neck chemoradiotherapy. *Int J Radiat Oncol Biol Phys.* 2012;83(1):210–219.

57. Kotz T, Federman AD, Kao J, et al. Prophylactic swallowing exercises in patients with head and neck cancer undergoing chemoradiation: a randomized trial. *Arch Otolaryngol Head Neck Surg.* 2012;138(4):376–382.

58. Starmer HM, Yang W, Raval R, et al. Effect of gabapentin on swallowing during and after chemoradiation for oropharyngeal squamous cell cancer. *Dysphagia.* 2014;29(3):396–402.

59. Fingeret MC, Hutcheson KA, Jensen K, Yuan Y, Urbauer D, Lewin JS. Associations among speech, eating, and body image concerns for surgical patients with head and neck cancer. *Head Neck.* 2013;35(5):354–360.

60. Fingeret, MC. Body image and disfigurement. In: Duffy JD, Valentine AD, eds. *MD Anderson Manual of Psychosocial Oncology.* New York: McGraw-Hill; 2010:271–288.

61. Institute of Medicine Committee on Psychosocial Services to Cancer Patients/Families in a Community Setting, Adler NE, Page AEK, eds. *Cancer Care for the Whole Patient: Meeting Psychosocial Health Needs.* Washington, DC: National Academies Press; 2008.

SECTION III
SPECIAL POPULATIONS

CHAPTER 12

BODY IMAGE IN CHILDREN AND ADOLESCENTS WITH CANCER

Clinical Considerations for Assessment and Intervention

Amanda L. Thompson and Lori Wiener

Consider, for a moment, the nine9-year old girl known for her pigtails, watching as her signature curls fall out, feeling scared and worried that her classmates will make fun of her when she returns to school. Or the 13-year-old boy with a gift for playing the violin, being told that doctors will have to amputate his arm below the elbow in order to prevent spread of his osteosarcoma. Or the 15-year-old girl who identifies first and foremost as an athlete, as she struggles to cope with significant weight and muscle loss after prolonged complications secondary to her diagnosis of leukemia and wonders whether she will ever be able to get her strength back to be competitive on the soccer field. Consider the 17-year-old young man whose treatment-induced growth hormone deficiency has kept him at 5'2" while his peers are soaring toward 6 feet; he can't imagine that a girl would ever be interested in him as more than just a friend. Or the 18-year-old survivor, in her first serious relationship, fearful of intimacy as a result of multiple surgical scars and radiation burns that have left her skin patchy and discolored.

These stories are far from unique, as each year more than 150,000 children are diagnosed with cancer around the world[1] and must cope with the impact of disease and treatment on their physical appearance and developing body image. Body image is a multifaceted construct that encompasses perceptions, thoughts, and feelings about the entire body and its functioning. Perception of and satisfaction with one's physical appearance is ultimately subjective, influenced by societal and cultural norms, environmental experiences, individual and biological factors, cognitive development, and psychological well-being. Overall, body image develops over the course of childhood and adolescence, as preteens become more aware of how their body compares to their peers and are increasingly conscious of pubertal changes. In middle adolescence, as teens explore their identity, they may experiment with different images and looks. This often continues into late adolescence, when body image can be powerfully influenced by cultural messages and societal standards of appearance and attractiveness.[2]

Common childhood cancers include leukemias, lymphomas, brain tumors, and solid tumors like neuroblastoma and osteosarcoma. A diagnosis of cancer in childhood or adolescence has the potential to influence body image development, as disease and treatment have direct effects on physical appearance (e.g., hair loss, weight gain or loss, physical scars, limb amputation) and may have a lasting impact on self-perception and comfort in one's own skin. At a time in development when children and adolescents may already feel awkward and self-conscious about their bodies, they must cope with significant unpleasant physical changes, lack of physical privacy that is inherent to the patient role, loss of control over their own bodies, and ongoing uncertainty regarding long-term impact of disease and treatment on their physical appearance and functioning. As such, clinicians have a responsibility to assess potential body image concerns in their patients and support the development of a healthy body image by providing developmentally appropriate education about anticipated physical changes (both permanent and temporary) and strategies to minimize disruptions to how young people perceive their body over the cancer trajectory and into survivorship. In this chapter, we first describe existing research, albeit fairly limited, about body image in children and adolescents with cancer and then discuss implications for clinical assessment and care. We present a case study throughout to illustrate key concepts and principles.

Case Study: Sarah

Sarah is a 14-year-old Asian female with lymphoma. She is an honors student and an active member of her school's dance team. At the time of diagnosis, Sarah was mildly underweight as a result of early disease symptoms. While treatment for lymphoma is typically short compared to treatment for other pediatric malignancies, Sarah's disease has been resistant and physicians have yet to be able to obtain full remission. Treatment has been ongoing for almost two years and has included several chemotherapy combinations, radiation, and an upcoming stem cell transplant. Over the course of treatment, Sarah has gained close to 30 lbs. Contributing factors include decreased activity, treatment steroids, taste aversion to some previously enjoyed healthy food options, and behavioral changes in eating habits (e.g., increased snacking when bored, emotional eating). She is increasingly concerned and focused on her weight gain, noting changes in her body shape (e.g., decrease in muscle tone, increase in belly fat) and impact on her mood, self-esteem, and social interactions.

IMPACT OF CANCER ON THE DEVELOPING BODY IMAGE ON CHILDREN AND ADOLESCENTS

While cancer and its treatment would be expected to have adverse consequences for one's body image, empirical evidence, to date, has been inconsistent.[3] In a systematic review of studies from 1980 to 2008 (18 quantitative, 7 qualitative, and 7 mixed-methods), Fan and Eiser[4] concluded that there was no consistent evidence pertaining to differences in body image between children and adolescents with cancer and healthy controls. The authors did, however, report correlations between body image and gender, specific disease characteristics, and psychological adjustment, particularly self-esteem being negatively affected and increased depression, somatization, withdrawal, and social stress. A separate meta-synthesis of qualitative research findings[5] reported that children and adolescents with cancer experience various problems associated with changes in their body image (e.g., significant body difference between the past and present, loss of self-identity, trying to maintain normalcy with an altered body appearance), with repeated courses of treatment potentially leading to loss of a "normal" life and changes in interpersonal interactions.

The majority of other individual studies (both qualitative and quantitative) have identified adverse effects of cancer and its treatment on young people's body image. Compared to other illness groups (e.g., cardiology, cystic fibrosis) and healthy peers, oncology patients and survivors have reported greater concerns about body image.[6,7] Enskar et al.[8] reported that major appearance changes due to treatment or the disease have been described as "very hard to live with," especially for girls. Qualitative interviews have revealed negative perceptions of one's body image through participant comments such as, "I don't look normal"; "I look ugly and I look sick"; "people look at me."[9] Despite attempts to hide their physical changes, adolescents also reported avoiding social situations and romantic relationships and becoming more cautious around others. Findings also indicate that children and adolescents with cancer may feel socially undesirable, wish to change their physical appearance,[10] and experience lower self-esteem that impacts their peer relationships, social identity,[11] and future romantic and intimate relationships.[12]

OUTCOMES FOR CHILDREN AND ADOLESCENTS WITH CANCER WITH POORER BODY IMAGE

PSYCHOLOGICAL DISTRESS

Despite the theoretical implications of body image concerns for psychosocial adjustment, few controlled studies have empirically been conducted in pediatric cancer populations.[13–15] A relationship, however, between body image and psychological symptoms has been reported. Poorer self-image, for example, has been associated with depression,[8] decreased self-esteem,[8] and somatization, withdrawal, and social stress.[16] In a study with children, adolescents and adults living with gastrointestinal stromal tumor, concerns with body images were associated with sweating, trembling, racing heartbeat when thinking about their illness, or nightmares and bad dreams.[17] In contrast, more positive body image has been associated with lower anxiety and loneliness and greater self-worth.[15]

In a well-designed trial, Pendley et al.[15] examined body image and social adjustment in 21 adolescents who had completed cancer treatment approximately 17 months earlier and 21 healthy controls. Study participants completed questionnaires assessing body image and social adjustment and were videotaped during an interview. There were no significant differences found between those who had completed cancer treatment and healthy peers on the four objective ratings of attractiveness (overall, face, body, and mobility). The videotapes were also viewed by raters blind to the condition (cancer survivor vs. control). Those who underwent cancer treatment were not viewed as less attractive than healthy peers. The study hypothesis that adolescents with cancer would perceive their bodies more negatively than would objective raters was not confirmed, yet participants with cancer participated in less than half as many peer activities than their healthy peers. Body image was found to be correlated negatively with social anxiety and loneliness and positively with global self-worth. Overall, psychosocial adjustment was significantly related to adolescents' subjective rating of their overall appearance instead of objective ratings. In other words, how adolescents feel about how they look is more important to self-esteem than their actual appearance.

PEER AND PARTNER RELATIONSHIPS

An association between body image and the quality of peer relationships has been reported for children with cancer. Qualitative research has revealed that children and adolescents with cancer worry about how other people judge them and that lack of understanding and ridicule by peers might also lead to interpersonal problems.[18] Negative experiences with peers who tease them about their physical appearance have been described,[19] and feeling different or rejected can lead to withdrawal, losing touch with peers, feeling lost at school, and falling behind with schoolwork.[9,20] Finally, perception of physical changes affect their desires to interact with others and establish intimate relationships.[9,12,20,21] Larouche and Chin-Peuckert[9] have noted that teens often use friends as "peer shields" to help them cope with body image issues related to their cancer treatment, with most of their cohort acknowledging that concerns about body image impacted their desire to return to school.

RISK FACTORS FOR DEVELOPING POORER BODY IMAGE DURING OR AFTER TREATMENT

Research findings, supported by decades of the authors' clinical experience, has shown that some adolescents and young adults learn to live with the changes in their appearance whereas others struggle to accept their altered bodies. Risk factors for poorer body image may include premorbid overemphasis on appearance and weight (e.g., high body image investment), distorted body image perception (i.e., body dysmorphia), history of disordered eating (e.g., restricting, binge eating, purging), psychological inflexibility, perfectionism, obsessive/compulsive tendencies, and pre-existing anxiety disorders.

Disease and treatment factors also may play a role, as stage of treatment,[22] longer hospitalizations, visible physical impairment,[23] changes in physical functioning and appearance,[24] multiple relapses, frequent side effects,[8] and less chance of cure have been found to be associated with poorer body image.[25] Poorer body image has also been found for survivors of solid tumors compared to survivors of leukemia, likely due to resulting functional and physical impairment,[24] and for those who had not undergone bone marrow transplantation than those who had.[26] Whether underlying reasons for this high rate of concern about body image in survivors is due to the cancer treatment itself (e.g., chemotherapy or surgery), delayed maturity, or having endured a life-threatening disease is unknown and remains an area for future investigation.

Findings on the relationship between body image and demographic factors of age and gender are mixed. According to the review by Fan et al., the majority of studies found no relationship between body image and age.[15,26–31] One study[32] found female adolescent (16 years+) survivors of childhood leukemia had better body image than healthy controls matched for age, gender, social economic status, and residence area. Another study of children who completed treatment for childhood leukemia found that mothers perceived that five- to nine-year-old children had more concerns about body image than zero- to four-year-old children, and 10- to 14-year-olds who were concerned about body image were more likely to show social withdrawal.[21] While some studies with children had not found an association between gender and body image,[15,27,28,29,31,33] others described males as rating their body image as better than females.[8,34–37] Only one published study reported that females rated their body image better than males.[38,39]

Overall, methodological challenges in the available literature contribute to diverse and sometimes conflicting findings and make it difficult to draw robust conclusions about cancer's impact on the body image of children and adolescents. Available studies are limited in number and describe highly heterogenous samples that range in age, diagnosis, disease status (i.e., on active treatment vs. off), treatment intensity, and functional impairment. Measures used vary widely, ranging from specific quantification of degree of scarring and disfigurement[40] to general body image perception[41] and broader measures of quality of life that include physical appearance.[42] Few scales have been validated in pediatric or adolescent cancer populations. Additionally, measures used in the current studies are often limited to the attitudinal component of body image or body satisfaction,[43] not the social, emotional, and behavioral components.[44] In order to advance research and clinical care related to body image and how it impacts psychosocial functioning and health-related quality of life, more consistent measurement methodology is needed, as well as sample sizes large enough to evaluate risk factors for poorer body image. In addition to quantitative studies, there remains a key role for qualitative and longitudinal follow-up.

The rest of this chapter addresses key principles of clinical care as they pertain to body image issues in youth with cancer. First we discuss the need for a thorough assessment of pre-cancer body image, beliefs, expectations, and concerns, then consider the impact of treatment on appearance and perception of physical differences over the illness trajectory. Strategies to address body-altering side effects of cancer, including the role of social support, are discussed, and we conclude by discussing clinical interventions for more persistent and intrusive body image concerns that interfere with social functioning or cause significant emotional distress. Box 12.1 offers an overview of these principles of clinical care.

> **BOX 12.1 PRINCIPLES OF CLINICAL CARE FOR BODY IMAGE ISSUES OF YOUTH WITH CANCER**
>
> - Evaluate for pre-existing body image issues
> - Evaluate core beliefs about body pre-cancer
> - Know family culture about body expectations
> - Normalize worries and fears
> - Identify how treatment disrupts normal development of body image
> - Address body image changes over illness and developmental trajectory
> - Address multiple dimensions of body image
> - Address multiple domains of impact of body changes
> - Support exposure to body changes as patient can tolerate but educate against avoidance
> - Support grieving of changes
> - Give patients skills to communicate about changes
> - Actively use interventions to promote coping

ASSESSMENT OF BODY IMAGE CONCERNS

Assessment of body image concerns should happen early in treatment. As adolescents who have been off treatment longer have been found to have more negative body image perceptions,[15] assessment should be ongoing and extend into survivorship. Currently, there is no widely accepted or standard approach to clinical assessment of body image in youth treated for cancer. Appropriate tools for measuring body image are clearly needed. As such, the field would benefit from a broadly representative group of pediatric, adolescent, and young adult stakeholders including patients both on and off treatment, caregivers, clinicians, psychologists, social workers, and others to convene to define a core set of measures that takes into account stage of disease, time since diagnosis, and developmental stage to use not just in research but as part of a standard of psychosocial care.[45]

Discussions about body image can be difficult for both patients and providers. Adolescents, in particular, may be reluctant to bring up or divulge concerns, as the topic can be a sensitive one. As such, providers should bear the responsibility of bringing up the topic of body image during routine visits, regardless of patient gender or age and whether survival is expected to be short or long term. As a general rule, discussions about body image should occur separate from parents and caregivers, so that patients are less self-conscious and more inclined to be open about their thoughts and feelings. Providers should broach the topic matter-of-factly, letting the patient know that they ask everyone how they feel

- It is not uncommon for patients to have concerns about changes in their physical appearance during and after treatment. These changes can impact how you view yourself, so I'm hoping we can talk a little today about your body image.
- Can you tell me how you felt about your appearance before your cancer diagnosis? What aspects of your appearance did you like the most? Were there things you thought you'd like to change?
- What changes have you noticed in your body now? During treatment? Since treatment ended? What do you like/not like about these changes?
- How do you feel about your appearance now?
- How does your body image affect you? Your relationships? Your self-esteem? Your social life? Your sex life?
- Can you tell me whether you have noticed changes in your ability to get around, such as walk or run? How about changes in your speech, swallowing, hearing, eyesight? How have these affected the time you spend with peers?
- What are the expectations within your family and your culture for body appearance? Tell me how this impacts you.

about their body and appearance before, during, and after treatment, as it's not unusual for concerns to arise. This approach normalizes their thoughts and feelings and communicates that their experience is not atypical. Open-ended questions encourage richer discussion than closed-ended ones. Finally, providers are encouraged to ask openly to be informed of how a patient's culture impacts his or her body image perception. Examples of conversational prompts and questions are provided in Box 12.2.

Following a diagnosis of cancer, clinicians should pay attention to whether a patient expresses unrealistic expectations of physical changes posttreatment, has difficulty making treatment decisions based on concerns about appearance and functionality (amputation, external catheter,[46] colostomy bag), difficulty with or avoidance of viewing oneself in the mirror, expression of a high degree of dissatisfaction with appearance, avoidance of social situations due to appearance/functional changes, distress and challenges with peer and romantic relationships due to appearance/body image concerns, considerable time spent in appearance-fixing behaviors, or persistent distress, depression, or anxiety due to appearance/body changes. There are specific risk factors for the emergence of body image issues in youth with cancer such as pre-illness eating or anxiety disorders, pre-existing body dissatisfaction and limited coping strategies, avoidance of social situations due to body changes during treatment and beyond, and lack of acceptance of permanent changes posttreatment. See Table 12.1 for additional considerations.

TABLE 12.1: Risk Factors for Body Image Issues in Youth with Cancer

Pre-illness	Pre-existing body dissatisfaction
	History of eating disorder
	Psychological inflexibility
	Limited coping strategies
	Significant anxiety about appearance
	Anxiety disorder
	High appearance investment
Diagnosis/Treatment	Treatment choices weighted heavily on unwanted appearance changes
	Avoidance of viewing body changes
	Avoidance of social situations due to body changes
	Relationship disruptions due to body changes (friends and intimate relationships)
	Taking responsibility for changes that cannot be controlled
	Seeing emotional distress as related to body changes alone
	Needing significant reassurance about appearance
	Criticism from close others
	Depression
Survivorship	Lack of skill for communicating about body changes to others
	Avoidance of social situations due to body changes
	Relationship disruptions due to body changes (friends and intimate relationships)
	Expectation to return to pre-cancer self
	Lack of understanding of permanence of changes
	Lack of acceptance of permanent changes
	Inability to grieve changes
	Lack of attention to body health (exercise and nutrition)

Case Study: Assessment

In discussion with her psychosocial provider, separate from her parents, Sarah reported that, prior to her cancer diagnosis, she was proud of her long, lean muscles and "dancer's body." She felt that she fit in with her peers and had confidence in her appearance. Since diagnosis, that confidence has disappeared. While she knows her hair will grow back, she feels that her bald head is a constant reminder to everyone around her that she is sick. Her weight gain has been the most distressing reminder, and it's reportedly "all [she] thinks about." Dance practices have grown emotional for her, as she is surrounded by her peers who are lean and muscular, while wearing unforgiving spandex uniforms, surrounded by wall to wall mirrors. Sarah is often tearful, noting that she "hates" her body, that she's "disgusting," and that she "can't stand" to look at herself in the mirror or to view photos of herself before diagnosis. She stated that her clothes no longer fit well, so she's resorted to wearing baggy sweats; she reports significant shame and embarrassment during dance performance, as she's the "biggest and least toned" girl on the floor. She's dreading summertime, as friends tend to have pool parties and her family has planned several beach vacations. Sarah states that her thoughts about her body have impacted her mood and her interest in going out in public. She notes that her self-esteem is "nonexistent" and that she is convinced that no boy would find her attractive at her current size. Sarah indicates that most women in her family are thin and that she previously enjoyed sharing clothes with her same-aged cousin. She notes that her parents haven't said anything about her weight gain, other than telling her "not to worry about it; you're beautiful." She jokes that her mother tends to bring her cookies and snacks on treatment days because "she doesn't know what else to do." Sarah feels responsible for her weight gain because she "enjoys food," finds that sweet and salty foods taste better since the start of treatment than healthier options, and hasn't "pushed" herself to maintain her previous level of physical activity. While she denies engaging in any concerning behaviors like food restriction or purging, she reports that she is "holding out hope" that she'll lose the weight during transplant.

Sarah denies any history of eating disorder or disordered eating behaviors. She reports a pre-existing history of anxiety and depression, which prior to diagnosis she feels was being well-controlled by medication prescribed by a psychiatrist. She notes that she's been crying more often about her appearance and worries that her depression may be recurring. Sarah indicates that she feels lonely because no one (family or friends) could understand.

STRATEGIES TO ADDRESS BODY-ALTERING SIDE EFFECTS

Body-altering side effects from cancer and repeated courses of cancer treatment can exacerbate developmentally typical concerns about one's body. In fact, the body-altering side effects of cancer have been reported by adolescents to be the most devastating aspect of their disease.[47] Hair loss, presence of a venous catheter, weight gain or loss resulting from treatment, amputation, growth disorders, surgery scars, and the unpredictability of health status are some of the major changes that can place adolescents with cancer at risk for poor body image and can threaten body integrity and functioning.[13,48] These appearance changes are visible and obvious indications of illness and can be challenging to adolescents, particularly those who work hard to fit in and prefer not to be identified as different. Table 12.2 describes specific body-altering side effects, potential impacts on patients, and possible coping strategies that youth may find helpful.

The support of parents/caregivers, immediate and extended family, classmates and peers, and healthcare professionals is vital to child and adolescent adjustment to physical changes. For example, strong relationships with friends and positive experiences with peers (e.g., receiving encouraging comments about their appearance; being a "peer shield" to protect against psychological distress) are central factors related to satisfaction with appearance and important to image-related interactions with potential partners.[49,50] Table 12.3 provides examples of sources of support for positive body image in youth with cancer.

CLINICAL INTERVENTION BY PROVIDERS

Figure 12.1 illustrates the trajectory of distress that patients may experience related to their body changes and subsequent body image concerns, ranging from mild (with little impact on functioning) to more severe (with significant impact on functioning). While support from family and friends is critical for all youth, some children and adolescents may require intervention by their healthcare or psychosocial providers. This is particularly the case for children and adolescents who experience more persistent and intrusive body image

TABLE 12.2: Specific Body-Altering Side Effects

Side Effect	Impact	Strategies for Minimizing Impact	Notes to Clinicians
Hair thinning and loss due to chemotherapy	- Often the first recognizable effect of chemotherapy treatment - "It changes the image you display."[9]	- Shaving of head as the hair begins to fall out (provides a sense of control) - Wearing hats or scarves - Use of wigs or hair extensions - Using makeup to fill in eyebrows - Use of accessories (e.g., earrings) to draw attention away from hair loss	- Do not assume that male patients will not be distressed by hair loss - While emphasizing the temporary nature of hair loss can be helpful for some patients, adolescents in particular are most concerned with the here and now and may not be comforted (yet) by the notion that "it will grow back"
Venous catheter	- Visible whether implanted or externalized - May cause a scar - Often located in a precarious place for adolescents (e.g., chest) - May cause self-consciousness in bathing suits, tank tops, dresses, etc. - May impact ability to participate in physical activities	- Consideration of lifestyle factors in decisions regarding type of catheter - Purchase of new clothes that cover the catheter and/or scar	- Assess for self-esteem issues and avoidance of baths/showers despite the dressings provided by the medical team - Advocate for having a private place to change clothes for gym class or other programs
Weight loss due to changes in food taste, decreased appetite, nausea and vomiting, food aversions,	- Distress over new appearance, loss of strength, muscle tone, their "normal" body - For some who considered themselves overweight prior to cancer treatment, weight loss could result in happiness at new body weight/shape	- Working with dietician to maintain appropriate caloric and nutrient intake - Medical management of nausea and vomiting - Medical intervention (e.g., TPN, NG tube) if weight loss is substantial	- Do not assume weight loss is welcomed, even in patients who may be of normal body weight or overweight - Consider cultural norms of body shape and physical appearance

Side Effect	Impact	Strategies for Minimizing Impact	Notes to Clinicians
Weight gain due to steroid treatment, decreased physical activity, changes in eating habits	- Distress over weight gain - Increased comparison to healthy peers - May impact adherence to medications causing weight gain, which has the potential to impact disease outcomes[54,55]	- Working with dietician to manage cravings and address changes in eating habits - Working with physical therapy to discuss options for increased activity	- There is no data to suggest that eating disorders that are triggered or reawakened during or following cancer treatment during childhood or adolescence. Nevertheless, assess for food restriction and other unhealthy eating behaviors
Amputation	- Clearly visible and significant change in physical appearance - Fear of stigmatization by peers - May avoid looking at the limb or in a mirror - May impact participation in social and physical activities - May impact future career aspirations (e.g., as an athlete, artist, surgeon) - May be hesitant to pursue dating or romantic interests. Alternatively, may engage in promiscuous behaviors in the hopes of gaining acceptance.[56]	- Give patient permission to grieve - A supportive home environment is critically important - Classmate support can help buffer some of the stress of returning to school following surgery - Meeting and talking with other amputees and engaging in activities that promote independence can increase self-esteem and improve coping and adaptation.[57] - Participating in adaptive sports	- It is important to prepare the child or adolescent for the psychosocial impact of losing a limb prior to surgery. - Assess for depression and behavior changes following surgery (e.g., avoidance of peers)
Growth disorders due to high-dose steroid therapy, radiation therapy	- Poor quality of life, often due to feelings of anxiety, depression, and social isolation[58] - May be hesitant to pursue dating or romantic interests - Others may view patient as younger, less mature despite chronological age	- Treatment with growth hormone might be recommended - Participating in activities where height is not an issue and where self-esteem can be increased (e.g., yearbook club, certain sports)	- Assess for psychosocial adaptation - Assess for stressed family relationships (e.g., parents more concerned about height than the teen; younger and taller siblings) - Assess for perceived and real social reputation

TABLE 12.3: Sources of Support for Positive Body Image in Youth with Cancer

Adolescent Cancer Survivors	• Provides similar-aged peer with common experience[5] • Comfortable asking questions without concern about being judged[5] • Offers opportunity to obtain meaningful and valuable advice[5] • Provides companionship[59] • Improves social gaps (i.e., provides transitional support from treatment to re-entry to school/work)
Family	• Provides safe emotional space and environment • Encourages maintenance of peer relationships[5] • Reduces child's sensitivity to his or her physical appearance by demonstrating comfort with child's changing appearance[5] • Deflects unwanted attention from others[50] • Diffuses awkward social situations that might arise[50] • Documents physical appearance changes (photos/videos) to show friends and family to prepare them[50]
Peers[49]	• Provide gentle encouragement to take their wig off, if desired • Help them improve their appearance (e.g., go shopping with them, help with make-up, etc.) • Boost their morale (simple compliments, encourage them to go out in public) • Answer questions from others when they do not want to • Be by their side and protect them from others' negative reactions (i.e., act as a "peer shield")
Hospital Professionals	• Talk to them about body image and related problems and challenges[21] • Be the one to start the conversation[21] • Communicate that they can ask any questions free of judgment[50] • Offer time to talk to another patient or someone who went through cancer treatment and understands similar body image concerns • Consider intervention modalities as indicated (e.g., psychoeducation, CBT, ACT; individual, group, family)

concerns that interfere with social functioning or cause significant emotional distress. In these situations, aforementioned strategies to minimize impact of body changes may not be sufficient. Currently, however, there are no evidence-based interventions for negative body image/body dysmorphia specific to youth with cancer. Providers, then, must rely on approaches that have been shown to promote adaptive coping, address distorted or dysfunctional thought patterns, and promote acceptance of one's appearance.

Cognitive-behavior therapy (CBT),[51] for example, can be used to understand the relationship between negative thoughts about appearance (e.g., "I'm ugly"), subsequent feelings (e.g., despair), and behaviors (e.g., social withdrawal). CBT can identify patterns of maladaptive thinking, target automatic negative thoughts about appearance (e.g., "Romantic partners will reject me when they learn of my prosthesis"; "Everyone is judging how I look"), evaluate the validity of those thoughts, and ultimately address core beliefs about appearance. An acceptance and commitment therapy (ACT)[52] approach may be helpful in promoting acceptance of body image changes by using mindfulness-based strategies[53] to promote psychological flexibility, clarify personal values, set goals, and take actions that are in line with those goals. In contrast to CBT's focus on changing maladaptive thought patterns, ACT teaches patients to be aware of and receptive to unpleasant feelings (i.e., just notice them rather than

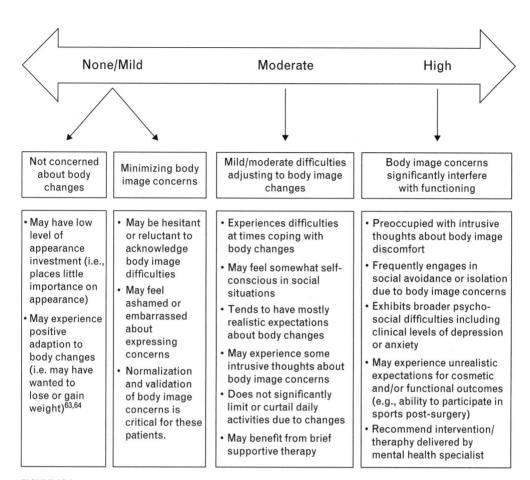

FIGURE 12.1: Trajectory of distress related to body image.

Credit Michelle Fingeret.

struggle against them) without overreacting to them or avoiding the situations that invoke them. Exposure-based approaches are appropriate when body image concerns result in social anxiety, withdrawal from peers and social interactions, and avoidance of looking in mirrors. Table 12.4 outlines these and other intervention approaches that may be helpful in youth with significant body image concerns.

TABLE 12.4: Summary of Clinical Interventions

Issue	Possible Clinical Tools
Misconceptions about body changes (e.g., causes, permanence)	Psychoeducation and anticipatory guidance to promote realistic expectations
Maladaptive thinking	Cognitive-behavioral therapy
Rigid focus on/preoccupation with body changes	Acceptance and commitment therapy
Stress due to others' lack of sensitivity	Communication/assertiveness training
Avoiding social situations/social withdrawal	Exposure; peer shield
Lack of control; feelings of helplessness	Problem-solving skills training[60]
Disordered eating	Family-based treatment[61]

Case Study: Intervention

Support for Sarah included strategies for minimizing the impact of her physical changes in combination with evidence-based interventions to address her emotional distress, preoccupation with weight, and maladaptive thoughts. Psychosocial and medical providers provided Sarah with education regarding the impact of disease and treatment on weight and appearance, helping her to understand that some factors contributing to her weight gain (e.g., steroids, fatigue due to low blood counts) are not under her control. Although reluctant at first, Sarah participated in a hospital program, Look Good Feel Better, focused on improving adolescent patients' self-esteem through instruction in use of makeup, wigs, scarves, jewelry, and other accessories. She was encouraged to meet other adolescent patients, which had a powerful impact on her feelings of loneliness and helped her to recognize that she was not alone in her experience. A referral was made for Sarah to meet with one of the hospital's registered dieticians, who emphasized "food as fuel"' for regaining strength and stamina in dance rather than a specific weight loss strategy. She suggested Sarah keep an electronic food log and worked with her to review choices and consider healthier alternatives.

Sarah's psychologist took an integrative approach, using strategies from CBT, ACT, and problem-solving skills training. Cognitive-behavioral strategies were used to address Sarah's negative thoughts about herself and her body (e.g., "I'm ugly"; "The weight gain is my fault," "No boy will ever like me like this"). She developed skills in identifying these negative thoughts and challenging their validity by evaluating evidence for and against her stated beliefs. She understood the clear connection between her negative thought patterns, her feelings (e.g., helplessness, anxiety, and sadness), and her behaviors (social withdrawal, emotional eating). ACT was incorporated to address her preoccupation with her weight and help her to explore her core values. Sarah was able to identify "being a good person," "helping others," and "making a difference" as the values most important to her, which helped her to refocus on what is most important in her life. She set goals in line with her values, including resuming volunteer efforts at school and in her community, which had a notable positive impact on her mood.

To combat her feelings of helplessness and provide a sense of control, problem-solving skills were introduced. Sarah easily identified her problem (weight gain) and was able to generate a number of solutions including eating less, exercising more, "letting it go," and waiting until after transplant to make any changes. She evaluated the pros and cons of each option and over the course of treatment and implemented action plans for several solutions. Through this problem-solving work, Sarah decided to have a conversation with her mother about her tendency to provide her with unhealthy food options during clinic visits and inpatient stays, to resume her group exercise classes (with physician approval), and to identify a close friend as her "peer shield" during potentially uncomfortable social situations. As a result, Sarah reported increased feelings of control, a heightened sense of self-efficacy, and a more positive mood. Finally, providers on Sarah's medical team collaborated with her community psychiatrist to monitor and maximize the role of medication in managing her depression.

CONCLUSION

Body image is a complex, dynamic construct that develops during childhood and adolescence and is strongly associated with self-esteem and psychosocial adjustment. Childhood cancer can have a significant impact on body image, as disease and treatment alter physical appearance in visible, and sometimes lasting, ways. Adverse effects can be moderated by skilled and ongoing clinical assessments, psychosocial interventions that include integrated approaches, and social support. Body image in youth with cancer is an area in need of clinical and research attention, specifically the development of valid and reliable body image measures, evidence-based interventions, and longitudinal follow-up.

Case Study: Disposition

While Sarah is still not pleased with her weight gain, she has learned to cope more effectively with negative thoughts about her body, to focus less on her appearance and more on skills in line with her personal values, and to actively problem-solve strategies for tacking challenges within her sphere of control. She continues to dance in front of crowds in what she perceives as unforgiving outfits, with mindful effort to enjoy the moment; she's proud of her efforts to regain her strength and stamina and has adjusted her expectations to account for the ongoing and cumulative impact of two years of treatment. At times, like most adolescent girls, she still struggles to feel pretty and not compare herself to her peers, but she is no longer avoiding social interactions.

REFERENCES

1. World Health Organization. http://www.who.int/cancer/iccd_2016/en/

2. Croll J. Body image and adolescents. In: Stang J, Story M, eds. *Guidelines for Adolescent Nutrition Services.* Rockville, MD: U.S. Department of Health and Human Services; 2005:155–166. http://www.epi.umn. edu/let/pubs/img/adol_preface_materials.pdf

3. White CA. Body image dimensions and cancer: A heuristic cognitive behavioural model. *Psychooncology.* 2000;9:183–192.

4. Fan SY, Eiser C. Body image of children and adolescents with cancer: a systematic review. *Body Image.* 2009;6:247–256.

5. Lee MY, Mu PF, Tsay SF. Body image of children and adolescents with cancer: a metasynthesis on qualitative research findings. *Nurs Health Sci.* 2012;14:381–390.

6. Zeltzer L, Kellerman J, Ellenberg L, Dash J, Rigler D. Psychologic effects of illness in adolescence. II. Impact of illness in adolescence—crucial issues and coping styles. *J Pediatrics.* 1980;97:132–138.

7. Madan-Swain A, Brown, RT, Sexson SB, Baldwin K, Ragab A. Adolescent cancer survivors: psychosocial and familial adaptation. *J Psychosom Res.* 1994;35:453–459.

8. Enskar K, Carlsson M, Golsater M, Hamrin E. Symptom distress and life situation in adolescents with cancer. *Cancer Nurs.* 1997;20:23–33.

9. Larouche SS, Chin-Peuckert L. Changes in body image experienced by adolescents with cancer. *J Pediatr Oncol Nurs.* 2006;23:200–209.

10. Eapen V, Revesz T, Mpofu C, Daradkeh T. Self-perception profile in children with cancer: self vs parent report. *Psychol Rep.* 1999;84:427–432.

11. Woodgate RL. A different way of being: adolescents' experiences with cancer. *Cancer Nurs.* 2005;28:8–15.

12. Thompson AL, Marsland AL, Marshal MP, Tersak JM. Romantic relationships of emerging adult survivors of childhood cancer. *Psychooncology.* 2009;18(7):767–774.

13. Cull A. Invited review: Psychological aspects of cancer and chemotherapy. *J Psychosom Res.* 1990;34:129–140.

14. La Greca AM. Social consequences of pediatric conditions: fertile area for future investigation and intervention. *J Pediatr Psychol.* 1990;15:285–307.

15. Pendley JS, Dahlquist LM, Dreyer Z. Body image and psychosocial adjustment in adolescent cancer survivors. *J Pediatr Psychol.* 1997;22:29–43.

16. Moore IM, Challinor J, Pasvogel A, Matthay K, Hutter J, Kaemingk K. Behavioral adjustment of children and adolescents with cancer: teacher, parent, and self-report. *Oncol Nurs Forum.* 2003;30:E84–E91.

17. Wiener L, Battles H, Zadeh S, et al. Gastrointestinal stromal tumor: psychosocial characteristics and considerations. *Support Care Cancer.* 2012;20:1343–1349.

18. Stegenga K, Ward-Smith P. On receiving the diagnosis of cancer: the adolescent perspective. *J Pediatr Oncol Nurs.* 2009;26(2):75–80.

19. Wasserman AL, Thompson EL, Wilimas JA, Fairclough D. The psychological status of survivors of childhood/adolescent Hodgkin's disease. *Am J Dis Child.* 1987;141(6):626–631.

20. McCaffrey CN. Major stressors and their effects on the well-being of children with cancer. *J Pediatr Nurs.* 2006;21:59–66.

21. Earle EA, Eiser C. Children's behaviour following diagnosis of acute lymphoblastic leukemia: a qualitative longitudinal study. *Clin Child Psychol Psychiatry.* 2007;12:281–293.

22. Hedstrom M, Skolin I, von Essen L. Distressing and positive experiences and important aspects of care for adolescents treated for cancer: adolescent and nurse perceptions. *Eur J Oncol Nurs.* 2004;8:6–17.

23. Anholt UV, GK. Fritz GK, Keener M. Self-concept in survivors of childhood and adolescent cancer. *J Psychosoc Oncol.* 1993;11:1–16.

24. Calaminus G, Weinspach S, Teske C, Gobel U. Quality of survival in children and adolescents after treatment for childhood cancer: the influence of reported late effects on health related quality of life. *Klin Padiatr.* 2007;219:152–157.

25. Beardslee C, Neff EJ. Body related concerns of children with cancer as compared with the concerns of other children. *Matern Child Nurs J.* 1982;11:121–134.

26. Puukko LR, Hirvonen E, Aalberg V, Hovi L, Rautonen J, Siimes MA. Impaired body image of young female survivors of childhood leukemia. *J Psychosom Res.* 1997;38:54–62.

27. Kopel SJ, Eiser C, Cool P, Grimer RJ, Carter SR. Brief report: assessment of body image in survivors of childhood cancer. *J Pediatr Psychol.* 1998;23:141–147.

28. Kyritsi H, Matziou V, Papadatou D, Evagellou E, Koutelekos G, Polikandrioti M. Self concept of children and adolescents with cancer. *Health Sci J.* 2007;11:1–11.

29. Puukko LR Sammallahti PR, Siimes MA, Aalberg VA. Childhood leukemia and body image: interview reveals impairment not found with a questionnaire. *J Clin Psychol.* 1997;53:133–137.

30. Stern M, Norman SL, Zevon, MA. Adolescents with cancer self-image and perceived social support as indexes of adaptation. *J Adolesc Res.* 1993;8:124–142.

31. Varni J. W, Katz ER, Colegrove R Jr, Dolgin M. Perceived physical appearance and adjustment of children with newly diagnosed cancer: a path analytic model. *J Behav Med.* 1995;18:261–278.

32. Maggiolini A, Grassi R, Adamoli L, et al. Self-image of adolescent survivors of long-term childhood leukemia. *J Pediatr Hematol Oncol.* 2000;22:417–421.

33. Zebrack BJ, Chesler M. Health-related worries, self-image, and life outlooks of long-term survivors of childhood cancer. *Health Social Work.* 2001;26:245–256.

34. Eapen V, Revesz T, Mpofu C, Daradkeh, T. Self-perception profile in children with cancer: self vs parent report. *Psychol Rep.* 1999;84:427–432.

35. Langeveld NE, Grootenhuis MA, Voute PA, de Haan RJ, van den Bos C. Quality of life, self-esteem and worries in young adult survivors of childhood cancer. *Psychooncology.* 2004;13:867–881.

36. Mullis RL, Mullis AK, Kerchoff NF. The effect of leukemia and its treatment on self-esteem of school-age children. *Matern Child Nurs J.* 1992;20:155–165.

37. Wu LM, Chin CC. Factors related to satisfaction with body image in children undergoing chemotherapy. *Kaohsiung J Med Sci*. 2003;19:217–224.

38. Jamison RN, Lewis S, Burish TG. Psychological impact of cancer on adolescents: self-image, locus of control, perception of illness and knowledge of cancer. *J Chronic Dis*. 1986;39:609–617.

39. Sheng-Yu F, Eiser C. Body image of children and adolescents with cancer: a systematic review. *Body Image*. 2009;6:247–256.

40. Kinahan KE, Sharp LK, Seidel K, et al. Scarring, disfigurement, and quality of life in long-term survivors of childhood cancer: a report from the Childhood Cancer Survivor study. *J Clin Oncol*. 2012;30:2466–2474.

41. Hopwood P, Fletcher I, Lee A, Al Ghazal S. A body image scale for use with cancer patients. *Eur J Cancer*. 2001;37:189–197.

42. Varni JW, Burwinkle TM, Katz ER, Meeske K, Dickinson P. The PedsQL in pediatric cancer: reliability and validity of the Pediatric Quality of Life Inventory Generic Core Scales, Multidimensional Fatigue Scale, and Cancer Module. *Cancer*. 2002;94:2090–2106.

43. Smolak L. Body image in children and adolescents: where do we go from here? *Body Image*. 2004;1:15–28.

44. Cash TF. A negative body image: evaluating epidemiological evidence. In: Cash TF, Pruzinsky T, eds. *Body Image: A Handbook of Theory, Research and Practice*. New York: Guilford Press; 2002:269–276.

45. Pruzinsky T, Cash TF. Assessing body image and quality of life in medical settings. In: Cash TF, Pruzinsky T, eds. *Body Image: A Handbook of Theory, Research and Practice*. New York: Guilford Press; 2002:171–179.

46. Batista Mdo R, Rocha FC, da Silva DM, Júnior FJ. [Self-image of clients with colostomy related to the collecting bag]. *Revista Brasil Enfermagem*. 2011;64(6):1043–1047.

47. Abrams, A, Muriel, AC, Wiener, L, eds. *Pediatric Psychosocial Oncology: Textbook for Multi-disciplinary Care*. Cham, Switzerland: Springer International; 2016.

48. Fritz GK, Williams JR. Issues of adolescent development for survivors of childhood cancer. *J Am Acad Child Adolesc Psychiatry*. 1988;27:712–715.

49. Jones DC, Vigfusdottir TH, Lee Y. Body image and the appearance culture among adolescent girls and boys: an examination of friend conversations, peer criticism, appearance magazines, and the internalization of appearance ideals. *J Adolesc Res*. 2004;19:323–339.

50. Williamson H, Halliwell E, Wallace M. Adolescents' and parents' experiences of managing the psychosocial impact of appearance change during cancer treatment. *J Pediatr Oncol Nurs*. 2012; 27:168–175.

51. Beck JS. *Cognitive Behavior Therapy: Basics and Beyond*, 2nd ed. New York: Guilford Press; 2011.

52. Hayes, SC, Kirk D, Strosahl KD, Wilson KG. *Acceptance and Commitment Therapy*, 2nd ed. New York: Guilford Press; 2012.

53. Jones P, Blunda M, Biegel G, Carlson L, Biel M, Wiener, L. Can mindfulness-based interventions help adolescents with cancer? *Psychooncology*. 2013;22(9):2148–2151.

54. Butow P, Palmer S, Pai ALH, Goodenough B, Luckett T, King M. Review of adherence-related issues in adolescents and young adults with cancer. *J Clin Oncol*. 2010;28:4800–4809.

55. Bhatia S, Landier W, Shangguan M, et al. Nonadherence to oral mercaptopurine and risk of relapse in Hispanic and non-Hispanic white children with acute lymphoblastic leukemia: a report from the children's oncology group. *J Clin Oncol*. 2012;30:2094–2101.

56. Kahle A. Children and limb loss. http://www.healio.com/orthotics-prosthetics/prosthetics/news/online/%7B20bb0ac6-5ae1-4c65-b8e7-281ca1821228%7D/the-psychology-of-losing-a-limb

57. Loucas CA, Brand SR, Bedoya SZ, Muriel AC, Wiener L. Preparing youth with cancer for amputation: a systematic review. *J Psychosoc Oncol*. 2017;35(4):483–493. doi:10.1080/07347332.2017.1307894

58. Stabler B. Impact of growth hormone (GH) therapy on quality of life along the lifespan of GH-treated patients. *Hormone Res*. 2001;56(Suppl. 1):55–58.

59. Pinquart M. Body image of children and adolescents with chronic illness: a meta-analytic comparison with healthy peers. *Body Image.* 2013;10:141–148.

60. Sahler, OJZ., Fairclough DL, Phipps S, et al. Using problem-solving skills training to reduce negative affectivity in mothers of children with newly diagnosed cancer: report of a multisite randomized trial. *J Consult Clin Psychol.* 2005;73:272.

61. De Benedetta G, Bolognini I, D'Ovidio S, Pinto A. Cancer and anorexia nervosa in the adolescence: a family-based systemic intervention. *Int J Fam Med.* 2011;2011:769–869.

62. Mattsson E, Ringner A, Ljungman G, von Essen L Positive and negative consequences with regard to cancer during adolescence: experiences two years after diagnosis. *Psychooncology.* 2007;16:1003–1009.

63. Wallace ML, Harcourt D, Rumsey N, Foot A. Managing appearance changes resulting from cancer treatment: resilience in adolescent females. *J Psychosoc Oncol.* 2007;16:1019–1027.

CHAPTER 13

AGE-RELATED CONSIDERATIONS FOR TREATING BODY IMAGE ISSUES IN CANCER PATIENTS (OLDER ADULTS)

Tammy A. Schuler, Andy Roth, and Jimmie Holland

PURPOSE AND OVERVIEW

"To lose confidence in one's body is to lose confidence in oneself."

—*Simone de Beauvoir*

An understanding of the relationship between cancer and body image is integral to oncology clinical care and research. The impact of body image distress on emotional distress, sexual functioning, and quality of life (QoL) outcomes is well-documented. This chapter describes complex interactions of cancer and body image in older women and men (defined as 65 years and older) and provides clinical recommendations for approaching body image concerns in this group, about which less is known. Improving our knowledge in this area is important as more than half of all cancers occur in patients 65 years and older.[1]

As limited work in body image and related constructs has been done for certain cancer sites,[2] and as different diagnostic sites are linked with variable biopsychosocial histories and postdiagnostic trajectories, we divide the chapter broadly by diagnosis (and gender as appropriate). We bring attention to both patient groups for which body image is frequently studied (e.g., patients with breast cancer)[3] and those for which it is less studied (e.g., patients with bladder or gastric cancers). Finally, as body image symptoms are identified as some of the most distressing in cancer and palliative care populations worldwide,[4] care was taken to include relevant research from all over the globe. In addition to research findings, we offer anecdotal commentary from our experiences in working with older patients.

HYPOTHESES ON THE POTENTIAL IMPACT OF CANCER DIAGNOSIS ON BODY IMAGE ACROSS THE LATTER PART OF THE LIFESPAN

As described in previous chapters, body image is a multidimensional construct involving thoughts, emotions, and behaviors related to the entire body and its functioning.[5] Cash's model delineates attitudes that impact overall body image, including body image evaluation (i.e., the degree to which one is satisfied with one's appearance and whether there is a discrepancy between self-perceived physical characteristics and desired characteristics), and body image investment (i.e., the importance one places on appearance).[6]

By far, the majority of body image studies among the general population have drawn samples from healthy college students. The smaller collection of literature that describes body image across the lifespan notes that one might expect the marked changes in appearance across the adult lifespan to lead to concomitant changes in body image. However, reports in the literature with regards to body image and aging are mixed. While some facets of body image may change across time, others appear to remain stable. For example, cross-sectional data from women ages 20 to 84 have indicated that body dissatisfaction (i.e., body image evaluation)[6] is remarkably stable across the adult lifespan. In contrast, for women, other thoughts and behaviors such as self-objectification, habitual body monitoring, appearance anxiety, disordered eating, and the importance of body shape, weight, and appearance (i.e., body image investment)[6] seems to decrease with aging.[7,8]

As some of the attitudes that impact overall body image change across the lifespan, we hypothesized that cancer and its treatment would interact differently with body image at different points during the lifespan. We believed that this phenomenon could occur for several different reasons:

1. *"I don't recognize the stooped-over body looking back at me from store windows, but I am happy that the figure is alive enough to look back."* As shown, some body image-related attitudes and behaviors tend to evolve in general as people grow older.[7,8] In contrast, anthropologist Sharon Kaufman writes about an "ageless" core identity that holds throughout life and irrespective of events, writing about the "me" that integrates the past and present, bringing comfort and a sense of continuity.[9]

2. Different cohorts or generations may be exposed to different historical and proximal factors that would lead them to relate differently to body image than other cohorts or generations.[6] Social media is a relevant example. Many individuals are

exposed to social media as young adults today, but previous generations were not exposed to social media as young adults. It is thought that social media can significantly influence body image concerns though social comparisons, transportation, and peer normative processes.[10]

3. Younger cancer patients are thought to experience greater distress from cancer and its treatment than older patients, both at diagnosis/initial treatment and across the survivorship period.[11] However, it should be noted that supporting evidence has been equivocal, as some research groups have reported that cancer experiences may induce a similar level of distress across the lifespan.[12] At least one study reported that perceived changes in body image following diagnosis did not differ in younger versus older gynecologic cancer patients,[13] although we note that studies contrasting body image in younger patients versus patients aged 65 years and older were infrequent at the time of our literature review.

    In addition, Kaur and colleagues' retrospective chart review of mental health concerns among cancer patients indicated complexities in the distress experiences of cancer patients across the lifespan. While both younger and older groups reported high levels of distress, body image disturbances and self-blame tended to be common in the younger sample. By contrast, difficulties adjusting to cancer, sleep disturbances, and reminisces of the past and existential concerns tended to be common in the older sample.[14]

4. Some cancers with treatments that tend to drastically alter physical appearance, such as penile or gastric cancer, are more prevalent in patients aged 65 years and older.[15]

5. Medical providers sometimes approach cancer and its treatment differently depending on a person's age, which may have consequences for body image. For example, women with breast cancer who are 60+ are sometimes not offered the option of breast reconstruction. This practice may be due to a number of factors, including physician/surgeon bias regarding the safety or relevance of breast reconstruction in older women.[16]

In general, patients do not agree with this practice. In fact, Bowman and colleagues surveyed 75 older women who underwent various forms of breast reconstruction during an eight-year period.[16] Over 90% felt that age should not be a determining factor for breast reconstruction. Only 16% of patients who had a delayed reconstruction reported that the option of breast reconstruction was presented to them at diagnosis, although 100% felt that it should have been. Moreover, reviews have shown receiving treatment concordant with preferences about body image to be associated with better QoL in older women.[17] Nevertheless, women who choose breast reconstruction do tend to be younger than women who opt not to have breast reconstruction.[18] Thus, even though older patients may not opt for conserving surgery, research suggests that they still wish to be informed of their options. We also note here that large trials have indicated no survival difference for older women who undergo radical mastectomy versus breast-conserving surgery in those with histologically or cytologically confirmed operable breast cancer.[19]

CANCER AND BODY IMAGE
IN OLDER WOMEN

Most literature on body image in cancer has focused on female patients. Anecdotally, female participants of all ages in body image–focused support groups at our cancer institution regularly report relief at having an open forum to discuss body image. Although visible changes in appearance are frequently discussed, women also seem to universally note that even when their outward appearance seemed unchanged, they felt quite changed on the inside. Body image for them is not merely about outward appearance. They described an inner sense of loss of an aspect of femininity that is deeper than appearance. We did not detect these themes in many research papers during our literature review of body image in cancer patients aged 65 years and older, so we revisit these ideas at the end of the chapter when we describe future directions for research.

BREAST AND GYNECOLOGIC CANCERS

Up to one-third of breast cancer patients report body image disturbances, which tend to persist into the survivorship period.[5] In older patients, body image distress is strongly tied to surgery and reconstructive treatment. Unsurprisingly, patients treated with more conservative surgery tend to report better body image outcomes. Although research in this area has been variable and complex, older women with histologically or cytologically confirmed operable breast cancer who were more conservatively treated (tumor excision plus Tamoxifen) reported a trend toward better body image during the year after surgery compared to women who underwent radical mastectomy in one large trial.[19] Significantly better body image was present up to two years after surgery in a follow-up study.[20] In the follow-up study, body image significantly predicted two-year mental health.[20] Similar findings were reported for women in a large study of outcomes following mastectomy versus breast-conserving surgery when comparisons were cross-sectional, but the report indicated that age did not predict body image outcomes and body image did not improve across the five-year follow-up period for either treatment group.[21]

In a recent prospective study of older early stage breast cancer patients who had begun radiotherapy, axillary node dissection patients reported a notable six-point decline in body image on a breast cancer specific measure of QoL by the end of the follow-up period when radiotherapy had finished.[22] Finally, cross-sectional data from breast cancer patients, aged 60 years and older, treated at a German university hospital indicated that chemotherapy patients tended to report higher body image–related distress compared with those who had not received chemotherapy.[23] Perhaps this related to side effects of chemotherapy interfering with sexual activity.

Gynecologic cancer, while it produces no visible loss of overall external appearance, the feelings of loss of sexual options, and loss of libido and orgasm are common "invisible" losses with potent images of being no longer sexually capable. Ovarian cancer is one gynecologic cancer which is more common in older women than middle-aged or younger women.[24] A trend we noted across ovarian cancer studies was that body image distress became more apparent later in treatment. In a study of Chinese ovarian cancer patients, women reported body image disruptions both at the beginning of postsurgical chemotherapy and later in chemotherapy, but disruptions became more severe later in treatment.[25] Similarly, American gynecologic cancer patients reported significant declines in body image and other areas of health-related QoL (HRQoL) one month after surgery, but this decline persisted only among women specifically with ovarian cancer.[26] Australian ovarian cancer patients described chemotherapy-induced alopecia as an especially powerful disruptor of body image.[27]

CANCER AND BODY IMAGE IN OLDER MEN

As mentioned, much of the body image in cancer literature has focused on women and there is less discussion on men. However, cancer also takes a toll on men's lives in many ways—it threatens life, compromises QoL, and can result in physical appearance and functional changes to the body. Cancer and cancer treatment impacts work, relationships, family, and social activity for all patients. Older men, already experiencing changes in body function and image from aging, may find added distress from the consequences of cancer treatment. To put these issues in context, even healthy men may be unhappy with their body image. Gay men may be at even higher risk than straight men for developing body dissatisfaction and feel more vulnerable to social pressures regarding their appearance. To illustrate, one study reported that perceptions of media influence were higher among gay men compared with straight men and significantly mediated the relation between sexual orientation and body image concerns.[28]

Not all cancer treatments cause noticeable physical changes. However, many do. Whether in appearance or function, this secondary bodily remodeling may be temporary or permanent. Men may even feel insecure about distortions that others cannot see but which they know are there. These transformations can include loss of sexual interest; difficulty with erectile or ejaculatory function; and whether or not the man is in an active sexual relationship, interested in dating, or merely interested in masturbation. Sexual difficulties may be present in men with prostate cancer, bladder cancer, or cancer located or treated in the pelvic region.

Qualitative data regarding body image and self-esteem have indicated that men describe themselves as "abnormal," "ugly," "disgusting," "like a cripple," and a "half man," and some of them described shame, especially with a body transformation such as Peyronie's disease, a penile deformity from plaque buildup or scar tissue related to surgical procedures or injections. Many men reported that they lost their sexual confidence, interest, or ability to initiate sex with a partner. Additionally, many men expressed a sense of stigmatization and isolation. This led to difficulties in speaking about their disease with sexual partners or healthcare professionals.[29]

Nonetheless, there are few studies about how older men with cancer cope with body image changes or interventions about how to help them and the impact of changed body image on QoL. About two-thirds of 200,000 men diagnosed yearly with prostate cancer are over the age of 65; it may therefore be some indication of how older men cope with a particular cancer that has significant impact on body image, with suggestions that body image has a meaningful association with QoL for older survivors of prostate cancer.[30]

PROSTATE CANCER

"Since my prostate cancer treatment, my penis has shrunk and I can't get an erection. I don't feel, or look, like a man anymore."

"I don't go to the beach or the gym anymore—my breasts have grown so large from the hormones I take for prostate cancer. It is embarrassing to take my shirt off in public."

"My scrotum is blown up like a balloon. It is heavy and it hurts to walk around and is uncomfortable even while sitting."

The average age of onset for prostate cancer in the United States is 66 years old.[15] As it is a diagnosis conferring extended long-term survival, prostate cancer represents a significant health problem among older men. Men who pursue active treatment for prostate cancer face important psychosocial consequences of their treatment.[31] Body image is related to many of these sequelae. Unfortunately, the focus on clinical symptoms of QoL does not always spotlight attention to body image changes that adds to the burden of therapy. Clark and colleagues found that body image was a valid and reliable indicator of prostate-specific QoL in men after prostate cancer treatment.[31] Hopwood and colleagues found a significant negative relationship between body image dissatisfaction and overall QoL.[32]

Bodily changes from endocrine therapy are particularly well-recognized as impacting sexuality and masculinity.[33] Adjuvant androgen deprivation therapy (ADT) is associated with depression, sleep problems, worse QoL, and altered self body image in prostate cancer patients.[34–37] Another study reported no difference in QOL based on ADT status but noted a significant negative correlation between body image dissatisfaction and QoL.[38]

Regret can be related to treatment decisions and outcome in terms of QoL. Among men studied who had been treated with either surgical castration or chemical castration for metastatic prostate cancer, most reported complications of hot flashes, nausea, and erectile dysfunction, yet most were satisfied with their treatment decisions. However, 23% expressed regret about those treatment decisions. Regretful men more frequently reported having surgical (vs. chemical) castration, and nausea in the past week, but less frequently reported erectile dysfunction. Regretful men indicated poorer scores on every measure of generic and prostate cancer-related QoL.[39] When looking at men receiving ADT versus those who did not, a significant difference in body image dissatisfaction existed. No relationship was identified between age and body image dissatisfaction or between duration of therapy and body image dissatisfaction. A significant positive relationship was found between body mass index and body image dissatisfaction for the sample overall. A greater degree of body image dissatisfaction existed in the men who received ADT as compared to those who were ADT naïve, perhaps indicating that any significant change in body image could impact dissatisfaction in treatment choice.[35]

TESTICULAR AND PENILE CANCER

Though germ cell cancers are thought to be a disease of younger men, about 7% of cases occur in men 55+. Men with germ cell tumors undergoing orchiectomy may have body image issues related to look and feel of their testes afterwards. More than one-quarter of germ cell tumor patients wish to have a testicular prosthesis. Overall satisfaction with implants is high in more than 80% of men. Specific items of dissatisfaction include shape, size, and consistency of the implant and inconvenient high position of the implant within the scrotum. Appropriate preoperative counseling to inform the patient of the effects of the procedure and possible body image-relevant sequelae is important.[40] Seventeen percent of the long-term testicular cancer survivors reported changes in body image significantly associated with sexual dysfunction. Yet, when comparing treatments, only the retroperitoneal lymph node dissection was associated with sexual dysfunction in the form of ejaculatory dysfunction.[41] Thus, in this study, body image changes could not be fully accounted for by ejaculatory dysfunction. In a study of older men with penile cancer undergoing penile-sparing surgery versus partial penectomy and lymphadenectomy, partial penectomy and lymphadenectomy were associated with problems with orgasm, body image, life interference, and urination.[42]

CANCER AND BODY IMAGE IN OLDER PERSONS OF ANY SEX OR GENDER

COLORECTAL AND ANAL CANCER

Although recent findings show that the average age of diagnosis for colorectal cancer may be decreasing in the United States,[43] the average age of diagnosis in 2016 was 72.[15] The diagnosis and treatment of colorectal cancer entails detailed discussions of bodily functions, invasive procedures, and a reorientation of life around bowel habit. Furthermore, people with stomas undergo a second experience of toilet training to adapt to a stoma, which is embarrassing. Inability to assure that "accidents" or uncontrollable noises from the stoma do not happen in a public place make it difficult to feel secure in accepting social invitations. Narrative interviews with colorectal cancer patients indicate embarrassment in the loss of dignity, privacy, independence, and sexual confidence as well as a compromised ability to work, travel, and socialize. Body image loss has been shown to be a significant predictor of adjustment among Chinese colostomy patients.[44] It is important for the oncology treatment team to be aware of these sensitivities and reactions.[45] Ostomy nurses and support groups provide important practical help, especially for the person learning to navigate stomas.

A prospective analysis of colorectal cancer patients assessed within nine weeks of surgery and again at the end of adjuvant treatment indicated that those who received stomas had poorer body image, which worsened over time. Although there were no differences between stoma groups on anxiety or depressive symptoms, those who received a late stoma were most depressed. Body image was a strong predictor of initial levels of anxiety, depression, and distress and subsequent anxiety and distress. For rectal cancer patients with poorly functioning loop ileostomies, reversing the ileostomy resulted in improvements across many HRQoL domains, but this was not the case for body image. Moreover, there was a significant negative correlation between defecation-related problems, global QoL, and body image.[46] These results underscore the importance of assessing and treating body image disturbance in colorectal patients who receive a stoma.[47,48] This general result of patients with stomas showing greater problems with decreasing body image, feeling unattractive, experiencing discomfort in clothing, and suffering emotional distress and difficulties with sexual functioning across time compared with non-stoma patients has been replicated across numerous studies of patients in the United States and other countries[47,49–51] and unfortunately also in their caregivers.[50]

Unfortunately, body image difficulties tend to persist over time among older colorectal cancer patients undergoing radiation and chemotherapy as well.[51] In fact, body image difficulties may actually increase over time. In a study of colorectal cancer patients treated with bifractionated radiation therapy followed by surgical resection, the sexual dysfunction score increased significantly, particularly in men, and a trend toward a lower body image score was observed one year after beginning radiation.[52] Another study describing the impact of short-course radiation and long-course chemoradiation for patients with operable rectal cancer reported a similar decrease in regard to male sexual functioning and sexual enjoyment.[53] Other reports have indicated that, although male sexual problems persisted, body image returned to baseline levels in rectal cancer patients who were candidates for presurgical chemoradiotherapy one year after baseline assessment.[54] Similar findings have been shown for anal cancer patients in Germany. One study showed the global HRQoL of anal cancer patients to be generally comparable with that of the general German population, with the exception of sexual dysfunction, urological/gastrointestinal complaints, financial difficulties, fatigue, and a reduction in emotional and social well-being.[55]

GASTRIC CANCER

The average age of diagnosis for stomach cancer is 69 years old.[56] Patients with gastric cancer also experience significant body image disturbances. Loss of the social interactions around food, meals, and celebratory events become sad losses of sociability. Fears of nausea, inability to eat, or spitting up or drooling saliva are dreaded occasional side effects. Compared with healthy controls, Korean gastric cancer patients who underwent open distal subtotal gastrectomy showed QoL deterioration in the 36 months afterward, which was thought to be due to financial difficulties, eating restrictions, and body image concerns.[57] In a follow-up study of the same patients, five-year survivors still showed worse QoL compared to the control group in terms of functioning, physical symptoms, financial difficulties, and body image.[58] Functional status may, in particular, impact body image outcomes in gastric cancer patients. In northeast Iran, upper-gastrointestinal cancer patients admitted to the oncology/radiotherapy departments were assessed for HRQoL. Patients who had the ability to care for themselves had better HRQoL across many domains, including body image.[59]

Although more research is needed, body image disturbances may be more universal, regardless of surgery type, in gastric cancer patients compared with other oncology populations who undergo appearance-altering surgeries (e.g., breast and colorectal). In a different study of Korean gastric cancer patients, patients with total gastrectomy reported worse QoL in terms of functioning and physical symptoms than those with subtotal gastrectomy during the follow-up. However, all patients reported problems with fatigue, digestive symptoms, cognitive functioning, and body image which persisted at one year.[60]

BLADDER CANCER

The average age of bladder cancer diagnosis in the United States is 73.[15] Shame and embarrassment may affect patients who need to deal with cystostomy or who have to self-catheterize several times a day, which limits activities substantially. Both men and women suffer from fears of spillage of urine from bags which are strapped to the leg. Patients have described changes in body function, body image, sexual relationships, and intimacy as particularly challenging.[61]

In one study, bladder-cancer patients reported themselves to be more likely to curtail their social activities, compared with the patients with incontinence or bladder dysfunction, following ileal conduit urinary diversion. Appliance-related problems were described by half of the patients who reported decreased social activity, and one-third of the patients considered accidental leakage or fear of such leakage as the most negative aspect of surgery. Factors related to an altered body image were the most common negative aspect reported by females.[62] In this same sample of patients who underwent ileal conduit urinary diversion, females with the diagnosis of incontinence or bladder dysfunction (i.e., not cancer) were actually more likely to increase their sexual activity after the operation whereas females with bladder cancer did not.[63] However, systematic review data (1996–2008) examining the impact of cystectomy and urinary diversion types on QoL indicated that family, relationships, health, and finance tended to be the most important determinants of QoL, not body image.[64]

LUNG CANCER

About two out of three people diagnosed with lung cancer are aged 65 years and older. The average age at the time of diagnosis is about 70.[65] After the association with smoking and lung cancer was established in the late 1960s, the first question asked of patients with lung cancer was "Did you smoke?" The self-image of a person was already affected by guilt, despite the fact that the danger of smoking had not previously been widely recognized and most adults smoked. Medical providers have noted over the years, "We don't ask patients with heart disease 'did you eat a lot of red meat?' Why do we single out cancer patients to blame?" Thus, a lung cancer diagnosis has for decades been complicated by stigma, shame, and blame for a particular behavior—smoking—which is taken to imply lack of willpower and weakness of character, and hence the implication that "it is your fault," which adds to the burden. Today, more people who *never* smoked are getting lung cancer, and they find themselves defensively saying "and I never smoked!"

For those with lung cancer, stigma has a powerful, deleterious impact on body image.[66] Stigma has been shown to be higher in men than women and higher in those with lung cancer compared with other patient groups—perhaps even more than those with head and neck cancers. It is also more profound in people have been highly disfigured by cancer and/or its treatment. On top of being a stigmatizing diagnosis, lung cancer is a site of cancer that is known to have a poor prognosis. Thus, due to a combination of factors, many patients struggle with "whom do I tell?" since responses of others can be awkward and hurtful. Similar to ovarian cancer, the physical body of the lung cancer patient may look normal but an internal organ—what we use to breath with—is damaged, in actuality, and so is body image. Decreased functional status is known to affect body image in other oncology populations,[59] and it is thus possible that symptoms such as breathlessness, and decreased ability to engage in daily activities, increase body image distress in lung cancer patients as well. Feelings of vulnerability are great and can be heightened by what people say, such as "how are you, *really*?" Many patients say "I feel people will pity me and so I don't tell acquaintances—I only tell my family."

HEAD AND NECK CANCERS

Head and neck cancers are most frequently diagnosed in men aged 50 and older.[67] The body image impact of head and neck cancer persists in both older men and women, as the physical sequelae of treatment tends to be more externally observable as scars and permanently altered anatomy. Cigarette smoking, cigars, and chewing tobacco increase risk, leading to similar issues of stigma, shame, and blame as those experienced by lung cancer patients. These difficulties are especially profound in people who were highly disfigured by the cancer and/or its treatment.

Another stigmatized group, emerging more recently, are patients with head and neck cancer related to human papilloma viruses (HPV). A rise in incidence of HPV-mediated oropharyngeal squamous cell cancer in men younger than age 50 years (who have no history of alcohol or tobacco use) has been recorded during recent years.[68] This oral transmission through sex is becoming more widely known. We theorize that, as this information becomes more common knowledge among the general public, this specific group of patients may also find themselves grappling with additional stigma, shame, and blame related to a sexually transmitted disease–mediated cancer diagnosis.

Studies indicate that up to 75% of head and neck cancer patients undergoing surgical treatment acknowledge concerns or embarrassment about one or more types of bodily changes at some point following diagnosis.[69,70] Social problems are particularly frequent in head and neck cancer patients for whom very visible portions of the face, eyes, head, and neck are resected.[71] In US veterans treated for head and neck cancer and diagnosed an average of 30 months prior, most reported sexual arousal problems, over half did not participate in sexual intercourse, and over half had orgasmic problems. Notably, there was no correlation between sexual functioning and performance status or severity of disfigurement. Moreover, patients younger than 65 years of age had more advanced disease, lower performance status, and significantly poorer sexual functioning; those older than 65 years were more satisfied with their sexual partner and current sexual functioning.[72] We note that benefit finding has been found to buffer stigma's deleterious effects in lung and head and neck cancer patients.[73]

Poignantly, perhaps more telling than our review of the literature, head and neck cancer patients have told us:

> *"Kids look at me with this electric vocalizer and they think I am some video game character."*
>
> *"My face is central to my interactions with people and society. I am grateful for the remarkable reconstruction that lets me teach my class every day."*
>
> *"I lost my left eye to cancer and I could never feel the same confidence in looking at people. The sense that the artificial eye would fall out worried me as a teacher."*
>
> *"I was embarrassed by the total paralysis of one side of my face. I could not smile or talk cleanly."*
>
> *"I lost part of my tongue and people have trouble understanding me now. It is very frustrating."*
>
> *"Losing my voice box was frightening and devastating, but I have learned to use my device and it works though people do stare at me."*
>
> *"I feel ugly when I think about the reconstruction I have had of my jaw. Though the plastic surgery was excellent, I feel it has changed my face, something deep in my feeling about myself."*
>
> *"It is difficult to look into a mirror. I can't imagine what others are thinking when they see my deformed face and neck. I don't want to know what others think. I look broken. I feel broken."*

MULTIPLE MYELOMA

In a research study of patients with multiple myeloma, patients diagnosed with multiple myeloma exhibited more concerns about body integrity than at-risk patients. Moreover, women reported more concerns about physical appearance than men. The researchers also noted that body integrity concerns were related to what they referred to as compulsive personality characteristics, whereas concerns about appearance were associated with histrionic personality characteristics. Higher body image investment (importance placed on appearance) was related to heightened symptoms of fatigue and stress.[74]

Anecdotally, older women with multiple myeloma have described to us that they were acutely aware of appearance and functional changes as a result of the disease. Reduced ability to walk, to climb stairs, and to use the subway or bus are real problems in sustaining work roles for older patients, which is often financially important. However, the women felt that the myeloma-related appearance and functional changes were less important to their happiness than other aspects of their lives, such as their families, friends, and activities they were still physically able to do. They noted to us that they placed less importance on appearance and function than they may have when they were younger.

Limb amputation, which can occur in the context of multiple myeloma is, in particular, a long and difficult adjustment process leading to changes in self-identity.[75] For patients who have had a limb amputation and use a prosthesis, body image has been shown to have particularly strong correlations with prosthesis satisfaction.[76] Individuals with amputations who engage in regular physical activity also tend to report better body image,[77] though we suspect that other forms of behavioral activation (such as going to a movie with a friend or taking a book to a coffee shop) would also lead to better body image among individuals with amputations.

ALOPECIA AND OTHER TREATMENT SIDE EFFECTS

"I think the hardest thing about breast cancer was losing my long, carefully grown locks. They were the signature of my appearance. I look in the mirror and see a different person and everyone immediately knows that [this person has] cancer."

"Thank God for the wigs of today, which are fabulous. Few people know I have cancer and the wig helps me keep it a secret. I don't want their pity."

"As a man, I think that baldness has less negative meaning than in women, but I still was not ready to lose my hair."

In one study, older men and women showed no differences in coping with alopecia from cancer or cancer treatment, although the body image of the male and female patients who had partial or complete alopecia was poorer than that in patients who had no alopecia; psychological well-being of women was lower than that in men, perhaps because the incidence of alopecia was higher in women.[78] When younger men and women with cancer were studied, hair loss made many of them acutely aware of their vulnerability and visibility as a "cancer patient." Both men and women described a sense of strangeness or shock when they lost their hair and experienced various negative reactions when people assumed their hairless appearance was a lifestyle choice. The most striking contrast in their accounts was that women spoke solely of the loss of hair from the head and face above the eye line, and men spoke about losing hair from wider body surfaces.[79] Anecdotally, many women also complain of loss of hair over the pubic area as a concern in sexual intimacy.

"Because of my pelvic surgery my leg is swollen from lymphedema. I'm supposed to wear a compression stocking—but I won't in the summer because it is too hot."

As described in detail in these quotes, surgical or radiation procedures leave scars, alter or destroy body parts, and cause lymphedema.[80] Chemotherapy and other medications such as steroids, pain medications, antidepressants, and mood stabilizers (to name only a few) can change appetite, taste, muscle tone, and body weight. These changes lead older patients to be more self-conscious and change routine activities and social interactions, leading to increased emotional distress.

A common sign of advancing cancer is loss of weight, strength, and appetite and heightened fatigue. Patients sense the association with poor prognosis and often do not want family members or others to see them in a compromised state. Research indicates that cachexia in particular has a detrimental effect on QoL and is an indicator of poor prognosis. Patients frequently discussed repeated attempts to re-adapt to disruptions of self caused by an altered body image due to cachexia.[81] Anecdotally, patients have lamented to us that they wonder where the body they had gotten to know over the last 70 or 80 years has gone.

"It doesn't feel like the same body though I know I am still me."

RECOMMENDATIONS

Based on our clinical observations and our review of the literature, we offer the following recommendations to mitigate the burden of body image distress in older patients:

1. Prompt providers to examine biases that may have regarding certain procedures for older patients when age does not actually impact the procedure's clinical outcome. To illustrate, recall that breast cancer patients aged 60+ are sometimes not offered the option of breast reconstruction.[16] However, 100% of older women surveyed felt that the option should have been offered.[16] If the option of breast cancer reconstruction is clinically indicated and deemed safe, it should be offered to older patients. We note once again that large trials have indicated no survival difference for older women who undergo radical mastectomy versus breast-conserving surgery in those with histologically or cytologically confirmed operable breast cancer.[19]

2. In line with the first recommendation, providers should ensure that older patients are informed as to all of their treatment and reconstructive options as well as each option's potential impact on body image via changes in appearance and function.

3. Providers should be trained to appropriately detect and communicate about body image concerns.[81] As patients may not volunteer this information, providers should have an awareness of which patient groups are at heightened risk for body image issues and to gently query these groups.[5] Patients at particular risk are those whose disease or treatment cause significant changes in physical appearance or functioning.[5] Examples include breast cancer patients who undergo radical mastectomy, colorectal patients who receive a stoma, and gastric cancer patients. Fingeret and colleagues also recommend asking about body image in patients treated for cancers affecting sexual organs (e.g., ovarian, penile), as these have strong symbolic significance related to masculinity and femininity.[5]

    Providers should also recall that some patient groups, such as those with ovarian cancer and colorectal cancer, tend to report the onset or worsening of body image difficulties as treatment progresses. Thus, it is important to ask questions about body image difficulties not only at diagnosis but also across the treatment and survivorship period.

    Unfortunately, some patients perceive communication difficulties with their providers. In a study of German rectal cancer patients, over one-third indicated that some aspect of the communication from their physician was unclear and nearly two-thirds wished to speak more with their physician. Younger patients and those in large hospitals were most likely to report communication difficulties. Ultimately, patients reporting unclear communication also reported worse body image.[82] Research of patients who underwent curative rectal cancer surgery indicated that patients seldom remembered being told about sexual risks preoperatively and most had never been treated for sexual dysfunction.[83]

    However, the beneficial effects of open patient–physician communication are well-documented.[61] Fingeret and colleagues emphasized the utility of patient-centered approaches to challenging conversations about body image.[5] The authors delineated patient-centered approaches as including the normalization of body image difficulties, asking patients about specific concerns using open-ended questions (i.e., questions that prompt dialogue and elicit a response other than yes or no), asking patients about the impact of body image problems on their day-to-day lives, and actively listening to patient responses.[5] It is also imperative to recall that these can be difficult topics. Thus, allowing for silence to give patients time to gather their thoughts and speak can be a poignant communication technique as well.

4. Providers should use patient-reported outcome measures as another tool to prompt conversation. Another study of colorectal cancer patients underscored the importance of QoL assessment to detect problems that could otherwise go unnoticed in the routine of follow-up care. Specifically, the researchers indicated that assessment would be useful to detect sensitive issues which may impact body image, such as defecation-related problems, sexual dysfunction, and emotional distress.[84] The literature emphasizes screening for body image distress with self-report measures as early as possible, particularly as patients may be reluctant to approach their healthcare team with such issues.[85] Care should be taken to select assessment tools which have empirical support for validity and reliability.

5. Providers should ensure that older patients who experience body image distress are referred to treatment and/or provided with other resources as appropriate. We underscore that this should be in addition to physical and occupational rehabilitation. Fingeret and colleagues reported that approximately one-third of patients undergoing reconstructive surgery were interested in obtaining counseling or additional information to assist with body image distress and that concern about future appearance changes was the single best predictor of counseling enrollment.[5]

Current scientific research most strongly supports the use of cognitive-behavioral therapy (CBT) interventions for addressing body image concerns, though most interventions have been tested in patients with breast cancer and in either a couples or group format.[5] We have no reason to believe that the basic tenets of CBT would be different for older patients compared with younger patients. Physical activity interventions are another format with some support in older cancer patients,[86] though not to the same degree as CBT. Older breast cancer patients have expressed preferences for physical activities that are gentle and tailored to age and cancer-related abilities, which involve other older breast cancer survivors, and which feature an instructor that is knowledgeable. Patients from the same study also identified body image difficulties as a specific factor which affects physical activity.[87]

Our anecdotal experiences are that older men with cancer-related bodily changes will feel better if they can start an exercise regimen and begin to feel stronger and more connected to their bodies. Walking, biking, swimming, elliptical or rowing, or easy strength training, perhaps with an experienced trainer who is used to helping older men after cancer treatment, would be a good option. Men have also reported to us anecdotally that they are able to see improvement in muscle tone after starting exercise programs even when they are receiving ADT.

For those patients experiencing sexual dysfunction after cancer treatment, seeing an experienced therapist familiar with cancer issues, either alone or with a partner, may be helpful. Sexual intimacy is more than just intercourse. Using sensate function techniques to focus initially on bodily touching without erotic expectations, including kissing, massage, and showers together, can be fun places to start and help reinsert intimacy into a relationship.[88]

Other types of interventions found to improve body image outcomes include education, cosmetic rehabilitation for oral cancer patients with flap reconstruction, beauty treatments for patients during the first week after breast cancer surgery, and massage therapy.[5]

Case Study

Ms. P is a 73-year-old advertising executive who developed a melanoma on the retina which required the total removal of her eye and replacement with an artificial eye. She finds the artificial eye uncomfortable and required several visits to reduce the pain and discomfort from wearing it. Ms. P. has to hold important meetings with clients and her staff and she reports constant anxiety from thinking that the eye might fall out in a social situation, which would embarrass her very much. She indicates that it had, in fact, fallen out once when she was sitting at home. Ms. P cannot overcome the feeling that people detect the difference between her two eyes, particularly as she moves her eyes from side to side. She reports thinking that there is something macabre and bizarre about the false eye which simply changes her sense of self, even though family and friends assure her that people do not see the difference. Her image of her own face is changed in a strange and irrevocable way by the artificial eye. She says, "I know it makes no sense, but I don't feel myself when I look people in the eye. It is as if a key part of my identity has been changed forever".

Ms. P. is seen in supportive psychotherapy. Attention is paid first to her thoughts and subsequent anxiety regarding what would happen if the artificial eye fell out—including realistic thoughts (e.g., the eye could fall out) and unrealistic thoughts (e.g., the eye is constantly likely to fall out at any moment, she will be harshly judged if the eye fell out, people can detect the difference between her two eyes). Consultation with and education by the prosthesis expert also helps ease Ms. P.'s anxiety. Ms. P. is able to vocalize her concerns about being the same person since the eye brings up issues from her childhood in which she was often criticized by her mother that she was not an attractive child. She gains in confidence across a year of sessions, reports less anxiety and a more stabilized sense of self, and shows improved adjustment to the prosthesis

CONCLUSIONS

In summary, it was our determination that the empirical literature does not (yet) provide enough evidence that attitudes affecting body image in cancer patients aged 65 years and older are unequivocally different than attitudes affecting body image in younger patients. However, there appears to be a trend, based on our clinical experiences and the research we reviewed, which parallels findings regarding attitudes toward body image in healthy populations[6–8]—namely that body image investment (i.e., the importance placed on appearance) decreases with age. In addition, anecdotes from our patients indicate that distress from internal changes that occur with such cancers as ovarian, uterine, and prostate may have a profound impact despite external normal appearance.

Most empirical studies of body image in older patients focus on body image outcomes following surgical and reconstructive treatment. Ultimately, patients who undergo treatments that drastically alter appearance or function tend to report worse body image outcomes than patients who undergo procedures which less drastically impact appearance or function. However, these findings appear to be universal across patient groups, regardless of age. It was also our observation that same-study age comparisons contrasting younger patient groups with patient groups aged 65 years and older were infrequent in the literature.

Future research should thus focus on the impact of other variables on body image in older cancer patients, comparisons between younger and older patient populations, the body image sequelae of internal changes (such as with ovarian, uterine, and prostate cancer), and the building of paradigms that explains age-related body image differences in oncology patients across the lifespan. We believe that mixed-methods research (which includes qualitative research) will be important to elucidate details that are not captured with paper-and-pencil measures.

Finally, additional evidence is also needed to support interventions targeting body image difficulties in older cancer patients. Replication studies of CBT interventions may be particularly appropriate as CBT interventions have received the most empirical support in other patient groups. Physical activity interventions should be appropriately tailored to age.

ACKNOWLEDGMENTS

We would like to acknowledge the medical librarians at Memorial Sloan Kettering Cancer Center for their assistance with literature search. We would also like to thank Rachael Goldberg, LCSW, and Meredith Cammarata, LCSW, for their commentary regarding their clinical experiences in patient body image groups at Memorial Sloan Kettering Cancer Center. Finally, we are grateful for expert comments from Anna O. Levin, PhD, at the University of California San Francisco.

REFERENCES

1. Howlader N, Noone A, Krapcho M, et al. SEER Cancer Statistics Review (CSR), 1975–2014. National Cancer Institute; April 2017. https://seer.cancer.gov/csr/1975_2014/.

2. Flynn KE, Jeffery DD, Keefe FJ, et al. Sexual functioning along the cancer continuum: focus group results from the Patient-Reported Outcomes Measurement Information System (PROMIS). *Psychooncology.* 2011;20(4):378–386. doi:10.1002/pon.1738

3. Rhondali W, Chisholm GB, Filbet M, et al. Screening for body image dissatisfaction in patients with advanced cancer: a pilot study. *J Palliat Med.* 2015;18(2):151–156. doi:10.1089/jpm.2013.0588.

4. Lazenby M, Sebego M, Swart NC, Lopez L, Peterson K. Symptom burden and functional dependencies among cancer patients in Botswana suggest a need for palliative care nursing. *Cancer Nurs.* 2016;39(1):E29–E38. doi:10.1097/NCC.0000000000000249

5. Fingeret MC, Teo I, Epner DE. Managing body image difficulties of adult cancer patients: lessons from available research. *Cancer.* 2014;120(5):633–641. doi:10.1002/cncr.28469

6. Cash TF. Cognitive-behavioral perspectives on body image. In: Cash T, Smolak L, eds. *Body Image: A Handbook of Science, Practice, and Prevention.* New York: Guilford Press; 2011:39–47.

7. Tiggemann M, Lynch JE. Body image across the life span in adult women: The role of self-objectification. *Dev Psychol*. 2001;37(2):243–253. doi:10.1037/0012-1649.37.2.243

8. Tiggemann M. Body image across the adult life span: stability and change. *Body Image*. 2004;1(1):29–41. doi:10.1016/S1740-1445(03)00002-0

9. Kaufman S. *The Ageless Self: Sources of Meaning in Late Life*. Madison: University of Wisconsin Press; 1986.

10. Perloff RM. Social media effects on young women's body image concerns: theoretical perspectives and an agenda for research. *Sex Roles*. 2014;71(11–12):363–377. doi:10.1007/s11199-014-0384-6

11. Härtl K, Schennach R, Müller M, et al. Quality of life, anxiety, and oncological factors: a follow-up study of breast cancer patients. *Psychosomatics*. 2010;51:112–123. doi:10.1016/S0033-3182(10)70671-X

12. Pashak TJ, Kracen A, Handal PJ. Developmental patterns in distress response to cancer experiences. *Psychooncology*. 2013;22(S2):78. doi:10.1111/j.1099-1611.2012.03245

13. Nordin AJ, Dixon S, Chinn DJ, et al. Attitudes to radical gynecological oncology surgery in the elderly: a pilot study. *Int J Gynecol Cancer*. 2000;10(4):323–329. doi:10.1046/j.1525-1438.2000.010004323.x

14. Kaur D, Chaturvedi H, Anand AK, et al. To understand mental health related issues and the importance of regular counselling in medical management of pediatric and geriatric patients undergoing cancer treatment: experience from a super speciality private hospital in North India. *Psychooncology*. 2011;20:207–208.

15. Siegel RL, Miller KD, Jemal A. Cancer statistics, 2016. *CA Cancer J Clin*. 2016;66(1):7–30. doi:10.3322/caac.21332

16. Bowman CC, Lennox PA, Clugston PA, Courtemanche DJ. Breast reconstruction in older women: Should age be an exclusion criterion? *Plast Reconstr Surg*. 2006;118:16–22. doi:10.1097/01.prs.0000220473.94654.a4

17. Mandelblatt J, Figueiredo M, Cullen J. Outcomes and quality of life following breast cancer treatment in older women: When, why, how much, and what do women want? *Health Qual Life Outcomes*. 2003;1:45. doi:10.1186/1477-7525-1-45

18. Boughey JC, Hoskin TL, Hartmann LC, et al. Impact of reconstruction and reoperation on long-term patient-reported satisfaction after contralateral prophylactic mastectomy. *Ann Surg Oncol*. 2015;22(2):401–408. doi:10.1245/s10434-014-4053-3

19. De Haes JCJM, Curran D, Aaronson NK, Fentiman IS. Quality of life in breast cancer patients aged over 70 years, participating in the EORTC 10850 randomised clinical trial. *Eur J Cancer*. 2003;39(7):945–951. doi:10.1016/S0959-8049(03)00149-7

20. Figueiredo MI, Cullen J, Hwang YT, Rowland JH, Mandelblatt JS. Breast cancer treatment in older women: Does getting what you want improve your long-term body image and mental health? *J Clin Oncol*. 2004;22(19):4002–4009. doi:10.1200/JCO.2004.07.030

21. Engel J, Kerr J, Schlesinger-Raab A, Sauer H, Hölzel D. Quality of life following breast-conserving therapy or mastectomy: results of a 5-year prospective study. *Breast J*. 2004;10(3):223–231. doi:10.1111/j.1075-122X.2004.21323.x

22. Arraras J, Manterola A, Asin G, et al. Quality of life in elderly patients with localized breast cancer treated with radiotherapy: a prospective study. *Breast*. 2016;26:46–53. doi:10.1016/j.breast.2015.12.008

23. Wuerstlein R, Burgmann M, Lotz A, et al. Life satisfaction and life quality in the elderly patient with breast cancer. *Oncol Res Treat*. 2016;39:51.

24. Mellon A. Vulval cancer. *Aust J Cancer Nurs*. 2009;10(2):7–11.

25. Huang J, Gu L, Zhang L, Lu X, Zhuang W, Yang Y. Symptom clusters in ovarian cancer patients with chemotherapy after surgery: a longitudinal survey. *Cancer Nurs*. 2016;39(2):106–116. doi:10.1097/NCC.0000000000000252

26. Minig L, Vélez JI, Trimble EL, Biffi R, Maggioni A, Jeffery DD. Changes in short-term health-related quality of life in women undergoing gynecologic oncologic laparotomy: an associated factor analysis. *Support Care Cancer*. 2013;21(3):715–726. doi:10.1007/s00520-012-1571-z

27. Jayde V, Boughton M, Blomfield P. The experience of chemotherapy-induced alopecia for Australian women with ovarian cancer. *Eur J Cancer Care*. 2013;22(4):503–512. doi:10.1111/ecc.12056

28. Carper TLM, Negy C, Tantleff-Dunn S. Relations among media influence, body image, eating concerns, and sexual orientation in men: a preliminary investigation. *Body Image*. 2010;7(4):301–309. doi:10.1016/j.bodyim.2010.07.002

29. Terrier JE, Nelson CJ. Psychological aspects of Peyronie's disease. *Transl Androl Urol*. 2016;5(3):290–295. doi:10.21037/tau.2016.05.14

30. Taylor-Ford M, Meyerowitz BE, D'Orazio LM, Christie KM, Gross ME, Agus DB. Body image predicts quality of life in men with prostate cancer. *Psychooncology*. 2013;22(4):756–761. doi:10.1002/pon.3063

31. Clark JA, Wray N, Brody B, Ashton C, Giesler B, Watkins H. Dimensions of quality of life expressed by men treated for metastatic prostate cancer. *Soc Sci Med*. 1997;45(8):1299–1309. doi:10.1016/S0277-9536(97)00058-0

32. Hopwood P, Fletcher I, Lee A, Al Ghazal S. A body image scale for use with cancer patients. *Eur J Cancer*. 2001;37(2):189–197. doi:10.1016/S0959-8049(00)00353-1

33. Ervik B, Asplund K. Dealing with a troublesome body: a qualitative interview study of men's experiences living with prostate cancer treated with endocrine therapy. *Eur J Oncol Nurs*. 2012;16(2):103–108. doi:10.1016/j.ejon.2011.04.005

34. Fowler FJ Jr, Collins MM, Corkery EW, Elliott DB, Barry MJ. The impact of androgen deprivation on quality of life after radical prostatectomy for prostate carcinoma. *Cancer*. 2002;95(2):287–295.

35. Harrington J, Jones E, Badger T. Body image perceptions in men with prostate cancer. *Oncol Nurs Forum*. 2009;36(2):167–172. doi:10.1188/09.onf.167-172

36. Driessche H, Mattelaer P, Oyen P, et al. Changes in body image in patients with prostate cancer over 2 years of treatment with a gonadotropin-releasing hormone analogue (Triptorelin): results from a Belgian non-interventional study. *Drugs Real World Outcomes*. 2016;3(2):183–190.

37. Saini A, Berruti A, Cracco C, et al. Psychological distress in men with prostate cancer receiving adjuvant androgen-deprivation therapy. *Urol Oncol*. 2011;31(3):352–358. doi:10.1016/j.urolonc.2011.02.005

38. Harrington JM, Badger TA. Body image and quality of life in men with prostate cancer. *Cancer Nurs*. 2009;32(2):E1–E7. doi:10.1097/NCC.0b013e3181982d18

39. Clark JA, Wray NP, Ashton CM. Living with treatment decisions: regrets and quality of life among men treated for metastatic prostate cancer. *J Clin Oncol*. 2001;19(1):72–80.

40. Dieckmann K-P, Anheuser P, Schmidt S, et al. Testicular prostheses in patients with testicular cancer—acceptance rate and patient satisfaction. *BMC Urol*. 2015;15(1):16. doi:10.1186/s12894-015-0010-0

41. Rossen P, Pedersen AF, Zachariae R, Von Der Maase H. Sexuality and body image in long-term survivors of testicular cancer. *Eur J Cancer*. 2012;48(4):571–578. doi:10.1016/j.ejca.2011.11.029

42. Kieffer JM, Djajadiningrat RS, van Muilekom EAM, Graafland NM, Horenblas S, Aaronson NK. Quality of life for patients treated for penile cancer. *J Urol*. 2014;192(4):1105–1110. doi:10.1016/j.juro.2014.04.014

43. Siegel R, Fedewa S, Anderson W, et al. Colorectal cancer incidence patterns in the United States, 1974–2013. *J Natl Cancer Inst*. 2017;109(8). doi:10.1093/jnci/djw322

44. Zhang J, Wong FKY, Zheng M, Hu A, Zhang H. Psychometric evaluation of the ostomy adjustment scale in Chinese cancer patients with colostomies. *Cancer Nurs*. 2015;38(5):395–405. doi:10.1097/NCC.0000000000000213

45. Dázio EMR, Sonobe HM, Zago MMF. The meaning of being a man with intestinal stoma due to colorectal cancer: an anthropological approach to masculinities. *Rev Lat Am Enfermagem*. 2009;17(5):664–669. doi:10.1590/S0104-11692009000500011

46. Camilleri-Brennan J, Steele RJC. Prospective analysis of quality of life after reversal of a defunctioning loop ileostomy. *Color Dis.* 2002;4(3):167–171. doi:10.1046/j.1463-1318.2002.00352.x

47. Ross L, Abild-Nielsen AG, Thomsen BL, Karlsen R V., Boesen EH, Johansen C. Quality of life of Danish colorectal cancer patients with and without a stoma. *Support Care Cancer.* 2007;15(5):505–513. doi:10.1007/s00520-006-0177-8

48. Sharpe L, Patel D, Clarke S. The relationship between body image disturbance and distress in colorectal cancer patients with and without stomas. *J Psychosom Res.* 2011;70(5):395–402. doi:10.1016/j.jpsychores.2010.11.003

49. Neuman HB, Patil S, Fuzesi S, et al. Impact of a temporary stoma on the quality of life of rectal cancer patients undergoing treatment. *Ann Surg Oncol.* 2011;18(5):1397–1403. doi:10.1245/s10434-010-1446-9

50. Cotrim H, Pereira G. Impact of colorectal cancer on patient and family: implications for care. *Eur J Oncol Nurs.* 2008;12(3):217–226. doi:10.1016/j.ejon.2007.11.005

51. Yang X, Li Q, Zhao H, et al. Quality of life in rectal cancer patients with permanent colostomy in Xi'an. *Afr Health Sci.* 2014;14(1):28–36. doi:10.4314/ahs.v14i1.6

52. Allal AS, Gervaz P, Gertsch P, et al. Assessment of quality of life in patients with rectal cancer treated by preoperative radiotherapy: a longitudinal prospective study. *Int J Radiat Oncol Biol Phys.* 2005;61(4):1129–1135. doi:10.1016/j.ijrobp.2004.07.726

53. McLachlan SA, Fisher RJ, Zalcberg J, et al. The impact on health-related quality of life in the first 12 months: a randomised comparison of preoperative short-course radiation versus long-course chemoradiation for T3 rectal cancer (Trans-Tasman Radiation Oncology Group Trial 01.04). *Eur J Cancer.* 2016;55:15–26.

54. Pucciarelli S, Del Bianco P, Efficace F, et al. Patient-reported outcomes after neoadjuvant chemoradiotherapy for rectal cancer: a multicenter prospective observational study. *Ann Surg.* 2011;253(1):71–77. doi:10.1097/SLA.0b013e3181fcb856

55. Welzel G, Hägele V, Wenz F, Mai SK. Quality of life outcomes in patients with anal cancer after combined radiochemotherapy. *Strahlentherapie Onkol.* 2011;187(3):175–182. doi:10.1007/s00066-010-2175-5

56. American Cancer Society. What are the key statistics about stomach cancer? https://www.cancer.org/cancer/stomach-cancer/about/key-statistics.html. Published 2017. Accessed July 1, 2017.

57. Lee SS, Chung HY, Kwon O, Yu W. Long-term shifting patterns in quality of life after distal subtotal gastrectomy: preoperative-and healthy-based interpretations. *Ann Surg.* 2014;261(6):1131–1137. doi:10.1097/SLA.0000000000000832

58. Lee SS, Chung HY, Kwon OK, Yu W. Quality of life in cancer survivors 5 years or more after total gastrectomy: a case-control study. *Int J Surg.* 2014;12(7):700–705. doi:10.1016/j.ijsu.2014.05.067

59. Esmaili RAH, Homai-Shandiz F, Motevallian A, Madjd Z, Solaymani-Dodaran M, Asadi-Lari M. Do clinical and demographic features of patients with upper-gastrointestinal cancer affect their health-related quality of life? *Int J Prev Med.* 2012;3(11):783–790.

60. Kim AR, Cho J, Hsu YJ, et al. Changes of quality of life in gastric cancer patients after curative resection: a longitudinal cohort study in Korea. *Ann Surg.* 2012;256(6):1008–1013. doi:10.1097/SLA.0b013e31827661c9

61. Fitch MI, Miller D, Sharir S, McAndrew A. Radical cystectomy for bladder cancer: a qualitative study of patient experiences and implications for practice. *Cancer Oncol Nurs J.* 2010;20(4):177–187.

62. Nordstrom G, Nyman CR, Theorell T. Psychosocial adjustment and general state of health in patients with ileal conduit urinary diversion. *Scand J Urol Nephrol.* 1992;26(2):139–147.

63. Nordstrom GM, Nyman CR. Living with a urostomy: a follow up with special regard to the peristomal-skin complications, psychosocial and sexual life. *Scand J Urol Nephrol.* 1991;138:247–251.

64. Somani BK, Gimlin D, Fayers P, N'Dow J. Quality of life and body image for bladder cancer patients undergoing radical cystectomy and urinary diversion: a prospective cohort study with a systematic review of literature. *Urology.* 2009;74:1138–1143. doi:10.1016/j.urology.2009.05.087

65. American Cancer Society. Key statistics for lung cancer. https://www.cancer.org/cancer/non-small-cell-lung-cancer/about/key-statistics.html. Published 2017. Accessed July 1, 2017.

66. Hamann HA, Ostroff JS, Marks EG, Gerber DE, Schiller JH, Lee SJC. Stigma among patients with lung cancer: a patient-reported measurement model. *Psychooncology.* 2014;23(1):81–92. doi:10.1002/pon.3371

67. National Cancer Institute. Head and neck cancers fact sheet. https://www.cancer.gov/types/head-and-neck/head-neck-fact-sheet. Published 2017. Accessed July 1, 2017.

68. Marur S, D'Souza G, Westra WH, Forastiere AA. HPV-associated head and neck cancer: a virus-related cancer epidemic. *Lancet Oncol.* 2010;11(8):781–789. doi:10.1016/S1470-2045(10)70017-6

69. Fingeret MC, Vidrine DJ, Reece GP, Gillenwater AM, Gritz ER. Multidimensional analysis of body image concerns among newly diagnosed patients with oral cavity cancer. *Head Neck.* 2010;32(3):301–309. doi:10.1002/hed.21181.

70. Fingeret MC, Yuan Y, Urbauer D, Weston J, Nipomnick S, Weber R. The nature and extent of body image concerns among surgically treated patients with head and neck cancer. *Psychooncology.* 2012;21(8):836–844. doi:10.1002/pon.1990

71. Bonanno A, Esmaeli B, Fingeret MC, Nelson D V, Weber RS. Social challenges of cancer patients with orbitofacial disfigurement. *Ophthal Plast Reconstr Surg.* 2010;26(1):18–22. doi:10.1097/IOP.0b013e3181b8e646

72. Monga U, Tan G, Ostermann HJ, Monga TN. Sexuality in head and neck cancer patients. *Arch Phys Med Rehabil.* 1997;78(3):298–304.

73. Lebel S, Castonguay M, MacKness G, Irish J, Bezjak A, Devins GM. The psychosocial impact of stigma in people with head and neck or lung cancer. *Psychooncology.* 2013;22(1):140–152. doi:10.1002/pon.2063

74. Lichtenthal WG, Cruess DG, Clark VL, Ming ME. Investment in body image among patients diagnosed with or at risk for malignant melanoma. *Body Image.* 2005;2(1):41–52. doi:10.1016/j.bodyim.2004.11.003

75. Senra H, Oliveira RA, Leal I, Vieira C. Beyond the body image: a qualitative study on how adults experience lower limb amputation. *Clin Rehabil.* 2012;26(2):180–191. doi:0.1177/0269215511410731

76. Murray CD, Fox J. Body image and prosthesis satisfaction in the lower limb amputee. *Disabil Rehabil.* 2002;24(17):925–931. doi:10.1080/09638280210150014

77. Wetterhahn KA, Hanson C, Levy CE. Effect of participation in physical activity on body image of amputees. *Am J Phys Med Rehabil.* 2002;81(3):194–201. pm:11989516

78. Can G, Demir M, Erol O, Aydiner A. A comparison of men and women's experiences of chemotherapy-induced alopecia. *Eur J Oncol Nurs.* 2013;17(3):255–260. doi:10.1016/j.ejon.2012.06.003

79. Hilton S, Hunt K, Emslie C, Salinas M, Ziebland S. Have men been overlooked? A comparison of young men and women's experiences of chemotherapy-induced alopecia. *Psychooncology.* 2008;17(6):577–583. doi:10.1002/pon.1272

80. Frid M, Strang P, Friedrichsen MJ, Johansson K. Lower limb lymphedema: experiences and perceptions of cancer patients in the late palliative stage. *J Palliat Care.* 2006;22(1):5–11.

81. Hinsley R, Hughes R. "The reflections you get": an exploration of body image and cachexia. *Int J Palliat Nurs.* 2007;13(2):84–90. doi:10.12968/ijpn.2007.13.2.23068

82. Kerr J, Engel J, Schlesinger-Raab A, Sauer H, Hölzel D. Doctor-patient communication: results of a four-year prospective study in rectal cancer patients. *Dis Colon Rectum.* 2003;46(8):1038–1046. doi:10.1007/s10350-004-7278-6

83. Hendren SK, O'Connor BI, Liu M, et al. Prevalence of male and female sexual dysfunction is high following surgery for rectal cancer. *Ann Surg.* 2005;242(2):212–223. http://www.ncbi.nlm.nih.gov/pubmed/16041212

84. Di Fabio F, Koller M, Nascimbeni R, Talarico C, Salerni B. Long-term outcome after colorectal cancer resection: patients' self-reported quality of life, sexual dysfunction and surgeons' awareness of patients' needs. *Tumori*. 2008;94(1):30–35.

85. Fingeret MC, Nipomnick S, Guindani M, Baumann D, Hanasono M, Crosby M. Body image screening for cancer patients undergoing reconstructive surgery. *Psychooncology*. 2014;23(8):898–905. doi:10.1002/pon.3491

86. Heislein DM, Bonanno AM. Effect of exercise on quality of life and functional performance for patients undergoing treatment for gastrointestinal cancer. *Rehabil Oncol*. 2009;27(1):3–8.

87. Whitehead S, Lavelle K. Older breast cancer survivors' views and preferences for physical activity. *Qual Health Res*. 2009;19(7):894–906. doi:10.1177/1049732309337523

88. Roth A. *Managing Prostate Cancer: A Guide to Living Better*. New York: Oxford University Press; 2015.

CHAPTER 14

MEN, BODY IMAGE, AND CANCER

Murray Drummond and Brendan Gough

INTRODUCTION

Body image research has traditionally focused on (young) women and, to some extent, gay men (e.g., Drummond, 2005; Rumsey & Harcourt, 2012). When men have been studied, the research tends to focus on younger men and the pursuit of the lean-muscular ideal (e.g., Grogan & Richards, 2002). Much of the literature explores lifestyle practices, for example pertaining to diet, exercise, or substance use, and their role in the pursuit and maintenance of aesthetic goals. Some of these practices, *in extremis*, can be deemed risky (e.g., overexercising; taking supplements), contributing to health consequences and illness, such as addiction and eating disorders. Just as the pursuit of dominant body ideals can lead to illness, so can illness provoke experiences of body dissatisfaction. Treatment for a range of cancers including testicular, prostate, and breast cancers, as well as colorectal, head and neck, and sarcoma, for example, can induce anxieties about the "masculine" body. Despite a growing body of literature around men's bodies and body image, it is important to recognize that there is a paucity of literature surrounding men and body image within the cancer literature. The literature in this field has tended to focus more on women with particular reference to breast cancers (Fingeret, Teo, & Epner, 2014). This chapter considers research on both topics (i.e., ill health caused by men's appearance-related practices and illness-induced body dissatisfaction in men), so that health professionals can be informed about particular body image issues relevant to male cancer patients. The way in which the chapter is set out is designed to guide the reader through information that highlights the broader issues facing men with respect to body image. It provides evidence to emphasize the need to understand men and their bodies in contemporary Western society generally and in the context of illness such as prostate cancer, which is the leading gender-specific cancer in men. Additionally, it is this illness that contributes to a significant degree of body image concern for those men who deal with the illness and the recovery process.

CONTEXT

With the rise of consumerism since the 1980s, and associated male-targeted mass-market media and marketing around style, health, and fitness, men have been increasingly positioned as body-conscious consumers (Coupland, 2007). Although there have been periods historically where groups of men have engaged with fashion and appearance, in recent times this phenomenon has acquired a global, relentless character, driven by myriad forces, including advertising, celebrity culture, social media, and reality television. Particularly in Western society we now live in a "somatic society" where the body is for display, a source of capital, identity, and esteem; for [young] men in particular, a lean, toned, muscular physique is cherished—and often pursued with enthusiasm and endeavor through diet and fitness regimes (Grogan, 2008). Older men are not immune; for example, increasing numbers of middle-aged and older men are participating in fitness programs and events, including marathons, "ironman" competitions, and bodybuilding (e.g., Phoenix & Sparkes, 2009). There is also some evidence that corporations are setting appearance-based expectations for male executives (Miller, 2005).

When partaking in appearance-related practices, especially those conventionally deemed feminine (e.g., dieting, cosmetic use), we have found that men are often careful to present their activities in "masculine" ways. Indeed, there is evidence to suggest that some men with clinically diagnosed eating disorders will mask their eating disordered behaviors behind excessive amounts of physical activity. It appears sport and physical activity are far more masculinized means of weight loss compared to that of dieting alone (Drummond, 2002). So, although men are conducting themselves in traditionally "feminized" ways, the way they explain or justify their activity frequently invokes markers of masculinity. For example, men may downplay the significance or extent of their body dissatisfaction or favor more pragmatic accounts of their appearance practices. They may use humor to signal a masculine approach to body image issues and related emotions and emphasize the masculine capital that may accrue from their endeavors. They may also prefer anonymous self-disclosure with peers online rather than face-to-face encounters with family, friends, or health professionals. Such masculine ways of reframing embodiment and appearance are relevant to illnesses such as cancer, the impact and treatment of which men may experience as emasculating (e.g., Seymour-Smith, 2013), not least because of the assault on body image. In the next section the relevance of masculinity to men's understanding and experiences of body image issues and practices is elaborated and illustrated. We draw on a range of qualitative research projects in which men's own voices and language are showcased. First, though, we touch on the relationship between the body and masculinity and the impact of body dissatisfaction on men's self-image.

THE BODY AND MASCULINITY

Often, men's anxieties about their masculinity relate, at least in part, to perceptions of physical size, shape, and capabilities of the body (Connell, 1983). Therefore, it is necessary to develop theoretical links between constructions of gender and constructions of the body and its processes (Hearn & Morgan, 1990). However, it is in the interests of gender studies to direct the study of gender and masculinities away from the ideological and the cultural and toward the bodily without falling into biological reductionism (Hearn & Morgan, 1990). That is to say arguments relating to the body should not be reduced to simply that of being male or female. Indeed, there are multiples forms of masculinities, which need to be taken into consideration in discussions surrounding men and their bodies (Drummond, 1996). To this end we draw on the groundbreaking work by Merleau-Ponty (1962) and Connell (1983), who explicitly connect embodiment with masculine identities. Merleau-Ponty claimed that the experiences of our bodies are related to our senses, how we relate to the world and to others around us. Connell suggested that to learn to be a man is to learn to project a physical presence that displays latent power. Empowerment is the key element in this line of argument. To be masculine is to embody force and competence (Connell, 1983).

The way in which a man's body looks and its potential to function, particularly with respect to force and skill, is critical to the formation of masculinity for many men. A critical point made by Connell (1983) with respect to these elements of force and skill is that when the two are combined, power is the ultimate product: "while women conventionally have an image of attractiveness, men conventionally have a presence dependent on the promise of power they embody" (p. 33).

Power and empowerment of the body constitute a major part of the development of "hegemonic masculinity" (Day, 1990; Foucault, 1981; Hargreaves, 1986; McKay, 1991). Hegemonic masculinity concerns the gender order more widely—it is not (only) about men and/or masculinity but encompasses gender identities, relations, and conflicts. As originally formulated, it referred to "the currently most honored way of being a man, it required all other men to position themselves in relation to it, and it ideologically legitimated the global subordination of women to men" (Connell & Messerschmidt, 2005, p. 832). For example, many men who have undergone treatment for prostate cancer return to work, attempt to conceal side effects (e.g. urinary leakage), and limit disclosure of their cancer as they manage their masculine identity (Grunfeld, Drudge-Coates, Rixon, Eaton, & Cooper, 2013).

A pluralistic and hierarchical perspective is presented by Connell (1983), where multiple masculinities (and femininities) exist and operate in relation to each other. Specifically, Connell highlighted the operation of power through masculinities, which are best understood as "configurations of practice;' at a given moment in a given context some men will enact and be privileged by locally "hegemonic" masculinities while women and other men will be marginalized or subordinated by these hegemonic practices. Opposition to and oppression of women and gay men (among others) are built into hegemonic masculinities. Disabled men may be marginalized through having limited access to material resources and valued masculinities. Similarly, gay men, oppressed by heterosexism and homophobia and judged to fall short of "masculine" standards, are subordinated in both representational and material terms. The discrimination, prejudice, and oppression faced by disempowered, alienated men will inevitably impact on health. There is some evidence, for example, that erectile dysfunction (ED) following prostate cancer is considered more threatening to masculine identity for black British and American men compared to other groups (see Rivas et al., 2016). More generally, the health of economically disadvantaged men, racial and ethnic minority men, and gay and bisexual men tends to be worse than that of more privileged groups of men (Griffith, Allen, & Gunter, 2011). We must consider then how masculinity intersects with issues of class, ethnicity, sexual orientation, and so on in order to explain the health of particular groups of men, and we return to this issue shortly. Individual men will experience a range of situations and relationships and in some contexts will take up (or are assigned) more powerful positions but are then placed in subordinated or marginalized positions in other contexts. In addition, those men who subscribe to certain traditional hegemonic ideals (e.g., emotional restriction, self-reliance) often experience worse illness outcomes compared to men who reject or rework such ideals—including men with prostate cancer, where bodily changes can be viewed in terms of weakness, embarrassment, and frustration (see Hoyt, Stanton, Irwin, & Thomas, 2013). So, material and cultural constraints often influence men's capacity to occupy hegemonic status; that is, engaging in particular configurations is not a matter of free choice.

The occupation of space to which Connell (1983) refers is a crucial element in the development of masculinity. He claimed that "to be an adult male is distinctly to occupy space, to have a physical presence in the world" (p. 33). Conversely, it could be argued that to be an adult female, one must attempt to conserve space. To be physically large and muscularly developed commands attention from both males and females. A disruption to this convention for men, particularly in the form of illness or age, can have significant implications for men and the ways in which they perceive themselves and their masculine identity (Drummond, 2003).

For many men, masculine identity is built around what the body can do, what it looks like, or both. Illness, whether in the form of cancer or other compromised health state, and/or age can influence the way in which the body looks and how it performs. As a consequence of illness or age men have to come to terms with their diminished site for the construction of masculine identification, but they must also attempt to come to terms with a body that can no longer "do" what it used to in terms of strength, endurance, flexibility, and speed. Losing the capacity to be in control of one's life physically and having to hand over physical tasks that would normally have been dealt with personally has significant implications for one's sense of masculinity. This notion is explored further in the next section of the chapter.

DOING VERSUS BEING

What has just been discussed with respect to size and space is related to a theoretical concept that challenges men's corporeality (i.e., the nature of one's physical body) as one that leans toward a *being* body or a *doing* body. The aesthetics of the male body with associated masculinized archetypal traits make up much of the theory surrounding the notion of the *being* body. Take for example the pursuit of bodybuilding amongst men. Bodybuilders are seen as the extreme form of the archetypal male insofar as displaying hypermasculinized archetypal traits. Construction of masculinity is through the occupation of space and *being* hypermuscular, that is, the overdevelopment of a perceived masculine attribute. Together with this development is the manifestation of power, which is displayed through physical prowess. Stronger and physically larger than any woman or average male, the male bodybuilder's physical presence is highly noticeable or prominent. Dominance is established over anyone who is smaller and weaker and unable to match his size or strength, including peers in the weight room. Through bodybuilding this athlete has ultimately constructed a static form of masculinity. He has the *power of being*. In terms of men with a debilitating illness such as cancer, the insidious nature of the disease coupled with the demanding treatment process can emaciate the body to a shadow of itself. For men who may have taken pride in their size and stature and placed a good deal of their masculine identity on the way in which their body is perceived by peers, coping with these types of changes can be quite debilitating.

The *doing* body is different. Using another analogy from sport, in a study conducted by Drummond (1996), the male triathlete, who has to swim, cycle, and run long distances, is likely to gain his perception of masculinity through the success of competition and knowing that his body has competed to its fullest capacity. Despite not possessing a large body that occupies space to the same extent as that of a bodybuilder, there is contentment with regard to masculinity. There is awareness that his body is capable of performing, or *doing*, physical feats of endurance that most men, including bodybuilders and women, are incapable of. Bodies that are hard, lean, and devoid of excess fat hold the endurance capacity to swim, cycle, and run long distances for extended periods of time. Proud of his physiological health, this athlete displays accepted health-like qualities that are desired contemporary societal traits. To the ironman triathlete, masculinity is perceived as a dynamic concept whereby masculine behaviors are developed through the performance and successful completion of regarded physical activities. In another study by Drummond (2003) that investigated physical activity and ageing men, some of whom had developed various illnesses over time including cancer, losing the capacity to *do* "ordinary, everyday things" as a result of pain, fatigue, or functional impairment impacted their masculine identity considerably. The way in which masculinity is socially constructed in Western society has influenced many men's perceptions of self in terms of what their bodies are supposed to *do*. In the event of not be able to do what they perceive it should, there ends up being a sense of loss that needs to be dealt and come to terms with.

The notion of *being* or *doing* is not meant to be a reductionist concept in which men are seen as one or the other. Indeed, it is somewhat fluid, and men will often move in and out as they progress through various timelines and circumstances in their lives. It becomes problematic when the choice is taken away from them over time, as in the case of (some) older or ill men. With age, and illness processes, musculature diminishes, and so too does the functionality of the body. Therefore the body no longer looks like it once did in terms of muscle definition. Similarly, as men age they find it difficult to do the same things they did when they were younger with the same element of vigor. As Drummond (2003) noted, while this may seem problematic, the aging process provides men with the time to come to terms with losses in aesthetics and functionality of their bodies, with less chance of negative implications for psychological well-being. The sudden changes that occur through illness, as in the case of men with cancer, is different. In many instances both *being* and *doing* aspects are affected. For these men, their notion of manhood is compromised and so too is their fulfillment in life. While no life should be compromised irrespective of age, it seems that for younger men, particularly who are physically active and for whom physical aesthetics are seemingly paramount, it is arguable that the changes are even more difficult.

THE IMPACT OF BODY
DISSATISFACTION ON MEN

Body dissatisfaction in men is now recognized as widespread, with estimates varying between 35%—for specific body issues (e.g. body fat, muscularity; see Liossi, 2003; Mellor, Fuller-Tyszkiewicz, McCabe, & Ricciardelli, 2010)—and up to 95% in studies where a range of body-related issues are included (e.g. height, weight, hair, skin. etc.; see Jankowski & Diedrichs, 2011). Research is increasingly indicating the impact of body dissatisfaction on their self-esteem and identities. For example, the development of excess tissue around male breasts—gynecomastia—can cause distress for men and attempts to conceal the condition and/or avoid social situations (see Singleton, Fawkner, White, & Foster, 2009). Gynecomastia is also a side effect of prostate cancer treatment (Chapple & Ziebland, 2002), and together with other symptoms (urinary incontinence, ED, hot flushes) will undoubtedly impinge upon masculine identities and cancer management (see Grunfeld et al., 2013). In fact, any symptom or side effect which can be perceived as feminizing may be construed as a threat to masculinity—and for men, being diagnosed with breast cancer may prove especially troubling (see Rabee & Grogan, 2016). Notions surrounding the social construction of masculinity underpin this ideology. Given that breast cancers are predominantly female oriented, and in the eyes of Western society are almost solely associated with women, contracting a perceived feminized illness is disconcerting for many men (Drummond, 1999). For example, a similar ideology was raised in Drummond's research with men and eating disorders, including anorexia and bulimia nervosa. The men in this research struggled to come to terms with living with an illness that was largely perceived by Western society as one that only women could develop. Given that eating disorders are also rooted in psychology, any association with mental illness was also perceived as a weakness and a threat to their own masculine identity. As one of the men stated in this research, "as a bloke I didn't like seeing a shrink because it made me feel weak" (p. 88). We cannot underestimate the concerns men have around socially constructed notions of masculinity in relation to illnesses they may possess. While the illness may be largely physical in nature, the psychological distress can be enormous in terms of the way in which they perceive themselves as a man. How their bodies *look*, as in the case with men and breast cancer, also plays a part in this.

More generally, weight gain can also be experienced as difficult for men. For example, in a qualitative interview study (Gough, Seymour-Smith, & Matthews, 2016), it was noted that many older overweight and obese men conveyed distress about their bodies:

> *I mean I do put a lot [ache and pains] down to my weight you know I mean I really do, I'm very conscious of my weight . . . hate it I'm not one of these happy fat blokes I really am not . . . absolutely not. (David, 63)*

Although little research has been conducted with older or ill men about body image, we suggest that weight gain (and indeed weight loss), which can occur with cancer and associated treatment, may well threaten masculine identities as the body deviates from normative lean, muscular, and fit ideals.

Few studies have addressed the issue of hair loss in men, but there is evidence that it can impact greatly on a man's identity, especially younger men. For example, in a study of younger men aged around 21 (Jankowski et al., submitted for publication), we found reference to hair loss and dissatisfaction;

> *I'm getting a receding hairline which is why I've actually not cut my hair for like 3 months or something because I'm just trying to get it to grow over the receding hairline . . . it does get to me . . . it's just the fact that you're losing your hair or going to lose your hair is just a demeaning thing. (Greg)*

As hair loss can occur as a result of cancer treatment, it is likely that men will experience this as emasculating, along with other bodily changes, although more research needs to be conducted into the range of body image issues experienced by men in relation to different forms of cancer.

MEN MAY MINIMIZE BODY IMAGE PROBLEMS

We have found that although men may admit to body-related difficulties, they often minimize the extent of the problem; overweight and obese men may compare themselves favorably with larger men, for example (Gough et al., 2016). We also see minimization at work with men suffering from illness, where they downplay the impact of bodily insults, even when symptoms are visible and severe. In one study (O'Hara et al., 2013), we found that male patients downgraded the effects of serious problems such as impaired vision and toe amputation, as if their bodies were mere objects devoid of feeling. One man stated:

> *You have it for life but it's not a massive disease. You can handle it. . . . I'm not really ill with it. I have never missed school with it. Probably missed one day at the start with it. I've never been sick with it. (Shane, 24)*

Another claimed:

> *It's not a disease. It's a nuisance. (Conor)*

While another man said:

> *I don't call this a major amputation. I call that a blip. All it was, that's the big toe, it must have chaffed somewhere, got a little blister, I shower everyday, but who looks underneath the feet? You know you're supposed to get the mirror but who does? Who does? And um, it was too late to save it. So, now I do use a mirror (laughs). (Michael, 60)*

We know that men with cancer often seek to limit disclosure of their illness and ongoing treatment-related problems (Grunfeld et al., 2013). However, they may also downplay the situation. For example, in a study analyzing how men with testicular cancer support each other online, Seymour-Smith (2013, p. 95) presented data highlighting how some men downgrade the issue of testicular implants:

> *Don't worry too much over this—it's not a big deal either way, not necessary, not ridiculous. Whatever decision you make will be fine, and the important thing is getting rid of the cancer.*

In addition, there is evidence that men use humor to help contain and manage bodily changes, including those associated with cancer or treatment (e.g., Chapple & Ziebland, 2002). For example, although men treated for testicular cancer and who have had one or both testicles surgically removed (orchiectomy) may feel inadequate, vulnerable, and body-conscious, they may joke about decisions concerning testicular implants (Seymour-Smith, 2013, p. 94):

> *I would have a hard time deciding as well. I'm trying to live as naturally as possible, so I would probably decide not to. But then again, the other one would get lonely!*

This extract is a response to an original post requesting advice about testicular implants within the online support forum. Other interview-based research focusing on men with penile cancer also highlights humor as a popular way of managing masculinity postsurgery (Branney et al., 2014)

In sum, we have found that men of all ages and across different contexts will often play down the impact of their bodily changes, whether prompted by illness or appearance-related practices. This does not mean that men will not talk about the extent or impact of body dissatisfaction, but they may well take care to protect their masculine identity when doing so. These considerations are relevant when we turn directly to men with cancer.

MEN, BODY IMAGE, AND CANCER

As noted, much of the research on male body image has focused on adolescent males as well as males in the later teens and early 20s. Consequently, the voices of middle-aged and older men are conspicuous in their absence. So too are the voices of sick and disabled men. Scholars such as Smith and Sparkes (2005) have attempted to highlight issues facing men with spinal cord injuries. However, these have tended to take a more "holistic life" perspective more so than body image.

This chapter is different. Now that we have foregrounded the issues facing men with respect to body image we can turn to the ways in which men with cancer come to view their bodies during and following cancer treatment. Within this section we use prostate cancer as means through which to understand body image given the data we have collected in this area of study. However, it should be recognized that irrespective of cancer site, cancer treatment processes impact men in significant ways. Indeed, prostate cancer is a male-specific disease and has the potential to impact a number of physical functions that are socially constructed as being archetypically masculinized. For example, treatment through surgery may leave a man with ED due to nerve damage, given the proximity of the prostate to the nerves involved in penis function (Filiault, Drummond, & Smith, 2008). This is also true of other sexual organ–related cancers including testicular and penile. Given the significance that many cultures place on sexual virility for men, any loss of sexual function is likely to severely impact a man's self-worth with respect to masculinity. Similarly, androgen deprivation therapy (ADT), which is said to "chemically castrate" men by reducing the amount of testosterone that is produced by the male body, can have enormous ramifications for men in terms of how they perceive themselves, their bodies, and their masculinity. One of the major side effects of ADT is the "feminization" of the male body due to the resultant chemical imbalance of male and female hormones. Therefore men can often develop breast tissue, known as gynaecomastia, as well as develop fat deposits around the hips and thighs; they may also experience reduced muscle mass and associated strength through decreased levels of testosterone. The combined bodily feminization can impact the way in which a man undergoing ADT perceives himself and his masculinity.

This feminization is compounded by the potential for ED and diminished sexual activity, which can be a significant determinant in terms of the way in which a man perceives himself and his masculinity. Drummond (2011) has argued previously that the way in which the body functions (*doing*) and the way it looks (*being*) is integral to the overall masculinizing process for men. When these issues are coupled with factors such as urinary and bowel incontinence, loss of libido and sensual touch as a result of sexual inactivity, potential partnership breakdown, and the prospect of death, it is conceivable that men with prostate cancer who confront some or all of these issues may struggle with their masculine identity.

In the following section we present major themes from men with prostate cancer that impact masculine identity and body image. While a number of themes revolve around dealing with medical professionals, understanding the illness, family issues, and notions of mortality, it was the treatment process and the impact on sexual functioning and the physical changes that was the dominant theme and clearly one of the most influential on men's body image and, hence, masculine identity.

EXPERIENCES OF MEN WITH PROSTATE CANCER

Over the past 15 years I (Drummond) have had the opportunity of being involved in a variety of men's body image projects, including around older men's bodies and men's bodies with illnesses. A number of the men that I have interviewed have had prostate cancer and have reflected on the ways in which they have come to terms with their perceived "failing" bodies.

In terms of methods, all data have been collected and analyzed in the same manner. All men were involved in either focus groups or individual in-depth interviews in which their voices and stories were recorded using a digital audio recorder. All of the interview data were thematically analyzed to identify recurrent themes using a social constructionist framework as a lens. Finally, institutional ethics approval was attained and the men were all provided information sheets about the research in which they were to participate as well consent forms to sign. They were free to withdraw from the research at any time.

"SEXUAL FUNCTIONING, LEAKING, AND ALL THOSE SORTS OF THINGS"

A significant aspect of the body image–based issues that men with prostate cancer face is centered on the way in which the body functions. As it was identified earlier, this notion was articulated as the "doing" element, which is arguably closely related to traditional, and often hegemonic, masculinities. Historically, sexual functioning has been integral to the way in which men perceive themselves, their bodies, and their masculinity. Virility, numbers of female sexual partners, and penis size has played a major part of many cultures' beliefs about men and perceived notions of manlihood (Drummond & Filiault, 2007). ED, which is s major obstruction to sexual functioning in men, is one of the main side effects of prostate cancer treatments, whether it is through radical prostatectomy, radiotherapy, or ADT (Elliott et al., 2010). Therefore prostate cancer treatment–induced ED can impact the way in which a man perceives himself and his masculinity. All of the men that I have the opportunity of interviewing on this issue have identified levels of concern ranging from mild through to severe and sometimes depression. This was dependent on a number of factors including the age of the man, whether they were in a sexual relationship, and their stage of cancer and treatment. One of the men who was in his late 40s and had only been diagnosed with prostate cancer after six months in a serious relationship with a woman claimed:

> It was the worst news of my life. I really had a thing for this woman and, still do, but I can't do anything because nothing works. I have had my prostate removed and nothing is working properly down there. They're not even sure if they got it all. So I am having to go through more "seed" therapy which makes things even worse. I sometimes think whether this was all worth it. You know, the doctors said "some people can wait and watch," but I was young so they said "let's get in and get it out." If I had waited I would still be able to use my pecker. (Jason, 42)

Another man, also in his 40s, was in a married relationship and he had the full support of his wife to eradicate the cancer whatever the consequences of sexual functioning. He claimed:

> You know, my wife is great and she said she wants me alive more so than being able to have sex. You know, that's all well and good, and I must agree with her. But it really does make you feel less of man when you can't get it up. Fortunately, I have been able to have some movement down there and the doctors say that this is really a good sign. I haven't had to use pads much either so

that's good too. I know a lot of guys who are still on pads in my support group and that's not great. (Pete, 48)

For Steve,

It's a massive thing. I know some guys that I've spoken to in the support group that I attend and they say that it's a big problem for them. You know getting an erection. It really affects them, especially how they feel about themselves. You know, their manhood. (Steve, 43)

While it was also claimed:

The thing is after surgery I was given different sorts of drugs to help me with erections and so on. But I never felt good using them. They made me feel sick. And really I never had too many problems in actually getting an erection, which was really good. But the thing was, and this was probably the most annoying part of it, I just couldn't keep the erection for a very long time. I mean, as a man, you feel like you have an obligation to satisfy your partner, as much as yourself when you're having sex. So yeah, that was annoying. . . . I mean sex is a massive a part of a relationship, and men play a pretty big role (laughs). (Dave, 52)

Clearly there are differences for men who are not in relationships and are somewhat older. That is not to say sexual functioning is less important for older men. However, there was certainly an air of pragmatism involved surrounding sexual functioning versus additional life. For example, one man stated:

You know, I had a good time when I was younger and was married for many years. Now I'm in my late 60s it doesn't matter too much how it works. I'm happy to be alive and not have too many other problems. (Ian, 68)

Interestingly, this type of claim coincides with type of attitudes espoused by older men in a study by Drummond (2003) on aging men and physical activity. They too claimed that once they had come to terms with their "failing" bodies, they were comfortable with things that "it could not do." As a result they were able to move on with their lives and be happy that they were alive. It is clear from these comments that men's bodies, and body image, are inextricably linked to their perceived and actual sexual performance. ED represents a failure of a bodily function that is integral to manhood and sense of masculinity. However, other bodily failures also impacted the way in which the men perceived themselves. Urinary incontinence following prostate cancer surgery was an embarrassing consequence for many men, which influenced the way they viewed themselves in terms of human frailty and their "bullet-proof" perception of self which made up a big part of their masculine self-identity. The following is typical of the types of comments made men in the aftermath of prostate surgery:

Leaking is a real massive issue for me, and for other men I know who have had prostate surgery. I can't even have a couple of drinks now when I'm out at a party or at dinner or something like that. I have to always head to the bathroom. It's quite embarrassing. I mean, sometimes I've had too many drinks and I suffered the consequences, you know. It was my own silly fault, but you just sometimes get lost in the moment, you know what I mean? (James, 53)

The same man also claimed:

It just makes you depressed and irritable all the time because you have to think about things so much. You know, where you're going, what you're doing, how far you have to drive. I mean, even the other day I had to stop a couple of times at petrol stations because I feel myself leaking. I knew I only had the one pad with me, which is also incredibly embarrassing. I feel really embarrassed about wearing them, even in front of my wife and we've been through this whole thing together. You never thought you'd be wearing these when you were a younger bloke. Makes you really think about your life. (James, 53)

Noteworthy is that several of the gay men involved in the numerous research projects have had prostate cancer. The words of one of the men in particular resonated strongly and typified the types of issues faced by many of the men, irrespective of sexuality, who continue to take long-term medication, have had radiotherapy, or are undergoing ADT:

You know, my body is what it is. Sure, I used to use it as a means of attraction to attract someone. Because if you feel good about your body and you look good then you should attract someone. I mean one thing leads to another. But the thing is now because of the side effects of all of the medication that I'm on my body is just not what it used to be. (Jason, 56)

Further he stated:

I've got lumps and bumps now in places that I shouldn't. At first I was really concerned and I hated the way I looked. It was quite distressing. But as I said before, I've gotten over that now and don't care anymore. I went through a period of thinking about what surgery I could have to help me look better. But there's nothing I can do without spending $1000s to have it medically fixed and I'm happy with myself now and the people I'm around are happy with me and that's the important thing. (Jason, 56)

It is clear from these claims that men are concerned about their bodies with respect to the changes that occur with prostate cancer treatment and medication. However, it is also evident that men ultimately come to terms with the changes and that mortality, quality of life, and supportive people around them are paramount.

CONCLUSION

In this chapter we have pointed to masculinity issues as central to understanding how men experience, understand, and cope with body dissatisfaction, whether in everyday life or in illness (cancer) contexts. Masculinity is a complex, multifaceted concept, and individual men will invest more in some elements compared to others. Traditionally, men may have been socialized to not to care (much) about their appearance, but because society is increasingly influenced by consumerist, body-conscious norms, men are now expected to take more interest in their bodies. Both traditional and modern ideals co-exist, with the result that men do spend more time and effort on their appearance but may be careful not to overdo it lest they are deemed *unmasculine*. Similarly, when men experience body image–related problems—they may think themselves too fat, too thin, too short—they are likely to minimize the issues but at the same time may talk about their problems in certain contexts. We have found, for example, that many men do open up in research interviews or when talking to peers (anonymously) online. It is clear that certain body image problems, whether aesthetic or functional, are particularly difficult for men; appearance-wise, masculinity-relevant issues include a lack of muscle and fat deposits around the breasts and hips, while in terms of capability, erectile problems and diminished sexual performance are key—all problems associated with cancer and treatment.

Masculinity interacts with other forms of identity, including social class, ethnicity, age, and sexual orientation, such that body image issues may vary by subgroup. In fact, much more research is required to examine how particular communities of men construct and negotiate cancer-related bodily insults. For example, the issues for boys and young men dealing with cancer may well be very different to those for older men, while bereaved or divorced men will likely experience cancer differently from those in relationships. Just as masculinity is multidimensional, we must acknowledge heterogeneity among individuals, recognizing that men from different backgrounds and positions will often present with different concerns, language, and coping strategies. Health professionals working with male patients should be mindful of this diversity while also being aware of some of the key masculinity-related themes covered in this chapter. It is important not to accept stereotypes around men being disinterested in their bodies or disinclined to talk about body image issues—if the environment is considered safe and welcoming, men are likely to engage. In terms of supporting men with cancer, it is clear that peer support can be important for many men, whether online or face to face. Male patients who have had successful outcomes may also be recruited to act as mentors or buddies for men at the start of their cancer journey, complementing formal, medical services. If men's voices and concerns are respected by medical staff and peers, quality of life with or post-cancer will be enhanced.

REFERENCES

Branney P, Witty K, Braybrook D, Bullen K, White A, Eardley I. Masculinities, humour and care for penile cancer: a qualitative study. *J Adv Nurs*. 2014;70(9):2051–2060. doi:10.1111/jan.12363

Chapple A, Ziebland S. Prostate cancer: Embodied experience and perceptions of masculinity. *Sociol Health Illness*. 2002;24(6):820–841.

Connell RW. Men's bodies. *Australian Society*. 1983;2(9):33–39.

Connell RW, Messerschmidt JW. Hegemonic masculinity: rethinking the concept. *Gender Society*. 2005;19(6):829–859.

Coupland J. Gendered discourses on the "problem" of ageing: consumerized solutions. *Discourse Commun.* 2008;1:37–61.

Day I. *"Sorting the Men Out from the Boys": Masculinity, a Missing Link in the Sociology of Sport.* Sheffield, UK: Pavic; 1990.

Drummond M. The social construction of masculinity as it relates to sport: An investigation into the lives of elite male athletes competing in individually oriented masculinised sports (Unpublished doctoral thesis). Edith Cowan University, Perth, Australia; 1996.

Drummond MJ. Men, body image and eating disorders. *Int J Mens Health.* 2002;1(1):79–93.

Drummond MJ. Retired men, retired bodies. *Int J Mens Health.* 2003;2(3):183–199.

Drummond MJ. Reflections on the archetypal heterosexual male body. *Aust Feminist Studies.* 2011;26(67), 103–117.

Drummond MJN. Men's bodies: listening to the voices of young gay men. *Men Masculin.* 2005;7:270–290.

Drummond MJ, Filiault SM. The long and the short of it: gay men's perceptions of penis size. *Gay Lesbian Issues Psychol Rev.* 2007;3(2):121–129.

Elliott S, Latini DM, Walker LM, Wassersug R, Robinson JW, ADT Survivorship Working Group. Androgen deprivation therapy for prostate cancer: recommendations to improve patient and partner quality of life. *J Sex Med.* 2010;7(9):2996–3110.

Filiault SM, Drummond MJ, Smith J. Gay men and prostate cancer: voicing the concerns of a hidden population. *J Mens Health.* 2008;5(4):327–332.

Fingeret MC, Teo I, Epner DE. Managing body image difficulties of adult cancer patients: lessons from available research. *Cancer.* 2014;5(120):633–641.

Foucault M. *Power/Knowledge: Selected Interviews 1972–1977.* Toronto: Random House; 1981.

Gough B, Seymour-Smith S, Matthews CR. Body dissatisfaction, appearance investment and wellbeing: how older obese men orient to "aesthetic health." *Psychol Men Masculin.* 2016;17(1):84–91.

Griffith D, Allen JO, Gunter K. Social and cultural factors influence African American men's medical help seeking. *Res Social Work Pract.* 2011;21:337–347.

Grogan S. *Body Image: Understanding Body Dissatisfaction in Men, Women, and Children.* London: Routledge; 2008.

Grogan S, Richards H. Body image: focus groups with boys and men. *Men Masculin.* 2002;4:219–232.

Grunfeld EA, Drudge-Coates L, Rixon L, Eaton E, Cooper AF. "The only way I know how to live is to work": a qualitative study of work following treatment for prostate cancer. *Health Psychol.* 2013;32(1):75–82. doi: 10.1037/a0030387

Hargreaves J. *Sport, Power and Culture.* New York: St. Martin's Press; 1986.

Hoyt MA, Stanton AL, Irwin MR, Thomas KS. Cancer-related masculine threat, emotional approach coping, and physical functioning following treatment for prostate cancer. *Health Psychol.* 2013;32(1):66–74.

Jankowski G, Gough B, Fawkner H, Diedrichs P, Halliwell E. It affects me, it affects me not: The impact of men's body dissatisfaction. Manuscript submitted for publication.

Jankowski GS, Diedrichs PC. Men's appearance dissatisfaction: An analysis of self-discrepancy index responses [Unpublished raw data]. University of Bath; 2011.

Liossi C. Appearance related concerns across the general and clinical populations. City University, London; 2003. Retrieved from http://ukpmc.ac.uk/theses/ETH/407535

McKay J. *No Pain, No Gain? Sport and Australian Culture.* Sydney: Prentice Hall; 1991.

Mellor D, Fuller-Tyszkiewicz M, McCabe MP, Ricciardelli LA. Body image and self-esteem across age and gender: a short-term longitudinal study. *Sex Roles.* 2010;63(9–10), 672–681. http://doi.org/10.1007/s11199-010-9813-3

Merleau-Ponty M. *The Phenomenology of Perception.* New York: Humanities Press; 1962.

Miller T. A metrosexual eye on queer guy. *GLQ J Lesbian Gay Studies.* 2005;11:112–117.

O'Hara L, Gough B, Seymour-Smith S, Watts S. "It's not a disease, it's a nuisance": men's personal definitions of and adjustment to life with Type 1 diabetes. *Psychol Health*. 2013;28(11):1227–1245.

Phoenix C, Sparkes AC. Being Fred: big stories, small stories and the accomplishment of a positive ageing identity. *Qualit Res*. 2009;9(2):219–236.

Rabee Z, Grogan S. Young men's understandings of male breast cancer: "pink ribbons" and "war wounds." *Int J Mens Health*. 2016;15(3):210–217.

Rivas C, Matheson L, Nayoan J, et al. Ethnicity and the prostate cancer experience: a qualitative metasynthesis. *Psychooncology*. 2016;25(10):1147–1156. doi:10.1002/pon.422

Rumsey N, Harcourt D, eds. *The Oxford Handbook of the Psychology of Appearance*. Oxford: Oxford University Press; 2012.

Seymour-Smith S. A reconsideration of the gendered mechanisms of support in online interactions about testicular implants: a discursive approach. *Health Psychol*. 2013;32(1):91–99.

Singleton P, Fawkner H, White A, Foster S. Men's experience of cosmetic surgery: a phenomenological approach to discussion board data. *Qualit Meth Psychol Newslett*. 2009;8:17–23.

Smith B, Sparkes A. Men, sport, spinal cord injury, and narratives of hope. *Social Sci Med*. 2005;61(5):1095–1105.

CHAPTER 15

BODY IMAGE AND COUPLES

Esther Hansen, Jennifer Barsky Reese, and Justin Grayer

The objective of this chapter is to describe both research and clinical interventions focusing on couples experiencing body image distress associated with cancer and its treatment. First, we provide an overview of the importance of attending to the relationship and the partner. Second, we review the research on couple-based interventions for body image. Third, we discuss clinical concepts and work with couples affected by body image concerns. Case examples are provided to elucidate theory and concepts. While we recognize that not all individuals treated for cancer identify with the term "patient," we use this term for clarity.

THE COUPLE RELATIONSHIP AND BODY IMAGE

Cancer can undermine the body's integrity and can bring about or amplify body image concerns through changes in appearance and functioning. Patients can experience reduced feelings of attractiveness, sexual desirability, and femininity/masculinity and often end up questioning their acceptability to their partner. This may be expressed as a worry that "my partner won't find me attractive anymore." Patients may attempt to manage this body image distress in various ways within the relationship, for example, avoidance of intimate contact (Clarke et al. 2014, study 9), seeking reassurance from their partner, or refraining from discussing body image distress. It is easy to see how an individual's body image concerns can affect the couple's relationship.

Body image distress can also be associated with poorer relationship quality (e.g., Baucom et al. 2009; Manne et al. 2016) and relationship processes, such as communication (Manne et al. 2006, 2010). However, this is not a unidirectional process. Instead, there is an interplay between individual level factors (e.g., patient's body image distress or the partner's own distress) and relationship factors, where they mutually influence one another.

Partners' reactions to patients' body changes and their associated distress influences the coping responses of the patient and vice versa. Seeing that a partner's thoughts, feelings, and behaviors toward the patient and his or her body have not changed can serve as reassuring evidence to a patient that these changes can be dealt with. Similarly, unhelpful partner responses (e.g., being dismissive) or changes in behavior toward and interest in the patient (e.g., does not touch the body) may serve to heighten body image distress and influence how the patient responds. In breast cancer, the partners' response has been shown to predict women's acceptance of their appearance and sense of femininity, adjustment, and self-esteem, underlining the importance of attending to the relational processes (Scott & Kayser 2009).

Similarly, relationship factors play a role in influencing how both partners respond to each other and can accommodate the physical changes, which may be distressing to both of them. In a poor relationship, partners often spend less time together, may not express their emotions, and can struggle to manage difficult matters as a couple due to poor communication and high levels of distress. In such a scenario, patients may feel alone or unsupported with their distress, and they may not know how to share feelings (e.g., shame) that leave them vulnerable. Unsuccessful attempts to emotionally engage can lead to high levels of distress that can reinforce feelings of loneliness and misunderstanding.

In contrast, a satisfying relationship, likely to be characterized by mutual trust, respect, and open communication, can improve body satisfaction (Falkner 2012). These relationship qualities make it easier for a partner to be more attuned to the patient, aware of his or her concerns and better able to respond to the distress. Consequently, they attempt to resolve the issues based on open dialogue, expression of their needs, and a basic assumption that it can be addressed.

The reciprocal association between individual and relationship factors in body image distress contributes to overall coping within the relationship. Coping interventions that address the individual have generally been less effective at improving body image distress, possibly because they do not fully address couple-level processes of coping with body changes (Scott et al. 2004).

RESEARCH ON COUPLES AND BODY IMAGE

In order to understand the relational impact of body changes and related concerns, research that examines both patients' and partners' experiences is important. Yet, due to challenges in recruiting and retaining couples for studies (Fredman et al. 2009; Dagan & Hagedoorn 2014), research examining body image and other quality of life concerns in couples affected by cancer is less common compared to research on individual patients, and sample sizes in couple-based studies tend to be relatively small. However, findings seem to suggest that body image concerns can benefit from a couple-based approach, particularly when they perceive such changes differently within a relationship and therefore have difficulty developing effective coping strategies as a couple.

In this section, we briefly review results of observational studies examining body image concerns and relationship outcomes in cancer populations. Then we describe in detail research examining couple-based interventions addressing body image concerns in cancer, followed by a discussion of the strengths and limitations of research in this area.

OBSERVATIONAL RESEARCH

STUDIES ON WOMEN

There have been mixed findings on the impact of body image distress on the relationship. Some studies have found that for women diagnosed with cancer, greater feelings of body image distress and perceptions of decreased attractiveness are associated with worse sexual relations or function (Benedict et al. 2016; Schover et al. 1995; Burwell et al. 2006; Fang et al. 2015; Boquiren et al. 2016) and poorer relationship adjustment (Abend & Williamson, 2002; Fobair et al. 2006; Fang et al. 2015). Additionally, greater body image self-acceptance has been associated with greater relationship adjustment (Zimmermann, Scott, & Heinrichs, 2010). In contrast, in several studies, body image scores were not significantly associated with either relationship status (Falk Dahl et al. 2010) or with empathy from one's intimate partner (Fang, Chang, & Shu 2015; Fang et al. 2015).

Qualitative findings in women who had mastectomy with immediate reconstruction for breast cancer (Loaring et al. 2015) support the notion of differences in patients' and partners' reactions to women's body changes, with patients remarking on the difficulties adjusting to their altered bodies and their partners expressing relatively greater acceptance of the patients' body changes. These differences could create challenges for the couple in coping with body changes, yet many couples also described coping in dynamic ways that allowed them to continue to express and feel intimacy.

Fang et al. (2015) found that, following breast cancer treatment, unhelpful marital coping efforts (such as avoidance and self-blame) negatively mediated the effect of body image (as measured by the Body Image Scale) on their sexual relationships. This finding suggests that body image is intertwined with the sexual relationship. For example, body image distress might reduce the opportunity for physical affection among intimate partners or create difficulties in talking about body changes. In contrast, self-acceptance on the part of women and perceived acceptance of their body by their partner following cancer treatment might facilitate a return to physical intimacy and affection and could also increase the likelihood for effective communication about these topics.

STUDIES ON MEN

Only a few research studies have focused on body image concerns in men and relationship factors. An older study conducted by Hannah et al. (1992) examined feelings of attractiveness in 58 married men with either testicular cancer or Hodgkin's disease and their spouses. One-third of the patients reported a decrease in attractiveness, with approximately

20% experiencing this change "on a long-term basis." In contrast, more than 80% of spouses reported no perceived decrease in the patient's attractiveness. As part of a study comparing the utility of several sexual function scales in 27 testicular cancer patients (Sheppard & Wylie, 2001), the researchers conducted qualitative interviews with a subset of participants. Analysis suggested that body image was of concern in the context of sexual relationships, and the authors speculated that partners might play an important role in helping patients adjust to body image changes following their surgery. Though these studies document signs of body image distress in men diagnosed with testicular cancer, very few studies have examined this across different types of cancer, and the sample sizes remain small.

CLINICAL IMPLICATIONS

There are several clinical implications of these findings. First, it would be helpful to establish to what extent there is a discrepancy between a patient's perceived acceptance of his or her body by the partner and a partner's actual acceptance of the patient's body. Second, it is also beneficial to attempt to understand the impact of body image distress on the relationship, including sexual intimacy, and vice versa. A good grasp of this would help focus a therapeutic intervention. Matters of discrepancy in perceptions may be amenable to cognitive restructuring. However, if there is significant relationship distress, then this is likely to undermine efforts solely focused on altering the couple's beliefs or coping responses. Third, avoidance of touch or contact with the body is a key matter that should be addressed to resolve relationship difficulties and as a treatment for body image distress.

INTERVENTION STUDIES

OVERVIEW OF COUPLE-BASED INTERVENTION STUDIES ADDRESSING BODY IMAGE IN CANCER

Intervention studies are included in this chapter if they used a couple-based approach and measured some construct related to body image. Many of these studies have been summarized in recent systematic reviews alongside other related outcomes (e.g. Scott & Kayser 2009; Nelson & Kenowitz 2013). However, body image was rarely a primary outcome in these studies; rather, the interventions usually used general psychosocial outcomes or sexual function outcomes as their primary targets.

COUPLE-BASED INTERVENTION STUDIES ADDRESSING BODY IMAGE IN WOMEN

The most commonly represented populations in couple-based intervention studies are either exclusively breast cancer patients or a mixed sample, heavily represented by women with breast cancer. A number of these studies have been described and are summarized in reviews (Scott & Kayser 2009; Collins et al. 2013; Taylor et al. 2011), though only Scott and Kayser focused on body image as a particular outcome of interest along with sexual outcomes. Most commonly, these studies offered education along with skills training to help couples in which the patient was treated for cancer (usually of the breast) to cope either specifically with sexual concerns or with general cancer-related changes. Body image was usually a secondary focus of the intervention under study. Most often, interventions in these studies were informed by cognitive-behavioral approaches. Overall, these studies found positive effects of the couple-based interventions on body image outcomes (Kalaitzi et al. 2007; Baucom et al. 2009), though they used differing measures and intervention approaches. We offer detailed descriptions of two frequently cited studies (Scott et al. 2004; Kalaitzi et al. 2007) that serve as examples of couple-based interventions that had a positive impact on the women's body image.

In the 2004 Scott et al. study, the authors compared the CanCOPE couple-based intervention with individual coping training for women or a control condition consisting of medical education across a sample of 94 married couples, where the patient had early stage breast or gynecological cancer. The CanCOPE intervention consisted of five two-hour face-to-face sessions and two 30-minute phone calls focused on coping with cancer. This included communication skills training, sexual counseling, and information on how to provide (mutual) support on a range of topics, including body image and self-confidence. Body image was assessed through the Self Image Scale, which assesses (a) women's perceptions of their appearance and femininity and (b) their perceptions of their partners' acceptance of their appearance, at baseline, postintervention, and at 6- and 12-month follow-up. Effects on this measure were mixed. Self-acceptance did not change significantly. However, women who were in the CanCOPE condition reported significantly higher scores on the Partner Acceptance scale and positive effects in other individual and dyadic measures. One interpretation of these findings is that the CanCOPE sessions may have provided a useful opportunity to openly discuss women's body image concerns and that in hearing partners' responses it may have altered women's perceptions of their partners' acceptance of their appearance, although feelings of self-acceptance may prove more challenging to change given the focus of the intervention.

In the 2007 study by Kalaitzi et al., the authors compared the impact of brief couples' sex therapy with no intervention, with outcomes measuring body image and sexual and psychosocial functioning. This intervention is noteworthy from a body image perspective because it began with an unveiling of the mastectomy surgical wound several days postsurgery to the patient and the partner with the surgeon and the intervention therapist present, followed by a discussion of feelings, as well as an entire session devoted to body image. The questionnaire on body image and sexuality was not formally validated, although the authors provide some validity data obtained during the study. Results demonstrated significant differences at post-intervention favoring the intervention group for items assessing satisfaction with body image when naked or when dressed and with feeling attractive, along with differences in satisfaction with the relationship, orgasm frequency, sexual initiation, and depression. Although this study has limitations, including a relatively small total number of couples and use of nonvalidated body image measures, the results suggest that for couple-based interventions to improve body image distress in women, it is important to have content specifically focused on body image. It is not clear whether both the viewing of and discussion of the scars and the body image session, or one of these, would be necessary to see improvements in body image outcomes.

As another example, Reese et al. (2016) adapted a telephone-based Intimacy Enhancement (IE) intervention for use in breast cancer (initially developed in colorectal cancer) by using findings of focus groups with women who were treated for breast cancer. The original skills-based intervention addressed a range of both physical and emotional intimacy targets, in particular improving adjustment to sexual changes and helping the couple to re-establish physical intimacy. The manualized intervention also included communication and problem-solving skills as well as cognitive restructuring. The qualitative data suggested that women's breasts play an important part in their intimate relationships. For instance, a number of women used strong negative words to describe their breasts, such as "deformed" and "ugly." Some women were quite distressed by changes to their breasts (e.g., appearance or loss of sensation) and had difficulty adjusting to these in the context of their intimate activity (e.g., trying to avoid being touched on their breasts by their partners). The IE intervention now includes material in all four sessions to cover body image as it relates to women's intimate relationships. The instructions for the sensate focus exercises (sensual touching) were modified to guide patients and partners on how to include breast touching and how to react when uncomfortable emotions follow this touching. Educational material was also included to normalize the feelings many women have about their bodies after breast cancer surgery. Other modifications included examples of effective or ineffective conversations about breasts and body changes in the communication skills training and examples of potential unhelpful cognitions related to women's body image that affect intimacy in the cognitive restructuring material. Finally, by providing a nonjudgmental context in which to explore bodily touch, the sensate focus exercises could potentially help increase women's comfort with their own bodies through partnered touching. This intervention is currently being tested in a randomized pilot study for feasibility, acceptability, and preliminary efficacy. With promising preliminary findings, a larger randomized controlled trial is planned.

COUPLE-BASED STUDIES ADDRESSING BODY IMAGE IN MEN

Although body image measures are commonly included in couple-based intervention studies in women with cancer, similar measures are much less frequently used in comparable studies with male patients (Wootten et al. 2014, Nelson et al. 2015). Even when included in the intervention content, body image seems to take on a fairly peripheral role, and results from couple-based interventions are not consistent. Research in men links body image to function, as opposed to appearance, making other studies relevant to review here.

In Chambers et al.'s (2015) sample of 189 men with prostate cancer and their intimate partners, the authors found no significant effects of either of two active interventions (peer-led couple-based intervention vs. nurse-led couple-based telephone counseling) on men's appraisals of their masculinity or on sexual, relationship, or psychosocial outcomes, when compared to usual care. However, the intervention altered the use of erectile function medications. The authors surmised that the lack of effectiveness of either intervention on sexual function could be accounted for by the timing of the intervention being too early in the prostate cancer patients' recovery. Longer term follow-up could also have considered whether the use of medications lead to an improvement in masculine self-esteem, assuming such medications were generally effective in addressing erectile dysfunction for patients.

A pilot study by Wittmann et al. (2013) evaluated whether a couple-based one-day group intervention for 26 surgically treated men with prostate cancer could be feasible and acceptable and preliminarily efficacious for enhancing sexual recovery. Alongside several significant positive effects of the.intervention on sexual outcomes, findings of the study revealed that, six months after the intervention, partners viewed erections as being less critical to a man's sexual relationship and for sexual pleasure, although men's own perceptions of its importance did not change. In other words, partners' beliefs about the importance of erections for men's sexual relationships and pleasure may have been more susceptible to intervention as compared to men's own beliefs, suggesting that perhaps such beliefs may be more entrenched for the men who participated. Interestingly, these finding echoes that from the CanCOPE intervention in breast cancer survivors in that, in both cases, the couple-based intervention was effective at altering *partners'* perceptions of the patients' body changes or patients' perceptions of their *partners'* acceptance of these changes, whereas improvements in patients' own body image were less responsive to the intervention.

STRENGTHS AND LIMITATIONS OF CURRENT INTERVENTION STUDIES

Results from these studies suggest that couple-based interventions can be effective in reducing body image distress, although the findings are stronger in studies in which the woman is the identified patient. Interestingly, these intervention studies demonstrate that body image outcomes may be operationalized differently in intervention studies in women and men, focusing more on appearance in women and on function in men. The examination of different aspects of body image distress is a strength of the literature given that discomfort with either the appearance or performance of parts of one's body can lead to discomfort with and avoidance of sexual activity (Nelson et al. 2015) and thereby negatively impact the relationship. Moreover, interventions focused on the couple demonstrate that positive effects on patients' body image outcomes occur alongside improvements in other areas of the relationship, at least for women, such as relationship adjustment and sexual satisfaction. These studies used validated measures of body image, and some employed randomized controlled designs to test the efficacy of the intervention, which are strengths.

However, there are limitations that leave open opportunities for future research. First and foremost, the largest number of interventions has been conducted in breast cancer, leaving a wide gap in the availability of evidence-based interventions for those with other cancers. Second, although some of the studies were methodologically rigorous randomized controlled trials (Scott et al. 2004; Chambers et al. 2008), the findings from other studies are limited by the fact they used small sample sizes and/or were pilot trials (Kalaitzi et al. 2007; Baucom et al. 2009; Jun et al. 2011; Wittman et al. 2013). Third, the interventions are limited in their effectiveness of altering self-perceptions, so it may be helpful for interventions to be adapted to target this area. Fourth, the number of interventions using couple-based approaches to address body image have been relatively few in number, perhaps because couples' studies are resource-intensive and come with substantial challenges in recruitment and retention (Fredman et al. 2009; Dagan & Hagedoorn 2014). Fifth, the studies are conducted in Western countries, making it difficult to glean information about potentially important cross-cultural factors. For instance, gender roles within intimate relationships can vary across cultures, and women or men may seek support differently from within and outside of the relationship. However, cross-culturally there are a range of "normal" body types and levels of comfort with discussing body changes that can help explain potential cultural differences in how couples cope with body image changes following cancer (e.g., Odigie et al. 2010). Lastly, studies do not consider contextual factors such as patients' age and their life stage, which are likely to be influential on body image distress and its effect on the couple relationship. For example, avoidance of sexual activity due to body discomfort could cause particular distress and interference in couples seeking to have a child.

CLINICAL IMPLICATIONS

A key clinical implication of findings from the couple-based intervention studies is that they can be helpful in improving both patients' and partners' perspectives on the patients' body changes and related outcomes and improve relationship functioning. Poor pre-existing relationship functioning may undermine coping with body image distress, particularly if there are high levels of distress. Alternatively, the coping strategies used in response to body image distress by either partner can affect relationship functioning. Clarity on the main driver of body image distress (i.e. relationship vs body change) may help the clinician prioritize the different aspects of the interventions reviewed above. For example, it may be most helpful to address a poor relationship first and then proceed to view the scar, although with well-functioning couples starting with a focus on the body image itself may be appropriate.

Given that some interventions seemed to have less robust effects on patients' own body image as compared with their partners' perceptions of body image changes (Wittman et al. 2013; Scott et al. 2004), it would suggest that interventions could be usefully adapted to focus on self-acceptance. To assess this possibility, clinicians could monitor progress of both patients and their partners during treatment in learning appropriate body image coping skills and use individual sessions when necessary to help bolster patients' improvement, with the partner as a source for alternative views or facilitator for change (as discussed in the clinical section that follows).

Finally, the findings suggest that body image distress may be driven by changes in function or appearance or both. It would be helpful to clarify this for both partner and patient to optimize the likely effectiveness of treatment. For instance, a clinician should be aware whether a prostate cancer patient after treatment with androgen deprivation therapy is concerned about his appearance (e.g., gynaecomastia) or about the function of his genitals for sexual activity. In this way, intervention can focus on the concern the patient and the partner have to help them cope with these to maintain emotional and relationship well-being.

CLINICAL APPLICATIONS OF COUPLE-BASED INTERVENTIONS

In the sections that follow, we offer guidance for the assessment and management of body image distress within the couple. The research on couple-based interventions for body image distress is heavily influenced by cognitive-behavioral therapy (CBT). This approach has a focus on how each person's thoughts, emotions, and behaviors influence the interactional process, which includes communication skills training (Epstein, Baucom & Daiuto 1997). The CBT-informed research interventions reviewed earlier have provided education about the cancer experience and taught effective coping skills, such as goal-setting, engagement in adaptive behaviors, communication skills training, and evaluation of beliefs (Epstein & Baucom 2002). Prior to addressing the use of this within body image–based couple work, two intrapersonal concepts that can help clinicians make sense of the couple interactions in general and when focused on body image changes are introduced. These concepts inform our clinical practice, which draws on emotionally focused therapy (EFT; e.g., Johnson 1996) and second-order systemic couples therapy (e.g. Jones & Asen 2000). While EFT has not been explicitly tested in the area of body image, Naaman et al. (2009) write about its use in breast cancer to support couple adjustment processes. These concepts facilitate an understanding of interactions that generate intense emotions and unhelpful appraisals of the self or other and therefore produce unhelpful behavioral responses, which are not always explained by communication skills or beliefs per se.

CONCEPTUAL PRINCIPLES RELEVANT TO COUPLE WORK

MENTALIZATION

Mentalization is comprised of the ability to differentiate our own and others' minds and to perceive both affective and cognitive states, which is essential for effective relationships (Allen, Fonagy, & Bateman 2008). It is a concept that is similar to but differentiated from both mindfulness (being aware of one's *own* cognitive and affective state in the present moment) and empathy (the process of stepping into *another* person's shoes and feeling what he or she feels). The ability to mentalize is central to the ability to form secure attachments as it impacts how individuals relate to one another. In the context of body image, the extent of physical change does not always correspond to the degree of distress experienced (Rumsey & Harcourt 2004). A partner who is able to engage with the process of mentalizing can go beyond his or her own thoughts and feelings, hypothesize about the patient's internal state, and determine how to respond in order to match the response to the needs of the patient.

> *Tracy had a lumpectomy and her surgeon told her in their latest consultation that he was very pleased with her scar and that it will fade over time. She expressed that she is unhappy with how her breast looks and the asymmetry between her breasts; the surgeon said that she had a very*

good outcome and that the shape was much like her other breast so he wasn't sure why she was so distressed. When Tracy got home she told her partner Shelley about the consultation, in the hope that Shelley would be able to support her. Unfortunately, Shelley agreed with the surgeon and told Tracy "you won't notice it soon." In this example, both the surgeon and Shelley were only able to see Tracy from the outside and from their own perspectives – their inability to see Tracy from the inside (i.e., to mentalize), in terms of her thoughts and emotions impaired their ability to empathize with her and to offer the support she needed.

Being aware of a person's capacity to mentalize should help clinicians determine where the focus of intervention may be best placed to commence. Couple therapy can promote mentalizing by asking questions that invite patients and partners to consider the other's thoughts and feelings. For example, a clinician may ask Shelley, *"What effect do you believe it would have on Tracy to agree with her view that the breasts are uneven?"* Questions that invoke a different context can be a powerful means to changing the meaning ascribed to (in)actions and helps a person to mentalize. Occasionally, it can also be useful to share research or other couples' experiences to show different perspectives relevant to the couple and invite them to respond.

ATTACHMENT NARRATIVES

A cancer diagnosis and treatment involving changes in physical appearance or function are inherently distressing experiences, and a patient often needs to feel a sense of safety and security. Applied to adult relationships, attachment theory contributes to understanding couple processes in terms of meeting the needs for support and closeness (Dallos & Vetere 2014; Johnson 1996; Shaver & Mikulincer 2009). Attachment theory (Bowlby 1982) is a developmental theory focused on the bond between a child and his or her primary caregiver that, if secure, allows a child to be soothed by the caregiver's emotionally engaging response. In contrast, an inconsistent or absent response over time may lead children to develop a negative view of others and/or themselves, which can reduce their ability to see their caregiver(s) as a safe haven and secure base. In turn, they may adapt their behavior as a way of self-regulating their emotional state and may pursue or withdraw from their caregiver. In adult relationships, an available and responsive partner would suggest secure attachment, and that the partner would be more likely to provide appropriate support and reassurance with respect to body image changes. An illustration of this is provided next.

Ryan attended an appointment recently as part of his care for the osteosarcoma in his leg, where the planned surgery was discussed in detail and he was cautioned that he could lose his leg. He is devastated and calls his partner, Jane, and leaves her a voicemail message telling her that he needs to meet her even though he knows she has a busy day at work. In spite of her busy schedule she phones Ryan back after 20 minutes. When they meet, he talks about how he cannot cope with losing his leg as well as the cancer and how disabled he will be in terms of function and activity. Jane is able to contain her own distress and so she listens and soothes him so that he feels supported. They are then able to begin to work out what their next steps will be to manage the situation.

Here, Jane demonstrates a sufficient level of emotional attunement and Ryan experiences a sense of safety, so that when he reaches out for Jane, she is available and responds in an emotionally engaging way. Ryan's felt sense of security is a mind-body experience: when a patient can turn to his or her partner and feel safe, the parasympathetic nervous system relaxes the body; concurrently, cognitive capacity is enhanced and fosters a more coherent sense of self as well as communication and problem-solving skills.

In contrast, when the need for emotional connection and safety is not (perceived as) available, a person may either (a) angrily demand contact to facilitate connection or (b) pull away and avoid contact to limit hurt feelings. In both instances, there is a greater sense of disconnection, abundance of strong emotions, and limited opportunities for support of body image distress. We return to the same example about Jane and Ryan to illustrate these attachment styles.

> *Insecure anxious attachment: Ryan calls his partner, Jane, and leaves her a voicemail message telling her that he needs to meet her even though he knows she has a busy day at work. He waits a few minutes and when she hasn't called back he calls again and texts her, and he repeats this process a number of times. While he waits he gets more anxious and upset and when he eventually reaches Jane he shouts at her for not calling him back. When they meet, he shares his news and his distress, particularly about the likely change in his appearance. Jane struggles to contain her own distress as she is being shouted at and is worried about Ryan, which makes it hard for her to let Ryan talk. He becomes agitated and demands that she listen to him. Jane tells him she will call the office and take off the rest of the day so that they can be together.*

> *Insecure avoidant attachment: Ryan does not call his partner, Jane, as he knows she has a busy day at work. He goes back to work and stays late to finish off a task. When he gets home, Jane asks what he has done during the day. Ryan is unsure how to respond—he wants to tell Jane what has happened, but he is also worried that if he tells her she will either get too upset about it and/or get angry that he did not tell her earlier and ask her to come to the appointment. He quickly decides that he won't take the risk of upsetting her and decides to tell her over the weekend.*

Couples are encouraged to use therapy as an opportunity to slow down their interactions so that they can observe and directly experience (rather than avoid) their attachment needs, name these needs, and voice their fears in a safe environment. A focus on vulnerable (e.g., scared, ashamed) rather than reactive (e.g., anger) emotions facilitates an environment that is less blaming and invites the couple to communicate in a way which enhances the likelihood that their emotional needs will be met. It also enables couples to gain a better sense of unhelpful patterns of interactions and communication and how this influences the beliefs they have about the other's behavior.

ASSESSMENT OF BODY IMAGE CONCERNS IN THE COUPLE

The remainder of this chapter focuses on assessment and implementation of partner-supported or couple work, rather than couple therapy per se. Readers interested in couple therapy are referred to Johnson (1996) or Jones and Asen (2000). The examples provided here are included to help mental health practitioners ask questions that can help make evident the relational impact of the disease and to identify how they as a couple may wish to work together on managing body image distress. This can be particularly important as healthcare providers and our cultural environment tends to be "individualistic" and to focus on the patient rather than the couple

Table 15.1 offers some examples of questions to include in a couple-based assessment of body image concerns, though a general body image assessment is discussed in Chapter 3 and is not repeated here.

Inviting the couple to attend the session together provides the therapist with an opportunity to see how each person conceptualizes the body image issue and identify the cycle that the couple gets stuck in with respect to the physical changes that one of them has experienced (see the later case example of Andrew and Martha). Breaking down the cycle into its component parts helps the couple to see both the intra- and interpersonal nature of their conflicts. Occasionally, the patient may attend alone and the absence of the partner can be indicative of both real external demands and/or ambivalence toward addressing difficulties. Therapists may also be interested to meet each partner individually. In both circumstances, it is important to negotiate how content from such meetings is treated within the joint sessions.

Individual sessions may be particularly helpful if one partner tends to dominate the conversation (to foster therapeutic alliance), to identify factors that reduce the safety of the relationship so it would be potentially unethical to encourage either partner to become emotionally vulnerable (e.g., ongoing affair, intention to leave the relationship, domestic violence) or to discuss issues that perpetuate body image distress, which a person may find difficult to raise with his or her partner. For example, the partner may have a strong emotional reaction (e.g., disgust) to the patient's body changes. The following case example illustrates the concepts discussed in this section.

Case Example

Andrew has recently finished treatment for colon cancer, which was treated with surgery and radiotherapy. Although his cancer has been successfully treated, a consequence of treatment is that Andrew has a colostomy bag, which he is struggling to adjust to in terms of appearance and function. Andrew is in a relationship with Martha; they met while both of them were with their former partners and quickly ended their other relationships to move in together six months prior to Andrew's diagnosis. A strong part of their attraction to each other was their enjoyment of the outdoors, cycling, and their overall fitness levels. They are both in their 50s and neither of them have children. The extract of the assessment shows how the therapist works to identify Andrew and Martha's cycle of conflict, linking perceptions of each other's behavior to their own emotions and behavior with a focus on verbal and nonverbal communication. By tracking the circular interaction, it shows Andrew's evaluation of and investment in his physical appearance and function. He may have had little prior awareness of this as his previous body image closely matched his ideal body image. Concurrently, the therapist's task is to begin to identify any underlying vulnerability and to reframe the problem. The reframe used here is of the primary emotions and unmet attachment needs (the insecurity that Andrew feels about the relationship), which moderates his body image distress.

Stages/Questions	Intention
Understanding more about the body image concern	
• Has your partner seen this part of your body? What do you think your partner thinks about your body? What has been your partner's reaction?	• This indicates the level of avoidance that may be present regarding the patient's body. The partner's reaction may have reinforced or challenged the patient's existing beliefs. Note distancing emotions such as disgust or queasiness.
• What effect has the change in your body had on what the two of you do together at home/outside/with friends?	• Look for the effects on the couple's relationship, particularly as it relates to their physical and emotional intimacy.
• How have other people reacted? What reactions do you find easier/difficult?	• Identifies broader relational influences that can impact the primary relationship
• How important is your physical appearance/sensation/function to the way you feel about yourself?	• Identify how invested each of them are in their body image and the effect it has on their self-image and confidence
• What types of things do you do to avoid/examine your body? If your partner notices, what can he or she do to support you?	• Normalize avoidance and surveillance. Asking how the partner would know this is happening puts the behavior back into the relationship and potentially provides the partner with an opportunity to intervene in a helpful way.
• How important is your physical appearance/sensation/function to your partner?	• Assesses how invested they think their partner is in body image.
• How important is your physical appearance/sensation/function to your relationship?	• Assesses how invested their relationship is in body image.
• How does your relationship affect how you feel about your body?	• Teases out the circularity of body image and relationship.
• (Asking the partner) What do you do that you think might be difficult for [your patient]? How do you think he or she may feel? How do you see him or her cope with this?	• Enables you to tie together the different information (perceptions/evaluations, importance, emotions, behaviors) you have elicited to make (if appropriate) explicit the cycle the couple gets stuck in around body image concerns.
The relationship history and context	
• How did the two of you meet? Who pursued whom? What attracted you to each other in terms of looks and personality and how has this changed over time?	• Listen for stories about what role/function their bodies and appearance played in their relationship formation and development. Couples who are more invested in body function and appearance will struggle more to adapt to changes.
• How satisfied are you with your sex life at the moment? How long has it been this way? Have you tried to improve your sex life in the past and if so how?	• People are often uncomfortable discussing sex; however, it is important to directly inquire about. You can return to this topic later if you encounter resistance.
	• Changes in body appearance and function can impact sexual confidence, desire, arousal and satisfaction.
• What strengths does your relationship have? When you have had difficult times in the past, how have you supported each other? What do the two of you value about your relationship?	• Spending time examining the couple's strengths so the assessment is not entirely problem focused.
	• Identifying values, or what is important to the couple, helps to provide a focus or direction.

Therapist: *Andrew, when you see Martha looking at your body when you are in the bathroom, in what you describe as a "disgusted way," what goes through your mind?*
[**rationale:** explicit naming of the interpersonal aspect of the cycle, that then encourages Andrew to identify intrapersonal factors]

Andrew: *I know that she doesn't want to be with me, that I'm not attractive to her anymore and that she wishes she had never ended her other relationship.*

Therapist, spoken slowly and in the first person: *And when you think this, that "she doesn't want me, that I'm not attractive anymore," how do you feel?* [rationale: speaking slowly reduces the cognitive load Andrew and Martha face and makes it more likely, in tandem with use of the first person, that they will experience more emotion. It can be helpful to heighten the emotion in the session to see how the person responds to it]

Andrew: *I feel so angry; everything that I have sacrificed to be with her, and now she wants to leave, all because she doesn't fancy me anymore.*

Therapist: *You feel angry, angry that she may leave you. And alongside the anger what else do you feel?* [rationale: asking Andrew if he feels any other emotions alongside anger is an attempt to identify any primary emotions. Anger can be a primary emotion, although it is often a secondary reactive emotion that is more comfortable to be with than the vulnerable primary emotion]

Andrew: *I don't know. All I can feel is anger and frustration.*

Therapist: *So much anger. Okay. And when you feel this anger, what do you do?* [rationale: linking feelings to behavior]

Andrew: *I get pretty critical. I tell her I know she doesn't find me attractive anymore.*

Therapist: *Anything else?*

Andrew: *I tell her that if she does still find me attractive then she should come and kiss me, and that she shouldn't stare at me in the way she does.*

Therapist: *And how does Martha respond when you say this to her?* [rationale: to help Andrew to see the effect of his behavior on Martha]

Andrew: *She doesn't do anything, she doesn't say anything. She just stands there and eventually leaves.*

Therapist: *And when you see Martha standing there not saying or doing anything* (turns to Martha), *I realize you may not see it this way Martha,* (turns back to Andrew), *what do you think and feel?* [rationale: addressing Martha at this point is a way of validating both partners, without invalidating the other]

Andrew: *It just proves the point—she doesn't even want to be in the same room as me—she's disgusted by what she sees. I don't blame her—I'm disgusted by it.*

Therapist: *"She doesn't even want to be in the same room as me"—that sounds so painful for you.* (Pause) *Is it okay if I check with Martha how she's doing?* (Andrew nods) *Martha, when you see Andrew's body and the colostomy bag when he is in the bathroom, what happens to you?* [rationale: it is important not to focus for too long on one partner to the exclusion of the other partner, and it is also helpful to let the couple know that the focus of attention is about to shift]

Martha: *I feel so sad for him, for us. Everything seems to be unravelling so quickly—I am worried how we'll get through this—our relationship is so new. And I don't know what to say. I rarely do in difficult situations.*

Therapist: *You're sad, and worried, and you don't know how to make it better for Andrew or for the relationship – is that right?* (Martha nods.) *It sounds overwhelming for you – what do you do?* [rationale: linking emotion to behavior again]

Martha: *It is overwhelming. I just stand there trying to think of something helpful to say. But before I can, Andrew starts getting angry and shouting at me, telling me I don't love him, that I've made a mistake being with him.*

Therapist: *That sounds difficult for you. You're trying to work out what to do or say that can be helpful, because you want to help Andrew, but it sounds like you feel you don't have time and that you get stuck, you freeze. Am I on the right track?* (Martha nods) *And then what happens for you before you walk out of the room—what happens in your mind and your body?* [rationale: the therapist reframes the behavior in the context of the importance of the relationship]

Martha: *It's just too much, I feel myself getting tense, and there's the sense that if I stay we'll have another argument, that whatever I say it won't be right, and that if I do go and kiss him, that he'll tell me I didn't really want to do it. So, I just leave. It seems safer that way.*

Therapist: *Okay, so you're concerned that whatever you do it won't be good enough, that by staying you'll somehow make the relationship worse, and so you leave. You leave to protect the relationship, as well as yourself. Thank you, Martha.* (turning to Andrew) *Andrew, when you see Martha leave, I guess, for you, that proves your point, that she doesn't want to be with you anymore?* [rationale: when Martha says she is worried that whatever she does will not be good enough, she is letting Andrew and the therapist know about one of her attachment needs: she wants to be good enough. When the therapist states that Martha walks out of the room partly to protect the relationship from an argument it is an attachment reframe]

Andrew: *Yes.*

COUPLE FORMULATION

At the end of the assessment, the therapist and couple should be able to explain how body image concerns function within the context of the couple's relationship and how the couple's interactions serve to maintain the body image distress or to cope effectively with body changes. The body image concerns are usually an issue when intrapersonal variables influence the patient's expression of, or the ability of a partner to respond to, concerns or where interpersonal processes (e.g., communication) are ineffective. The focus on emotion, communication, and circular responses should elucidate how body image concerns are perpetuated and affect couple functioning.

It is important that the therapeutic intervention fits with the couple's current emotional and cognitive capacities. Couples with greater emotional distress will likely have diminished cognitive functioning and will therefore be less able to process information; an emotional-focused intervention, with a possible referral for couple's therapy, is likely to be most appropriate. Conversely, couples who have a secure foundation and who are less distressed will likely be better placed to process psycho-education and to engage in behavioral tasks, as outlined later. Less distressed couples are not free from relationship difficulties; however, they tend to notice their unhelpful cycle earlier rather than later and to be able to repair their relationship more readily.

The therapist can also discuss with the couple the level of engagement they can commit to and obtain feedback about what aspects of the assessment were more or less helpful in creating an environment of safety and respect.

USING THE PARTNER IN INDIVIDUAL BODY IMAGE WORK

Chapter 4 discusses how to engage a person in individual psychological therapy for body image distress. This section focuses on how to include the partner in body image work in a number of ways. For example:

- The partner joins to witness the body image distress the patient experiences, which can foster empathic communication. This may be particularly helpful if the patient struggles to communicate distress and there is a significant element of shame which has led to withdrawal.
- The partner joins so the therapist can more easily explore, and the patient witness, alternative perspectives that may facilitate adjustments in body image–related beliefs. This may be particularly helpful in attempting to change avoidance behaviors related to "showing" the body part or when the patient holds strong beliefs about desirability within the relationship.
- The partner joins to become a facilitator of change outside of the therapy as he or she can provide support to the patient to make changes and provide feedback on change he or she has noticed.

It is helpful to discuss with the patient if the partner can be usefully involved in any of these roles. It is likely that partner involvement would be unhelpful if there is high relationship distress, for example, if the partner is described as disengaged, hostile, or critical of the patient or cancer-related changes. Attention to how the partner should be invited can help the joint session work well. This usually involves identifying the extent to which session content may be (un)familiar to the partner, whether the partner is keen to support the patient, whether the partner holds concerns about attending, and so on. This information guides who is best placed to make the invitation, how the partner is invited, and how to elicit concerns from the partner. When partners do join, it is important to check their understanding of their involvement and what they know about previous sessions.

The therapist needs to prepare the partner to be an empathic listener to the patient's distress. One way of doing this is to ask the partner to think of a time when he or she *really* felt listened to and understood. Once the partner has identified a memory, questions help identify the listener's body language, behavior, speech pattern (tone, pace, etc.) and language that helped the partner to feel listened to and understood. This helps the partner be alert to the behaviors and responses that may be helpful to embody when listening to the patient. Equally, it is also helpful to negotiate in advance how to remind the partner of his or her commitment to be a helpful listener during the conversation that follows, which can normalize its inherent difficulty.

PARTNER AS A LISTENER AND WITNESS

We find that witnessing is important and particularly powerful if patient have felt misunderstood, their body image distress has been dismissed, they have made helpful changes in how they respond to their distress, or they have reduced its interference in their life. We start by asking patients to discuss their position, thoughts, and feelings. We then interview partners about the conversation they observed which is particularly helpful if it is anchored in what the patient *said* and the focus remains on the effect of the patient's experiences on the partner. This is sometimes difficult to achieve as partners may be keen to share their experience. The following questions can be helpful to ask the partner to help keep the focus on the patient. For those interested in more detail, this process is informed by systemic and narrative concepts (e.g., outsider witness practice [White 2007]; reflecting team [Andersen, 1987]; with some sample questions informed by White 2007):

- What stood out for you when you were listening to [patient]?
- What do you feel it says about [patient]? (With such questions, we attempt to get at the value or principle behind what stood out to them.)
- What from your work or life helps us understand why this caught your attention?
- Knowing this, having witnessed this, how will it affect your life?

It is important to offer patients (who listened to their partner) an opportunity to respond to the conversation they witnessed by asking *"What does it mean to you to listen to what your partner said?"* These conversations make explicit the reciprocity of the relationship and the growth that couples can experience.

PARTNER AS A SOURCE OF ALTERNATIVE VIEWS

Partner involvement also facilitates the emergence of viewpoints different to the patient's beliefs that perpetuate his or her body image distress. In doing so a therapist asks questions of the partner, for example, *"Do you see it in a similar or different way?"* This can also locate the partner's view in context (e.g., his or her culture, gender, family, etc.) and considers how each contextual domain alters the partner's thoughts, emotions, and any subsequent actions (Jones & Asen, 2000). *"Do you think that as 'a man'* (context of gender) *you would see it similarly?"* or *"Do you think that 'as a person that is younger than you'* (context of age), *you would see it similarly?"* In the presence of multiple and different views, it is then helpful to follow up how this could lead to different behaviors, for example by asking *"If you were to see it in this way, what might you do next?"* This reciprocal process between meaning and action illustrates to the patient the implications of particular beliefs on behavior and the relationship. This process can also make explicit the ingrained cultural and societal values around appearance that can cause distress and to what extent partners or patients can resist subscribing to narrow appearance ideals. As couple-based interventions help patients to alter their perception of how their partner views them, this individual work around self-concept appears important in achieving a changed self-view and more acceptance of the actual self.

PARTNER AS A FACILITATOR OF CHANGE

In individual treatment, a patient can struggle with implementing some of the tasks planned. While each case may hold different explanations for this, a partner can be a useful person to recruit to apply in-session ideas in the real world. It is most useful that patients explain to their partners what the reasons are behind the task on a cognitive or behavioral level. The therapist then interviews the partner about what these changes could mean for the patient's life, which is intended to build motivation for the patient. The therapist also allows the patient to respond to what the partner has shared by asking questions such as "*Having heard this, how do you feel about the plan we had?*" The therapist also prepares partners for the possibility that their support may not lead to a change in the patient's behavior and discusses with patients how they would like their partner to respond in such circumstances.

Sunita had been able to see how her avoidance of particular situations perpetuated some of her distress about her body following a failed breast reconstruction. In particular, we had discussed how she does not get changed in front of her partner and locks herself in the bathroom. At some point during the session, which her partner attended, the following interaction took place:

Therapist: *Sunita, you have decided that you want to try to no longer lock yourself in the bathroom when having a bath or shower and also that you might get changed in front of your husband. How come?*

Sunita: *I think I hide my body away now, and I don't think it helps me.*

Therapist: *Is it helpful in any way?* (our attempt to help the partner understand the logic of her avoidance)

Sunita: *It helps because I don't end up feeling bad about him looking at me or worry about him feeling uncomfortable.*

Therapist: *And at the same time you want to stop hiding away. How would that be helpful?*

Sunita: *I know he is not bothered by how I look. He saw my chest when it all started to go wrong and it was much worse than it is now. If I was not hiding away I might realize that he is not bothered really.*

Therapist to husband: *What do you think these changes would mean to Sunita?*

Husband: *She might feel like she is getting back to normal, like doing things like she used to around me.*

Therapist: *Why do you think this is a good idea?*

Husband: *That might help her to feel better, like she is more like her old self.*

Therapist to husband: *Are you surprised this is what Sunita is planning on doing?*

Husband: *No, not really. She has managed a lot with the treatments and I have been humbled by this. It reminds me of something she said early on—I don't want the cancer to change us.*

Therapist to Sunita: *So how do you feel about doing some of this before our next meeting?*

Sunita: *I had forgotten how important it was to me to make sure that me and [husband] had each other and we didn't get lost in the cancer. I guess he is right; I should remember that I have done other hard things.*

COUPLE WORK WITH BODY IMAGE CONCERNS IN THE CONTEXT OF A SUPPORTIVE RELATIONSHIP

We now discuss several areas that clinicians can attend to in couple work since these have formed part of the research interventions reviewed that have been helpful at reducing body image distress. These may be most beneficial where there is low relationship distress and both partners report satisfaction with the relationship.

COMMUNICATION

Effective communication in the context of cancer-related challenges can reduce distress and is associated with relationship function/satisfaction (e.g. Barsky Reese et al. 2014; Manne et al. 2010). While definitions of effective communication in couples can vary, generally it is characterized by openness, trust, and respect and can help couples meet their needs (Epstein & Baucom 2002). Communication is a way for a person to feel heard and understood, and listening is central to this process. Communication can be a reciprocal process where an "act" invites a response from the other that shows that he or she is concerned, interested, and wants to understand. It includes more than just speech, for example, facial expressions, gestures, and touch. Working toward good communication is an important focus in couple work.

The therapist can helpfully focus on the couple's communication during other stressful times to allow the couple to reflect on what has helped in the past and consider whether this could assist them now. Therapy encourages the patient and partner to use "I" statements and questions aim to elicit the effect of (verbal and nonverbal) communication on the listener, knowing that its effects may be different to the communicator's intention. A focus on the detail of interactions where (either of) the couple felt they were interacting in a helpful way can show the couple what to do more of in the relationship.

Therapy also looks at the reported nonverbal changes in the couple's communication as these often have a distancing effect on emotional intimacy, which can perpetuate body image distress (as in the previous example of Martha and Andrew). Nonverbal changes often include hiding the body (e.g., showering in privacy) or less physical contact (e.g., going to bed earlier/later than the partner, fewer hugs). Therapy invites couples to determine other responses that may be more in keeping with what is important to them as a couple or that meet the needs of the other person more readily. Role-play and attention to barriers that prevent a person from using a particular style of communication is important to promote change.

In treatment, it is also helpful to look at any avoidance of communication in relation to cancer, which can be common (Henderson et al. 2002; Manne 1999). Alongside the influence of attachment patterns on interaction and avoidance, it is important for the therapist to consider other reasons, such as shame and humiliation (Gilbert & Miles 2002) that may render a patient less likely to want to raise body image concerns. This extract shows how useful it is to explore changes in communication.

Craig had radical surgery to remove a tumor, which involved losing the alar of his nose, part of the soft palate, and part of the upper mandible. He feels that his wife Annie has no idea about how upset he is about the way he looks and that he can't eat well or kiss properly. He feels that they have become distant which makes it harder to raise these difficulties.

> **Therapist to Annie:** *Before the cancer, when did you talk in a way that made you feel connected to Craig?*
> **Annie:** *In the evening, when we were sitting at the table we would chat, catch up, and provide moral support to each other and stuff.*
> **Therapist to Craig:** *Would you say that was the case for you too?*
> **Craig:** *Yes, and then watch some TV together and sometimes before we would go to bed we would chat some more.*
> **Therapist to Annie:** *How about now; what happens at dinner time or bed time?*
> **Annie:** *We don't talk at dinner time as Craig concentrates on eating and he often goes to bed early as he can get quite tired.*
> **Therapist to Annie:** *How come there is little time at dinner time or you go to bed later?*
> **Annie:** *We decided that we would try to keep things as normal as possible for the kids. So, I have continued to work, sort out the kids and household . . . which I usually do after dinner. I also do the cooking.* (turning to Craig) *I want to do this and wouldn't have it any other way.*
> **Therapist to Annie:** *So, this focus on keeping things as normal as possible has affected the couple-time that you used to have, your time to talk?*
> **Annie:** *We don't talk over dinner as it takes Craig all his effort to eat.*
> **Therapist to Craig:** *Is there a time where you would want to talk about the body changes?*
> **Craig:** *Yes, it would be good to do it when we used to do it.*
> **Annie:** (upset and crying) *I have been busy doing everything to help our family and life. I think that has been my focus and I don't think I have realized that it means that me and Craig just talk less or have less time for that moral support.*
> **Therapist:** *That sounds like a sad realization. What do you think might need to change to protect this talking time?*
> **Annie:** *Maybe dinner time needs to be longer so that I give Craig time to get involved in the talking. Maybe putting my hand on him.*
> **Craig:** *I could ask Annie to sit down or ask her to come to bed earlier.*
> **Therapist:** *What about the household stuff, that will still be there?*
> **Annie:** *Yes, we need to work something out.*

Here, the therapist's intention is to make transparent the unintended consequence of the changes made in response to the cancer and body changes. Inviting the couple to observe changes in their communication and closeness is likely to be experienced without blame and helps to foster change. Here, the couple is making plans on how to resume what used to work, acknowledging the complexities in doing so.

RELATIONAL COPING

The fact that distress levels in a dyad affected by cancer are highly interdependent suggests that couples may cope jointly with cancer-related challenges. The dyadic coping model in particular posits that a partner (in most cases the patient) shows signs of stress to which the other partner responds and which may also necessitate for him or her to manage his or her own distress (Revenson, Kayser, & Bodenman 2005). The partner's response in turn affects the patient's coping and ultimately relationship satisfaction. It is important to note that partners can experience similar or greater levels of distress than the patient (Northouse et al. 2000, 2005; Couper et al. 2006).

Relational coping builds on communication by ensuring a focus on circular patterns of interactions that increase the likelihood that the problem is located in the interactional process. Therapy should explore the beliefs a partner has about responses that would help the patient cope (better). It is not uncommon that partners are concerned that an acknowledgement or discussion about body changes may reinforce or exacerbate the patient's distress. Naming the (positive or logical) intention (e.g., a wish to protect the patient) can reframe the reason for the partner's apparent lack of support. In therapy, partners can also hear whether their concern that invites them to engage in such emotional protecting is helpful to the patient and potentially be given permission to discuss things, as their fear may be unfounded.

Tracy (previously discussed in the section on mentalization) *is unhappy about her breast reconstruction. Her surgeon had said that he failed to see why she was getting upset at her last consultation and her partner Shelley had said that her scars will look better soon.*

Therapist: *So do you talk about how unhappy you are about your breasts?*
Tracy: *Not really. I really appreciate what the surgeon has done. It is amazing what the surgery can do these days. I have not been bothered by looks before, and I guess keeping on at it is just vain and ungrateful.*
Therapist: *What does Shelley say if you talk about your breasts?*
Tracy: *She reminds me how good it is that the cancer is gone. That the treatment is over now. That we will get back to normal again.*
Therapist: *When Shelley says those things to you, that the cancer is gone, that treatment is over, that you will be back to normal again, what do you think Shelley is trying to achieve?*
(Our attempt is to logically connote Shelley's behavior even though it does not validate Tracy's concerns.)
Tracy: *She is trying to help me feel better.*
Therapist to Shelley: *What happens to Tracy's distress when you say those things?*
(We turn to Shelley, as we are more likely to invite criticism by asking this question to Tracy)

Shelley: *Tracey stops crying eventually but she still doesn't like her breasts. She always comes back to '"but they are not even."*

Therapist to Shelley: *What kind of things do you think might be unhelpful to say or talk about when Tracey is upset about the way she looks?*

Shelley: *I don't want to focus on things we can't change or get stuck on what is a problem. That won't help her.*

Therapist to Tracy: *What would it be like to hear Shelley talk about what can't be changed, if she said something like "I get it, how upsetting it is that your breasts are no longer the same."*

Tracy: *I would know that she got it.*

Therapist to Tracy: *And if she got it, how would that change the conversations you have?*

Tracy: *Maybe I wouldn't feel the need to keep trying to explain my unhappiness.*

In this extract, Shelley's response stems from lay beliefs about helping, such as "looking on the bright side" or "not dwelling on things." Discussing coping responses to distress might help the couple to work out how to best support each other with the appearance-related distress. This can include permission giving for particular responses, which for Tracy was an instruction to Shelley to *just listen*.

FOCUS ON THE AFFECTED PART OF THE BODY

Exploring coping responses and communication are helpful precursors to focusing on the affected body part as it provides the couple with a context to make sense of each other's reactions. This specific focus may also have contributed to the effectiveness of the intervention by Kalaitzi et al. (2007). Consider asking each partner *"How different does the body part feel or function?"* This implicitly suggests there has been a change and normalizes the change in sensation, appearance, and function. It can be helpful for the patient to connect to his or her direct physical experience, rather than to judge or evaluate the change, which can include asking the patient to run his or her finger or hand over it and really concentrate on what the fingers or hands experience, rather than what the mind experiences.

Most of the time the patient has been exposed to the body part more frequently than the partner, so consider asking the patient *"How have you adjusted to the change? What has helped you get to this point?"* This can help patients understand that they may be in a different stage of adjustment to their partner. Ask them, *"Has your partner had similar opportunities? What might help your partner adjust to it in a similar way?"* If it is appropriate, and the partner is likely to be able to stay with the direct experience (rather than judging), it can be helpful to encourage the partner to touch or look at the affected body part.

A partner may have only seen the affected body part in a medicalized way or not at all. For example, Annie had not touched Craig's lip or kissed him since he had surgery for his cancer, although she had been involved with dressings. If there has been (partial) avoidance we are particularly interested in asking the patient, *"What do you think [partner's] reaction might be? What kind of response would you like him or her to have?"* Attempts to look at responses and the meanings attributed to these are helpful to enable a couple to stop avoidance of touch or communication about the body changes.

The higher a person's disgust sensitivity, the more likely he or she will struggle to engage with wound care (Gaind, Clarke, & Butler 2011), so it may be useful to explain that different people may need more support in managing big changes to the body through graded exposure and taking a focus on "what is." The literature on sensate focus and creating boundaries for touch can help both partners make progress toward integrating the entire body into their relationship again. A couple like Annie and Craig may also need support to develop the skills to open up to challenging thoughts and feelings (e.g., sadness, concern to cause pain, etc.) that have prevented them from touching the body part, in particular kissing.

Craig described his lip as "tight, numb, okay, with a hard lump on the inside of his mouth" and that he can't open his mouth as wide anymore. Annie said that since changing Craig's dressings she had occasionally massaged his scar but essentially had not touched his face or kissed him properly since the surgery. She said his face felt soft except where the scar was.

Therapist to Craig: *How come you chose the word "okay"? What has helped you to get to "okay"?*

Craig: *My routine with the wound and also what I do to my face generally has helped me see it, so seeing it a lot must have helped. And it has also changed what it feels like, it's softer now.*

Therapist to Annie: *Are you still involved in touching Craig's face?*

Annie: *No, I might be around when he looks after his face, but not really.*

Therapist Annie: *So, there is no touching or kissing his face at the moment.*

Annie: *Not really.*

Therapist to Craig: *Do you think Annie is at "okay" or could get to "okay" to touch it or kiss it?*

Craig: *Yes, she could.*

Therapist to Craig: *What might it be like to kiss again?*

Craig: *Weird but good too, a sign that we are close.*

Therapist to Annie: *How do you think it would be for you to kiss again?*

Annie: *Weird too but I think it is important to do; it will change over time.*

SUMMARY AND FUTURE DIRECTIONS

Adjusting to changes to body integrity, functioning, or appearance following cancer and its treatment can be challenging for both patients and their partners. The context of the partnered relationship can play a critical role in determining how cancer patients cope with body image changes. Relationship distress may undermine the effectiveness of skills-based approaches to body image changes and, as such, warrants clinical attention to ensure that treatments can be effective. Couple-based interventions that incorporate education and the teaching of communication skills, alongside other skills and strategies, have demonstrated efficacy at addressing body image concerns and improving relationship functioning. Among the most critical aspects of successful interventions appear to be specific communication skills which help couples learn how best to communicate about patients' body image concerns and skills practice that serves to reduce body avoidance and increase acceptable, and even pleasurable, touching or viewing of the body. With this in mind, the clinical material included in this chapter focused on methods by which a therapist can bring patients' partners in to optimize individual work around cancer-related body image distress or couple work with the areas of focus on communication around body image changes, relational coping, and inclusion of the body part into treatment.

This chapter has led us to several interesting questions that remain to be studied in future work.

- As the body image target differs for men and women (i.e., focusing on body function versus body appearance, respectively), how can body image concerns be addressed in gender-mixed cancer populations?
- Is it necessary to match type of avoidance with type of exposure (i.e., visual exposure for appearance concerns and nonjudgmental partnered touching [e.g., sensate focus] for those with functional and appearance problems)?
- What are the key mechanisms behind the effectiveness of couple-based interventions, in particular, what behavioral skills discourage avoidance and increase exposure, and can these be parsed out into simpler interventions?
- How can couple-based interventions increase their effectiveness at improving patients' own self-acceptance, when effects appear to be greater for partners' perceptions?
- Can couple-based interventions be developed using different and innovative formats, such as those that are technology-based, in order to enhance dissemination and reach?
- Can causal relationships be teased out between body image concerns and relationship distress, and how might such causal effects be leveraged in the development of new couple-based interventions?
- How can couple-based interventions be developed to be maximally sensitive to cross-cultural concerns and/or nonheterosexual patients?

Mental health practitioners are in a unique position to implement couple-based interventions to address body image distress after cancer and its treatment. Taking a relational approach is respectful of the system of relationships that patients and their partner exist within and how these relationships influence the body image problems in a myriad of ways.

REFERENCES

Abend TA, Williamson GM. Feeling attractive in the wake of breast cancer: optimism matters, and so do interpersonal relationships. *Person Soc Psychol Bull.* 2002;28:427–436.

Allen J, Fonagy P, Bateman A. *Mentalizing in Clinical Practice.* Washington, DC: APPI; 2008.

Andersen T. The reflecting team: dialogue and meta-dialogue in clinical work. *Fam Process.* 1987;26:415–428.

Barsky Reese J, Porter LS, Regan KR, Keefe FJ, Azad NS, Diaz LA, Herman JM, Haythornthwaite JA. A randomized pilot trial of a telephone-based couples intervention for physical intimacy and sexual concerns in colorectal cancer. *Psychooncology.* 2014, 23, 1005–1013.

Baucom DH, Porter LS, Kirby JS, et al. A couple-based intervention for female breast cancer. *Psychooncology.* 2009;18:276–283.

Benedict C, Philip EJ, Baser RE, Carter J, Schuler TA, Jandorf L, DuHamel K, Nelson C. Body image and sexual function in women after treatment for anal and rectal cancer. *Psychooncology.* 2016;25:316–323.

Boquiren VM, Esplen MJ, Wong J, Toner B, Warner E, Malik N. Sexual functioning in breast cancer survivors experiencing body image disturbance. *Psychooncology.* 2016;25:66–76.

Bowlby J. *Attachment and Loss: Vol. 1. Attachment,* 2nd ed. New York: Basic Books; 1982.

Burwell SR, Case LD, Kaelin C, Avis NE. Sexual problems in younger women after breast cancer surgery. *J Clin Oncol.* 2006;24(18):2815–2821.

Chambers SK, Occhipinti S, Schover L, Nielsen L, Zajdlewicz L, Clutton S, Halford K, Gardiner RA, Dunn J. A randomized controlled trial of a couples-based sexuality intervention for men with localized prostate cancer and their female partners. *Psychooncology.* 2015;24(7):748–756.

Chambers SK, Schover L, Halford K, Clutton S, Ferguson M, Gordon L, Gardiner RA, Occhipinti S, Dunn J. ProsCan for couples: randomized controlled trial of a couples-based sexuality intervention for men with localized prostate cancer who receive radical prostatectomy. *BMC Cancer.* 2008;8:226.

Clarke A, Thompson A, Jenkinson E, Rumsey N, Newell R. *CBT for Appearance Anxiety.* London: Wiley Blackwell; 2014.

Collins AL, Love AW, Bloch S, Street AF, Duchesne GM, Dunai J, Couper JW. Cognitive existential couple therapy for newly diagnosed prostate cancer patients and their partners: a descriptive pilot study. *Psychooncology.* 2013;22:465–469.

Couper et al. J, Bloch S, Love A, MacVean M, Duchesne GM, Kissane D. Psychosocial adjustment of female partners of men with prostate cancer: a review of the literature. *Psychooncology.* 2006;15(11): 937–953.

Dagan M, Hagedoorn M. Response rates in studies of couples coping with cancer: a systematic review. *Health Psychol.* 2014;33:845–852.

Dallos R, Vetere A. Systemic therapy and attachment narratives: attachment narrative therapy. *Clin Child Psychol Psychiatry.* 2014;19(4):494–502.

Epstein NB, Baucom DH. *Enhanced Cognitive Behavioral Therapy for Couples: A Contextual Approach.* Washington, DC: American Psychological Association; 2002.

Epstein N, Baucom DH, Daiuto AD. Cognitive-behavioral couples therapy. In: Halford WK, Markman HJ, eds. *The Clinical Handbook of Marriage and Couples Interactions.* New York: Wiley; 1997:415–449.

Falk Dahl CA, Reinertsen KV, Nesvold IL, Fosså SD, Dahl AA. A study of body image in long-term breast cancer survivors. *Cancer.* 2010;116(15):3549–3557.

Falkner HJ. Gender. In: Rumsey N, Harcourt D, eds. *The Oxford Handbook of the Psychology of Appearance.* Oxford: Guilford Press; 2012:175–189.

Fang SY, Chang HT, Shu BC. The moderating effect of perceived partner empathy on body image and depression among breast cancer survivors. *Psychooncology.* 2015;24(12):1815–1822.

Fang SY, Lin YC, Chen TC, Lin CY. Impact of martial coping on the relationship between body image and sexuality among breast cancer survivors. *Support Care Cancer.* 2015;23:2551–2559.

Fobair P, Stewart SL, Chang S, D'Onofrio C, Banks PJ, Bloom JR. Body image and sexual problems in young women with breast cancer. *Psychooncology.* 2006;15:579–594.

Fredman SJ, Baucom DH, Gremore TM, et al. Quantifying the recruitment challenges with couple-based interventions for cancer: applications to early-stage breast cancer. *Psychooncology.* 2009;18: 667–673.

Gaind S, Clarke A, Butler PE. The role of disgust emotions in predicting self-management in wound care. *J Wound Care.* 2011;20(7):346–350.

Gilbert P, Miles J. *Body Shame: Conceptualization, Research and Treatment.* London: Routledge; 2002.

Hannah MT, Gritz ER, Wellisch DK, Fobair P, Hoppe RT, Bloom JR, Sun G-W, Varghese A, Cosgrove MD, Spiegel D. Changes in martial and sexual functioning in long-term survivors and their spouses: testicular cancer versus Hodgkin's disease. *Psychooncology.* 1992;1:89–103.

Henderson BN, Davison KP, Pennebaker JW, Gatchel RJ, Baum A. Disease disclosure patterns among breast cancer patients. *Psychol Health.* 2002;17(1):51–62.

Johnson SM. *The Practice of Emotionally Focused Couple Therapy: Creating Connection.* New York: Brunner/Mazel; 1996.

Jones E, Asen E. *Systemic Couple Therapy and Depression.* London: Karnac; 2000.

Jun EY, Kim S, Chang SB, Oh K, Kang HS, Kang SS. The effect of a sexual life reframing program on marital intimacy, body image, and sexual function among breast cancer survivors. *Cancer Nurs.* 2011;34:142–149.

Kalaitzi C, Papadopoulos VP, Michas K, Vlasis K, Skandalakis P, Filippou D. Combined brief psychosexual intervention after mastectomy: effects on sexuality, body image and psychological well-being. *J Surg Oncol.* 2007;96(3):235–240.

Loaring, JM, Larking M, Shaw R, Flowers P. Renegotiating sexual intimacy in the context of altered embodiment: the experiences of women with breast cancer and their male partners following mastectomy and reconstruction. *Health Psychol.* 2015;34(4):426–436.

Manne S, Badr H, Zaider T, Nelson C, Kissane D. Cancer-related communication, relationship intimacy, and psychological distress among couples coping with localized prostate cancer. *J Cancer Survivor.* 2010;4:74–85.

Manne SL. Intrusive thoughts and psychological distress among cancer patients: the role of spouse avoidance and criticism. *J Consult Clin Psychol.* 1999;67:539–546.

Manne SL, Ostroff J, Norton T, Fox K, Goldstein L, Grana G. Cancer-related relationship communication in couples coping with early stage breast cancer. *Psychooncology.* 2006;15:234–247.

Manne SL, Siegel SL, Siegel SD, Heckman CJ, Kashy DA. A randomized clinical trial of a supportive versus a skill-based couple-focused group intervention for breast cancer patients. *J Consult Clin Psychol.* 2016;84(8):668–681.

Naaman S, Radwan K, Johnson, S. Coping with early breast cancer: couple adjustment processes and couple-based interventions. *Psychiatry.* 2009;72(4):321–345.

Nelson CJ, Emanu JC, Avildsen I. Couples-based intervention following prostate cancer treatment: a narrative review. *Transl Androl Urol.* 2015;4(2):232–242.

Nelson CJ, Kenowitz, J. Communication and intimacy-enhancing interventions for men diagnosed with prostate cancer and their partners. *J Sex Med.* 2013;10:127–132.

Northouse L, Kershaw T, Mood D, Schafenacker A. Effects of a family intervention on the quality of life of women with recurrent breast cancer and their family caregivers. *Psychooncology.* 2005;14:478–491.

Northouse LL, Mood D, Templin T, Mellon S, George T. Patterns of adjustment to colon cancer. *Soc Sci Med.* 2000;50(2):271–284.

Odigie VI, Tanaka R, Yusufu LMD, Gomna A, Odigie EC, Dawotola DA, Margaritoni M. Psychosocial effects of mastectomy on married African women in northwestern Nigeria. *Psychooncology.* 2010;19:893–897.

Reese JB, Porter LS, Casale KE, Bantug ET, Bober SL, Schwartz SC, Smith KC. Adapting a couple-based intimacy enhancement intervention to breast cancer: a developmental study. *Health Psychol.* 2016;35:1085–1096.

Revenson TA, Kayser K, Bodenman G. *Couples Coping with Stress: Emerging Perspectives on Dyadic Coping.* Washington, DC: American Psychological Association; 2005.

Rumsey N, Harcourt D. *The Psychology of Appearance.* Oxford: Oxford University Press; 2004.

Scott JL, Halford WK, Ward BG. United we stand? The effects of a couple-coping intervention on adjustment to early stage breast or gynecological cancer. *J Consult Clin Psychol.* 2004;72(6):1122–1135.

Scott JL, Kayser K. Review of couple-based interventions for enhancing women's sexual adjustment and body image after cancer. *Cancer J.* 2009;15(1):48–56.

Schover LR, Yetman RJ, Tuason LJ, Meisler E, Esselstyn CB, Hermann RE, Grundfest-Broniatowski S, Dowden RV. Partial mastectomy and breast reconstruction: a comparison of their effects on psychosocial adjustment, body image and sexuality. *Cancer*. 1995;75(1):54–64.

Shaver PR, Mikulincer M. An overview of adult attachment theory. In: Obegi J, Berant E, eds. *Attachment Theory and Research in Clinical Work with Adults*. London: Guilford; 2009:17–45.

Sheppard C, Wylie KR. An assessment of sexual difficulties in men after treatment for testicular cancer. *Sex Relation Therapy*. 2001;16(1):47–58.

Taylor S, Harley C, Ziegler L, Brown J, Velikova G. Interventions for sexual problems following treatment for breast cancer: a systematic review. *Breast Cancer Res Treat*. 2011;130(3):711–724.

White M. *Maps of Narrative Practice*. New York: W. W. Norton; 2007.

Wittmann D, He C, Mitchell S, Wood DP Jr, Hola V, Thelen-Perry S, Montie JE. A one-day couple group intervention to enhance sexual recovery for surgically treated men with prostate cancer and their partners: a pilot study. *Urol Nurs*. 2013;33(3):140–147.

Wootten AC, Abbott JM, Farrell A, Austin DW, Klein B. Psychosocial interventions to support partners of men with prostate cancer: a systematic and critical review of the literature. *J Cancer Survivor*. 2014;8:472–484.

Zimmermann T, Scott JL, Heinrichs N. Individual and dyadic predictors of body image in women with breast cancer. *Psychooncology*. 2010;19(10):1061–1068.

CULTURAL CONSIDERATIONS IN BODY IMAGE AND CANCER

A Western Cultural Perspective

Kristina Harper and Hanne Konradsen

*K*elly was 32 years old when she was diagnosed with breast cancer. She was an avid runner, mother of a three-year-old daughter, and the author of a healthy lifestyle blog. She and her husband were actively trying to get pregnant when her obstetrician found a lump in her breast. Kelly underwent a radical bilateral mastectomy and an auxiliary lymph node dissection because the doctors believed her cancer was aggressive. Kelly described, "Over the past year, I have put my running life on hold, my blog has been discontinued due to time constraints, and I no longer connect to the fitness community of my former life. My daughter watches me cry and I struggle to have the energy to run after her. I have had several surgeries, including a mastectomy, portal placement, breast tissue expander placement, egg harvesting, removal of my fallopian tubes and ovaries, and breast implant placement and nipple reconstruction. I long to be outside, pushing my daughter in the running stroller and blogging about fitness to inspire others. But, well, now I spend my time at the physical therapist due to restricted movement in my arm and pain in my neck area from surgery. I went from a young, fit, toned mom to a woman in forced menopause, with weakened bones, thinned hair, and an "old-lady" body. I feel like my body is not my own . . . it has failed me. Why would my husband still want me? I cannot look in the mirror, and I cannot stop feeling like my femininity and sexuality have been taken away. I am mourning my old body, and hating this new one."

INTRODUCTION

Women with breast cancer, like Kelly, experience significant physical changes that can result in disfigurement or visible scarring, lymphedema, and hair loss. Further, physical functioning is impacted by chemotherapy, radiotherapy, and surgery often rendering the body unable to engage in previously enjoyed activities and potentially resulting in premature menopause or infertility. How do women like Kelly experience these consequences? What impacts one's adjustment at diagnosis and throughout treatment? What does the loss of youthfulness and breasts mean to Kelly? What does infertility at the age of 32 mean to a young woman in America or other Western cultures? To fully grasp the extent of cancer on one's life, cultural values must be considered, as they shape one's cognitions, medical decisions, and behaviors in response to the course of illness.

Culture can be defined as "a set of values, ideologies, traditions, beliefs, and ways of engaging in the world that can be transmitted through some type of communication over the course of time and place throughout generations."[1(p. 4)] Scholars attempt to understand cultural impact on body image by identifying beauty ideals and assessing the extent to which individuals in different societies are exposed to and assimilate to these pressures.[2] Cultural context influences various phenotypic features including, weight, shape, breast size, muscularity, and skin tone, which are areas frequently affected by cancer and its treatment. Western society emphasizes physical appearance and individual personal control over physical shape and attributes personal well-being and success to outward appearances. On a macro level, cultural factors often determine preferred body ideals which are then experienced at the individual level via influences such as mass media.

WESTERN BODY IMAGE IDEAL SHIFTS ACROSS TIME

Beauty ideals are fluid within a specific cultural society. Western culture can be defined according to beliefs, values, and norms that have their origin in the European culture and typically includes nations in Europe and nations such as the United States, Canada, Australia, New Zealand, and parts of Latin America. The Western perspective on the beauty ideal has shifted, changing in response to the cultural landscape and historical events. Until the 19th century, the preferred female physique in western Europe was full-bodied and soft with the use of the corset to exaggerate a curvaceous silhouette.[3] It was not until the late 19th century that we began to see a societal shift toward a leaner definition of femininity. By the 1920s, the "flapper" silhouette emerged, and women bound their breasts to appear boy-like and slender.[4] In the 1940s, Hollywood stardom and actresses like Marilyn Monroe shifted the ideal to a shape with larger breast sizes, while still retaining a slenderized figure. A review of Playboy centerfolds and Miss America pageant winners between 1967 and 1987 demonstrated that the average weight, bust, and hip size of women steadily decreased.[5] Analogous changes in body shape were apparent among English fashion models during this period.[6] Voracek and Fisher looked at temporal trends in Playboy centerfold models' body measurements through 2001 and found that bust size, hip circumference, and body mass index decreased, while waist size increased, creating a more androgynous look.[7] By the 21st century, Playboy centerfolds and Miss America pageant winners consistently exhibited body weights below normal weight, and the thin-ideal had become the stable, prominent goal of attainment for women of Westernized nations.[8] The thin-ideal remains a dominant social measure of female attractiveness, but images depicting women as athletic and muscular (i.e., the "fit-ideal") are increasingly evident in sociocultural messaging.[9] The cultural shift may initially seem like a healthier, more realistic ideal for women; however, women are often shown as achieving both ideals (i.e., thin and toned). Attainment of the fit-ideal physique would require most women to maintain a strict routine of weight training, caloric restriction, and exercise,[10] making it very difficult to achieve.[11]

Western cultural standards for the male physique also have shifted in the 21st century. Researchers analyzed images of Playgirl centerfolds and found that between 1970 and 1990, the average male physique became increasingly leaner with increased muscle mass. It was approximated that over time there was an estimated reduction of 12 pounds of fat and gain of 25 pounds of muscle on the male centerfold.[12] Other media suggests a similar male body ideal characterized by a v-shaped silhouette, with a defined muscular torso and narrowed waistline.[13,14] Research suggests that males report body dissatisfaction and identify increased muscle mass as a primary body goal.[15]

INTERNALIZATION OF THE WESTERN IDEAL

Fredrickson and Roberts suggested that women in Western culture are chronically sexualized and objectified (i.e., treated as a sum of their parts, such as breasts and legs), with the female body displayed for consumption by others.[16] Thus, objectification theory posits that in Western sociocultural contexts, the female is an object to be looked at evaluated based on conformity to the current beauty ideal.[17] As women are increasingly exposed to the objectified images, they internalize an observer's perspective of their own bodies (i.e., self-objectification), making external cues about standards of physical beauty one's own internal belief.[18] In other words, women begin to perceive themselves as an object to be evaluated based on appearance and garner their self-worth based upon one's ability to conform to the beauty ideal. Messages from various influential sources (media, family, and friends/peers) reinforce cultural ideals of attractiveness and the roles women are encouraged to adopt to gain societal approval. Internalization of cultural ideals has been a proposed causal variable between exposure to cultural messages (e.g., media) and body image dissatisfaction.[19]

Imagine now, Kelly from the start of our chapter, who has "lost" her breasts to surgery and her athletic body as she recovers from treatment. Kelly may be afraid or ashamed as she perceives the discrepancy between her body and the cultural ideal. Thus, conceivably she may view herself as having less worth as a woman.

FACETS OF WESTERN CULTURE THAT CAN AFFECT BODY IMAGE AND CANCER

Western culture is influenced and defined by the media, gender norms, and consumerism. Sociocultural models of body image maintain that these aspects impact the development and maintenance of one's view of their body. Research suggests that these facets also may impact cancer-related body image.

MEDIA

Western cultures are inundated with exposure to the thin ideal and muscular ideal across multiple forms of media, including television, magazine, advertisements, and social networking sites.[17] Western media is saturated with images depicting women as young and thin with large breasts[18] and men as tall, lean, and muscular.[20] Unfortunately, these beauty ideals presented are unattainable for most consumers.[21,22] There is extensive support that exposure to images of the thin or muscular ideal in the media is related to body dissatisfaction and body shame, and this relationship has been demonstrated in correlational, experimental, and longitudinal research designs.[23]

Newer forms of social media (e.g., Facebook and Instagram) allow immediate access to images of women who have either attained the beauty ideal or who or working on attaining the ideal (e.g., dieting, exercising). Statistics suggest that in Western nations, most adults report using social networking sites with daily activity.[24] Research has established an association between time viewing online images and body dissatisfaction among men and women.[25-27] Specifically, individuals look at and post idealized images to internet sites such as Twitter, Instagram, and Pinterest that typically present the ideal self, and certain platforms offer "filters" to enhance photo imaging.[28] Research suggests the images also promote the thin-ideal and objectification by showing isolated body parts, often sexual in nature.[29] Longitudinal research has shown that, among adult women, social network site use can result in increased body image concerns and maladaptive eating patterns.[30,31]

Recently, media images and campaigns (e.g., "strong is the new skinny") have advocated for the fit-ideal in opposition to the thin-ideal.[32] This trend has resulted in an increased presence of *fitspiration* (the integration of fitness and inspiration), or websites and hashtags that are purportedly intended to motivate and inspire people to engage in a "fit" lifestyle, primarily by viewing exercise and body-related images.[33] However, the fit-ideal is an unattainable figure for most women without considerable effort including excessive exercise and dietary restraint.[34] Thus, Internet-content promoted as healthy and "fit" often contains latent messaging that encourages overexercise behaviors and restrained eating. In fact, a content review of fitspiration websites and messaging revealed a heavy emphasis on the thin-ideal and appearance as the primary motivators to engage in healthy behaviors.[35] Research has shown that viewing fitspiration images increases one's aspirations to engage in exercise behaviors, it is also associated with increased body dissatisfaction and negative mood.[36] Purportedly, these images may convey that with enough effort, one *should* be able to attain the fit-ideal via exercise. Also, fit-ideal images often objectify bodies by showing snapshots of individual body parts (e.g., buttocks, abdominal muscles).[36]

Again, let's return to Kelly, who has created a profession by sharing daily images of her ideal self to inspire others to be fit (i.e., fitspiration blogger). Kelly is routinely exposed to and contributes to media advocating for others to engage in exercise and diet to attain the fit-ideal. She is at high risk for internalizing the Western belief that her value is based in part on her achievement of the fit-ideal. We can expect that adjusting to functional loss and appearance changes from breast cancer may be more difficult based on her investment in the Western culture.

MEDIA AND CANCER

Interestingly, media images of women with breast cancer may also perpetuate unrealistic Western beauty ideals. For example, an analysis of Canadian images used in breast cancer messaging found a large discrepancy between written content and visual depiction and that portrayals of breast cancer were largely inaccurate in terms of risk factors (e.g., age, body weight, ethnicity). Specifically, women in breast cancer-related media were portrayed as happy (e.g., smiling), healthy, attractive, and with minimal to no physical indicators of cancer.[37] Further, no images depicted physical "disfigurement" resulting from breast cancer such as missing or scarred breasts or lymphedema. These images seemed contrary to the written detail describing the physical impact of breast cancer (e.g., "my mastectomy flattened my chest and removed a nipple"; "I was bald and my chest burned"; "I now have a 10-inch scar from my underarm to my breastbone").[37] Even consumer cancer magazines, often provided at medical facilities, depict images of young, predominately white females, with few overt signs of the impact of cancer (e.g., nausea, fatigue) or treatment (e.g., scarring, loss of hair, scarring).[38] Imagine Kelly, sitting in her physician's waiting room, feeling nauseated and exhausted, losing her hair and recently finding out she has treatment-induced menopause, perusing through a consumer cancer magazine. She views the images of women smiling, appearing physically healthy with a full head of hair and no obvious changes to their breasts. Internalization of these images may increase shame and dissatisfaction, as she evaluates herself against these unrealistic ideals. There are similar concerns with messaging for skin cancer. A review of 154 articles (221 images) about skin cancer revealed that approximately 50% of the images conveyed attractive, tanned individuals; thus, providing conflicting messaging in text versus images (prevent skin cancer vs. be beautifully tanned).[39]

Others have argued that breast cancer–related media that exposes women's breasts (healthy or mastectomy with scarring) is in fact sexualizing and objectifying the experience.[40] Haines and colleagues assessed nine different messaging campaigns for breast cancer and found that women were often semi-nude in provocative poses.[40] The authors specifically discussed the ads featured in the "Expose the Truth" campaign by the Breast Cancer Research Foundation which features a young, thin, naked woman with thick hair, arching her back and covering her breasts with her hands. The authors suggest that this media image proliferates the idea that women's breasts are commodified products that need to be protected from deformity due to breast cancer, which renders one farther from the Western ideal. From this perspective, these images are similar to typical commercial advertising which uses women's bodies to attract attention and consumer interest in the "product."

While the expansion of the Internet increases proliferation of the thin-ideal in traditional media, it may be one medium in which cancer is presented in a more realistic manner. Blogs have become a vehicle for shared experience and day-to-day life for a variety of health topics. There are over 24,000 blogs with health-related themes, with several indexed for breast cancer.[41] Blogs often post images that are more transparent demonstrations of the visible bodily alterations associated with breast cancer, advocating for body acceptance.[41] For example, an Australian blogger participated in the project titled, Under the Red Dress, and posted an image online revealing her double mastectomy, hysterectomy, and navel reconstruction to raise awareness. Another project which combined photography and bloggers, The Scar Project, challenged the Western idealized imagery of breast cancer.[42] Photographs in the project capture women exposing postmastectomy breasts without shame or embarrassment. Bloggers also use their platform to bring attention to the media's incongruent messaging of women's body experience in relation to breast cancer. For example, one blogger cited in The Scar Project, criticized the media stating, "I think people prefer to pin a pink bow on us and package us up like a cuddly toy rather than see that cancer leaves its mark."[43(p. 271)]

GENDER

Gender roles in Western culture often emphasize stereotypes of feminism and masculinity. Thus, one may be at increased risk of marginalization when experiencing an illness associated with the opposite sex, such as men who are diagnosed with breast cancer. Qualitative research suggests that men who have breast cancer report perceived stigma and pressure to keep the experience concealed, often using more "masculine" words and avoiding the term breast cancer.[44] Further, men reported embarrassment, reduced attractiveness, and the need to hide their scars. Refer to Chapter 14 for further discussion of men, body image, and cancer.

CONSUMERISM

Western messaging also explicitly prescribes that with enough discipline, effort, and perhaps money, one can attain the thin and/or masculine ideal. Western media sells the body as a malleable project to be undertaken and altered by dieting, exercising, surgery, or other cosmetic procedures and products. Thus, the body ideal is marketed as a revered quality to be achieved, and failure to attain the ideal is perceived as a reflection of one's inner worth.[45,46] However, research suggests that the thin-ideal and muscular-ideal are overwhelmingly unattainable for most consumers and, consequently, many resort to cosmetic enhancement which is often marketed as an easy path to the ideal.[47]

The consumption of Western media as it spreads to new geographical areas has evident repercussions. A review of nine countries demonstrated that the import of Western media is associated with sociocultural shifts in body image and increased acceptance of the Western ideals.[48] Additionally, we see similar shifts among individuals who migrate to Western cultures and become new consumers of Western media. Migrants frequently report altering their appearance to match Western ideals[49] endorse increased body dissatisfaction compared to nonmigrants,[50,51] and have a thinner body ideal compared to nonmigrants still living in the country of origin.[52]

The consumption of Western messaging is reflected in the increasing acceptance and use of surgical procedures to "fix" perceived deviation from the cultural ideal.

Increased internalization of the cultural ideal and body dissatisfaction is associated with more positive attitudes toward cosmetic procedures[53] and one's reported probability of undergoing cosmetic procedures.[54] According to the American Society of Plastic Surgeons, there was a reported 59% increase in the total number of cosmetic procedures provided between 2003 and 2011.[55] During the same time frame, the British Association of Aesthetic Plastic Surgeons reported a 303% increase in surgical procedures.[56] In 2016, consumers spent $16.4 billion on cosmetic produces in the United Stated. The money was allocated between 1.7 million cosmetic surgical procedures (up 4% from 2015), 15.4 million cosmetic minimally invasive procedures (up 3% from 2015), and 5.8 million reconstructive procedures (no change compared to 2015).[55] The top procedures, breast augmentation and liposuction, parallel desired female attributes of the thin-ideal. Although both men and women in the United States have increasingly elected to have cosmetic surgery, women report more pressure, body dissatisfaction, and internalization of cultural ideals.[56] This suggests that there are still gender differentials in pressures to attain the ideal at any cost.

Let's now return to Kelly's experience as a woman who is experiencing the loss of her breasts amid a culture that is increasingly resorting to surgical procedures to attain bigger and more perfect breasts. One may suspect that these factors will impact her choice regarding treatment and reconstructive surgery. In the United States, there has been a significant increase (39%) in breast reconstruction from 2000 (78,832 procedures) to 2016 (109,256 procedures).[55] While breast reconstruction is known to significantly improve quality of life among breast cancer survivors, perhaps there is increased pressure for women to repair their perceived "defect" from breast cancer surgery because it has effectively taken them further from the ideal. Research has shown that women endorse body image concerns as a primary reason when deciding to undergo breast reconstruction following mastectomy.[57] Body image *investment,* or the value or importance placed on appearance and physical attributes, is a factor in the decisional process of undergoing breast reconstruction. Women who choose to have immediate breast reconstruction report more significant value on appearance and attractiveness to their partner in comparison to patients undergoing mastectomy only or breast-conserving therapy.[58] Additionally, body image investment may impact long-term adjustment in breast cancer patients. For example, appearance investment is associated with depression and quality of life outcomes for breast cancer survivors irrespective of treatment modality.[59] Further, throughout the course of treatment, body image investment predicts subsequent body shame, appearance dissatisfaction, and self-consciousness regarding one's looks.[60] Kelly, who placed significant investment and value on her physical attributes, may be at increased risk body image dissatisfaction and increased difficulty adjusting to her new body.

Women may also value and invest in appearance because it is part of their role in society. Women report that losing a breast creates insecurity about one's femininity and sexuality within the Western culture, thereby increasing body consciousness and beliefs that one does not belong.[61] Case studies even suggest that Western cultural expectations may hinder women's ability to conceptualize their bodies as feminine without breasts.[62] Women considering breast reconstruction, similarly report the perception that reconstruction is a way to restore lost femininity, sexuality, and even a sense of normalcy in one's body.[62]

BODY IMAGE IN WESTERN CULTURES AND HEAD AND NECK CANCER

While most of the chapter has focused on breast cancer, other cancers impact physical appearance in ways that may render someone further from the Western ideal. Head and neck cancers (HNC) are more likely to impact men and often encompass invasive treatment measures such as removal of tissue from the face, head, and neck, leaving the individual with significant disfigurement.[63] Unlike breast cancer in which scars are most likely hidden, those with HNC have visible disfigurement, placing them at increased risk for social stigmatization, especially in Western culture where outward appearance is highly valued. Patients with HNC regularly identify disfigurement as a primary treatment concern[64] and often feel socially isolated due to fear of stigma.[63,64] Isolation and difficulty adjusting to HNC is predicted by one's reported fear of negative evaluation.[65] Further, HNC treatment results in loss of functional abilities (e.g., eating, speaking) and impairments in being able to form certain facial expressions (such as a smile). Research has demonstrated that the reduced ability to smile among persons with HNC is associated with body dissatisfaction, increased discomfort in social situations, and avoidance as a body image coping strategy.[66] Smiling is a universal facial expression, but in Western culture it is an expected nonverbal form of communication in most sociocultural interactions; thus, individuals with HNC in Western cultures may be at high risk for body image distress.[67]

BODY IMAGE INTERVENTION IN THE ONCOLOGY SETTING

Addressing body image concerns among cancer patients seems particularly relevant in Western cultures that place extensive value on appearance and one's ability to conform to the current body ideal. A recent review suggests that there is limited research on empirically supported approaches to treating body image difficulties among various cancer patients, with most treatments focused on breast cancer.[68] Broadly, initial evidence suggests that addressing body image concerns has the potential to enhance comprehensive cancer care over the course of treatment, impacting treatment duration and adherence.[68,69] Returning to our patient Kelly, extensive shame and embarrassment about her body and its deviation from her previous Western ideal may lead to avoidance, increased negative emotionality, and social isolation. Further, although appearance is equated with worth in Western culture, research suggests that individuals like Kelly may be inhibited to spontaneously discuss body image concerns with their treatment team.[70]

Most treatments for cancer related body image have been within a cognitive-behavioral therapy framework which is typically goal-oriented and focused on maladaptive thoughts and behavioral patterns (e.g., avoidance, amotivation) that exacerbate distress. There are also programs that are community based and easily accessible to cancer patients. As we review a few select interventions, it is important to consider if the interventions specifically address sociocultural implications around body image. Do these programs attract women with different cultural values and backgrounds? Can cultural values be used to predict which program a person would find helpful, or can various programs be considered helpful for the same person? Finally, do some of these programs implicitly reinforce the message that self-worth and happiness are related to one's appearance?

Some community-based programs incorporate messaging that improving outward appearance can be a helpful means to enhance body image and quality of life. Look Good Feel Better[71] is a collaboration with the American Cancer Society and the Professional Beauty Association that offers free services to women to help manage the appearance-related side effects of cancer. Cancer patients can access information online, and they are encouraged to attend workshops where they receive a cosmetic kit and training on how to camouflage visible physical changes from cancer treatment. They provide information on makeup application, wig and head coverings, nail care, and clothing stylings to minimize noticeability of lymphedema and breast asymmetry. The premise of the program is that looking better on the outside can help women gain confidence, improve social interactions, and feel better throughout treatment. Feedback from participants who have participated in the program demonstrates that women appreciate the program and find it helpful. Changing Faces[72] is a registered charity that supports people who have a condition or injury that affects their appearance anywhere in the UK. The program includes counseling services, self-help guides, a skin camouflage service, and public awareness campaigns to raise awareness of unconscious beliefs about disfigurement that can result in prejudice and discrimination. These programs have wide-ranging positive impacts but are clearly impacted by and arise out of Western culture that emphasizes value based on appearance.

Interventions that focus on acceptance-based approaches to body image disturbance may allow individuals to adjust to cancer-related physical changes with awareness and nonjudgment, altering their own perceptions rather than focusing on how others perceive them. Research suggests that the way a woman perceives herself and the attitudes she adopts toward herself influence how she experiences cancer and treatment-related appearance changes.[73] One promising approach is self-compassionate mindfulness, which involves three primary components: self-kindness, mindful awareness, and a sense of common humanity.[74] Self-compassion emphasizes comforting oneself in response to distress and recognizing that suffering (e.g., cancer) is a shared experience.[74] Individuals who more readily engage in self-compassion are less likely to self-criticize, isolate, and overidentify with perceived flaws.[75] Thus, a self-compassion approach to body image promotes acceptance of one's present appearance, rather than a focus on achieving sociocultural ideals, and may even reduce cognitions that self-worth is based on appearance.[76] In non-cancer populations, self-compassion has been shown to be associated with reduced body shame and increased body positivity.[77] Among cancer patients, the literature reports that self-compassion is associated with reduced body image dissatisfaction,[73] less depression, and improved quality of life (Pinto-Gouveia et al., 2014). Research also suggests that self-compassion may facilitate exposure to aversive situations and thereby reducing avoidance.[78] Returning to our vignette, imagine the potential impact practicing self-compassion may have on Kelly's adjustment to breast cancer. Increased acceptance and kindness toward her body, reduced shame, and understanding her "suffering" within a larger broader context than Western ideals. With self-compassion, she may be able to treat herself kindness and patience and be more willing partake in treatment components that expose her body image-related distress.

Przezdziecki and Sherman developed a self-compassionate-focused writing intervention for helping women manage physical changes due to breast cancer and treatment.[79] Women were asked to recall and write about a negative body experience and were then given prompts to respond to the event from the three components of self-compassion (i.e., kindness, common humanity, and awareness). In comparison to a control group, the women who participated in the self-compassionate–focused writing reported lower negative affect and increased self-compassion cognitions during exposure to difficult memories related to body image. The intervention has been piloted as brief, one-time, self-administered, online intervention.[79] Both health professionals and breast cancer patients reported favorable opinions of the website and a moderate to high level of acceptability of the website. The program shows promise as an effective targeted intervention that could be easily disseminated at the community level.

CONSIDERATIONS IN INTERVENING ON BODY IMAGE ISSUES IN A WESTERN SETTING

Clinicians would benefit from screening for body image concerns and perceptions throughout the cancer experience. Assessing various facets of body image, including internalization, shame, investment, cognitions, and behaviors, can help the treatment team individualize treatment targets. Clinicians also need to consider that body image perception can influence treatment decisions, adherence to treatment, and long-term adjustment and quality of life.[80] Eliciting preferences about appearance and body image concerns from patients receiving treatment will increase treatment effectiveness.

Western medical practices has increased focus on patient participation and shared decision-making, which is related to greater patient satisfaction with treatment, greater self-efficacy, and more trust in one's provider.[81] Specific to breast cancer, female patients' perception of involvement in decision about treatment was related to long-term better health-related quality of life.[82] Age is another factor to consider as younger women are potentially facing greater discrepancy between self and ideal and the loss of child-bearing capabilities. Research suggests that younger women desire more information before decision-making in relation to breast cancer, including effect on family, sexuality, and body image.[83] Intervention techniques such as acceptance and mindfulness therapy and self-compassion focused treatment can help promote greater body image acceptance, and cognitive-behavioral–oriented therapy can help address maladaptive internalized cultural expectations and cognitions (e.g., I have control over my body). Tailoring these treatments in response to patient input can help women like Kelly adjust to their "new body" within Western culture.

CONCLUDING COMMENTS

This chapter focused on understanding body image and cancer through the Western cultural lens. The culturally expected body ideal has shifted over time, but Western culture consistently reveres the thin-ideal and fit-ideal as the dominant preferred body shape. Western culture also emphasizes the malleability of the appearance of the body and that, with sufficient effort, the ideal is attainable. Living within these cultural values may uniquely shape one's cancer experience, especially for those with cancers that result in physical alterations. Addressing body image concerns throughout the cancer diagnosis and treatment is implicated in several positive outcomes. Initial research indicates that frequent assessment and intervention to address body image can improve treatment adherence, reduce avoidance, and increase social connectivity. We encourage clinicians to explore and address potential body image concerns with cancer patients. Finally, extant research primarily focuses on breast cancer and HNC; thus, increasing the scope of body image research to other cancers may prove helpful in the future.

REFERENCES

1. Yam M. Does culture matter in body image? The effects of subjective and contextual culture on body image among bicultural women (Doctoral dissertation). University of Michigan; 2013.

2. Anderson-Fye EP. Body images in non-Western cultures. In: Cash TF, Smolak L, eds. *Body Image: A Handbook of Science, Practice, and Prevention,* 2nd ed. New York: Guilford Press; 2011:244–252.

3. Swami V, Gray M, Furnham A. The female nude in Rubens: disconfirmatory evidence of the waist-to-hip ratio hypothesis of female physical attractiveness. *Imagin Cogn Person.*, 2006;26(1):139–147.

4. Silverstein B, Perdue L, Peterson B, Kelly E. The role of the mass media in promoting a thin standard of bodily attractiveness for women. *Sex Roles.* 1986;14(9):519–532.

5. Garner DM, Garfinkel PE, Schwartz D, Thompson M. Cultural expectations of thinness in women. *Psychol Rep.* 1980;47(2):483–491.

6. Morris A, Cooper T, Cooper PJ. The changing shape of female fashion models. *Int J Eat Disord.* 1989;8(5):593–596.

7. Voracek M, Fisher ML. Shapely centrefolds? Temporal change in body measures: trend analysis. *BMJ.* 2002;325(7378):1447.

8. Wiseman CV, Gray JJ, Mosimann JE, Ahrens AH. Cultural expectations of thinness in women: an update. *Int J Eat Disord.* 1992;11(1):85–89.

9. Thompson JK, Roehrig M, Cafri G, Heinberg LJ. Assessment of body image disturbance. In: Mitchell JE, Peterson CB, eds. *Assessment of Eating Disorders.* New York: Guilford Press; 2005:175–202.

10. Homan K, McHugh E, Wells D, Watson C, King C. The effect of viewing ultra-fit images on college women's body dissatisfaction. *Body Image.* 2012;9(1):50–56.

11. Curioni CC, Lourenco PM. Long-term weight loss after diet and exercise: a systematic review. *Int J Obesity.* 2005;29(10):1168-1174.

12. Leit RA, Pope HG, Gray JJ. Cultural expectations of muscularity in men: THE evolution of Playgirl centerfolds. *Int J Eat Disord.* 2001;29(1):90–93.

13. Hargreaves DA, Tiggemann M. Muscular ideal media images and men's body image: social comparison processing and individual vulnerability. *Psychol Men Masculin.* 2009;10(2):109–119.

14. Morrison TG, Morrison MA, Hopkins C. Striving for bodily perfection? An exploration of the drive for muscularity in Canadian men. *Psychol Men Masculin.* 2003;4(2):111–120.

15. Frederick DA, Forbes GB, Grigorian KE, Jarcho JM. The UCLA Body Project I: gender and ethnic differences in self-objectification and body satisfaction among 2,206 undergraduates. *Sex Roles.* 2007;57(5–6):317–327.

16. Fredrickson BL, Roberts TA. Objectification theory: toward understanding women's lived experiences and mental health risks. *Psychol Women Q.* 1997;21(2):173–206.

17. Buote VM, Wilson AE, Strahan EJ, Gazzola SB, Papps F. Setting the bar: divergent sociocultural norms for women's and men's ideal appearance in real-world contexts. *Body Image.* 2011;8(4):322–334.

18. Thompson JK, Stice E. Thin-ideal internalization: mounting evidence for a new risk factor for body-image disturbance and eating pathology. *Curr Dir Psychol Sci.* 2001;10(5):181–183.

19. Moradi B, Dirks D, Matteson AV. Roles of sexual objectification experiences and internalization of standards of beauty in eating disorder symptomatology: a test and extension of objectification theory. *J Counsel Psychol.* 2005;52(3):420–428.

20. Hargreaves DA, Tiggemann M. "Body image is for girls": a qualitative study of boys' body image. *J Health Psychol.* 2006;11:567–576. doi:10.1177/1359105306065017

21. Tiggemann, M. (2011). Sociocultural perspectives on human appearance and body image. In T.F. Cash & L. Smolak (Eds). Body image: A handbook of science, practice, and prevention (pp. 12–19). New York, NY, Guilford Press.

22. Ridgeway RT, Tylka TL. College men's perceptions of ideal body composition and shape. *Psychol Men Masculin.* 2005;6(3):209–220.

23. Kilbourne J (Prod.), Jhally S (Dir.). Killing us softly 4: Advertising images of women [Motion picture]. 2010. Available from http://www.mediaed.org/cgi-bin/commerce.cgi?display=user1

24. Leit RA, Gray JJ, Pope HG. The media's representation of the ideal male body: a cause for muscle dysmorphia? *Int J Eat Disord.* 2002;31(3):334–338.

25. Grabe S, Ward LM, Hyde JS. The role of the media in body image concerns among women: a meta-analysis of experimental and correlational studies. *Psychol Bull.* 2008;134(3):460–476.

26. Sensis. Yellow social media report. May 2004. Retrieved from www.sensis.com.au/ content/dam/sas/ PDFdirectory/Yellow-Social-Media-Report-2014.pdf

27. Bair CE, Kelly NR, Serdar KL, Mazzeo SE. Does the Internet function like magazines? An exploration of image-focused media, eating pathology, and body dissatisfaction. *Eat Behav.* 2012;13(4):398–401.

28. Tiggemann M, Miller J. The Internet and adolescent girls' weight satisfaction and drive for thinness. *Sex Roles.* 2010;63(1–2):79–90.

29. Blond A. Impacts of exposure to images of ideal bodies on male body dissatisfaction: a review. *Body Image.* 2008;17:100–110. doi:10.1016/jbodyim.2016.02.008

30. Krämer NC, Winter S. Impression management 2.0: the relationship of self-esteem, extraversion, self-efficacy, and self-presentation within social networking sites. *J Media Psychol.* 2008;20(3):106–116.

31. Ghaznavi J, Taylor LD. Bones, body parts, and sex appeal: an analysis of #thinspiration images on popular social media. *Body Image.* 2015;14:54–61.

32. Boepple L, Ata RN, Rum R, Thompson JK. Strong is the new skinny: a content analysis of fitspiration websites. *Body Image.* 2016;17:132–135.

33. Abena. From thinspo to fitspiration: how social media could be affecting your body image. 2013. Retrieved from http://www.collegefashion.net/college-life/fromthinspo-to-fitspiration-how-social-media-could-be-affecting-your-bodyimage/

34. Krane V, Waldron J, Stiles-Shipley JA, Michalenok J. Relationships among body satisfaction, social physique anxiety, and eating behaviors in female athletes and exercisers. *J Sport Behav.* 2001;24(3):247–264.

35. Boepple L, Thompson JK. A content analysis of healthy living blogs: evidence of content thematically consistent with dysfunctional eating attitudes and behaviors. *Int J Eat Disord*. 2014;47:362–367. http://dx.doi.org/10.1002/eat.22244

36. Tiggemann M, Zaccardo M. "Exercise to be fit, not skinny": the effect of fitspiration imagery on women's body image. *Body Image*. 2015;15:61–67.

37. McWhirter JE, Hoffman-Goetz L, Clarke JN. Can you see what they are saying? Breast cancer images and text in Canadian women's and fashion magazines. *J Cancer Educ*. 2012;27(2):383–391.

38. Phillips SG, Della LJ, Sohn SH. What does cancer treatment look like in consumer cancer magazines? An exploratory analysis of photographic content in consumer cancer magazines. *J Health Comm*. 2011;16(4):416–430.

39. McWhirter JE, Hoffman-Goetz L. Coverage of skin cancer risk factors and UV behaviors in popular US magazines from 2000 to 2012. *J Cancer Educ*. 2016;31(2):382–388.

40. Haines RJ, Bottorff JL, Mckeown SB, Ptolemy E, Carey J, Sullivan K. Tobacco and breast cancer messaging for younger women: a gender analysis. *Psychooncology*. 2010;19:S150–S151.

41. Coll-Planas G, Visa M. The wounded blogger: analysis of narratives by women with breast cancer. *Sociol Health Illn*. 2016;38(6):884–898.

42. Jay D. The SCAR Project. Meridian Printing; 2011. www.thescarproject.com

43. Wilkinson S. Breast cancer: feminism, representations and resistance—a commentary on Dorothy Broom's "Reading Breast Cancer." *Health*. 2001;5(2):269–277.

44. Quincey K, Williamson I, Winstanley S. "Marginalised malignancies": a qualitative synthesis of men's accounts of living with breast cancer. *Soc Sci Med*. 2016;149:17–25.

45. Gimlin D. The absent body project: cosmetic surgery as a response to bodily dys-appearance. *Sociology*. 2006;40(4):699–716.

46. Levine MP, Smolak L. Cultural influences on body image and the eating disorders. In W. Stewart Agras (Ed.): *The Oxford Handbook of Eating Disorders*. New York: Oxford University Press; 2010: 223–246.

47. Muise A, Desmarais S. Women's perceptions and use of "anti-aging" products. *Sex Roles*. 2010;63(1–2):126–137.

48. Anderson-Fye EP, Becker AE. Sociocultural aspects of eating disorders. In Thompson JK, ed. *Handbook of Eating Disorders and Obesity*. Hoboken, NJ: John Wiley; 2004:565–589.

49. Tovée MJ, Furnham A, Swami V. Healthy body equals beautiful body? Changing perceptions of health and attractiveness with shifting socioeconomic status. In Swami, V., Furnham, A. (Eds.). *The Body Beautiful*. London: Palgrave Macmillan; 2007:108–128.

50. Becker AE, Fay K. (2006). Sociocultural issues and eating disorders. *Ann Rev Eat Disord*. 2006:35–63.

51. Swami V, Mada R, Tovée MJ. Weight discrepancy and body appreciation of Zimbabwean women in Zimbabwe and Britain. *Body Image*. 2012;9(4):559–562.

52. Bush HM, Williams RGA, Lean MEJ, Anderson AS. Body image and weight consciousness among South Asian, Italian and general population women in Britain. *Appetite*. 2001;37(3):207–215.

53. Calogero RM, Park LE, Rahemtulla ZK, Williams KC. Predicting excessive body image concerns among British university students: the unique role of appearance-based rejection sensitivity. *Body Image*. 2010;7(1):78–81.

54. Nabi RL. Cosmetic surgery makeover programs and intentions to undergo cosmetic enhancements: a consideration of three models of media effects. *Hum Comm Res*. 2009;35(1):1–27.

55. American Society of Plastic Surgeons. 2012 report of the 2011 statistics. National Clearinghouse of Plastic Surgery Statistics; 2012. Retrieved from https://www.plasticsurgery.org/documents/News/Statistics/2012/plastic-surgery-statistics-full-report-2012.pdf

56. British Association of Aesthetic Plastic Surgeons. 2011 annual audit. Retrieved from https://www.baaps.org.uk/baaps_annual_audit_results_.aspx

57. Duggal CS, Metcalfe D, Sackeyfio R, Carlson GW, Losken A. Patient motivations for choosing postmastectomy breast reconstruction. *Ann Plast Surg.* 2013;70(5):574–580.

58. Adachi K, Ueno T, Fujioka T, Fujitomi Y, Ueo H. Psychosocial factors affecting the therapeutic decision-making and postoperative mood states in Japanese breast cancer patients who underwent various types of surgery: body image and sexuality. *Japan J Clin Oncol.* 2007;37(6):412–418.

59. Moreira H, Canavarro MC. A longitudinal study about the body image and psychosocial adjustment of breast cancer patients during the course of the disease. *Eur J Oncol Nurs.* 2010;14(4):263–270.

60. Moreira H, Silva S, Canavarro MC. The role of appearance investment in the adjustment of women with breast cancer. *Psychooncology.* 2010;19(9):959–966.

61. Avis NE, Crawford S, Manuel J. Psychosocial problems among younger women with breast cancer. *Psychooncology.* 2004;13(5):295–308.

62. Crompvoets S. Comfort, control, or conformity: women who choose breast reconstruction following mastectomy. *Health Care Women Int.* 2006;27(1):75–93.

63. Callahan C. Facial disfigurement and sense of self in head and neck cancer. *Soc Work Health Care.* 2005;40:73–87.

64. Fingeret MC, Yuan Y, Urbauer D, Weston J, Nipomnick S, Weber R. The nature and extent of body image concerns among surgically treated patients with head and neck cancer. *Psychooncology.* 2012;21(8):836–844.

65. Clarke SA, Newell R, Thompson A, Harcourt D, Lindenmeyer A. Appearance concerns and psychosocial adjustment following head and neck cancer: a cross-sectional study and nine-month follow-up. *Psychol Health Med.* 2014;19(5):505–518.

66. Lee J, Teo I, Guindani M, Reece GP, Markey MK, Fingeret MC. Associations between psychosocial functioning and smiling intensity in patients with head and neck cancer. *Psychol Health Med.* 2015;20(4):469–476.

67. Arapova MA. A cross-cultural study of the smile in the Russian-and English-speaking world. *J Lang Cult Educ.* 2016;4(2):56–72.

68. Fingeret MC, Teo I, Epner DE. Managing body image difficulties of adult cancer patients: lessons from available research. *Cancer.* 2014;120(5):633–641.

69. Annunziata MA, Giovannini L, Muzzatti B. Assessing the body image: relevance, application and instruments for oncological settings. *Support Care Cancer.* 2012;20(5):901–907.

70. Hall EJ. Intensity-modulated radiation therapy, protons, and the risk of second cancers. *Int J Radiat Oncol Biol Phys.* 2006;65(1):1–7.

71. Look good, feel better, http://lookgoodfeelbetter.org/

72. Changing faces, https://www.changingfaces.org.uk/

73. Przezdziecki A, Sherman KA, Baillie A, Taylor A, Foley E, Stalgis-Bilinski K. My changed body: breast cancer, body image, distress and self-compassion. *Psychooncology.* 2013;22(8):1872–1879.

74. Neff KD. The development and validation of a scale to measure self-compassion. *Self Identity.* 2003;2(3):223–250.

75. Neff KD, Hsieh YP, Dejitterat K. Self-compassion, achievement goals, and coping with academic failure. *Self Identity.* 2005;4(3):263–287.

76. Albertson ER, Neff KD, Dill-Shackleford KE. Self-compassion and body dissatisfaction in women: a randomized controlled trial of a brief meditation intervention. *Mindfulness.* 2015;6(3):444–454.

77. Breines J, Toole A, Tu C, Chen S. Self-compassion, body image, and self-reported disordered eating. *Self Identity.* 2014;13(4):432–448.

78. Thompson BL, Waltz J. Mindfulness and experiential avoidance as predictors of posttraumatic stress disorder avoidance symptom severity. *J Anxiety Disord.* 2010;24(4):409–415.

79. Przezdziecki A, Sherman KA. Modifying affective and cognitive responses regarding body image difficulties in breast cancer survivors using a self-compassion-based writing intervention. *Mindfulness.* 2016;7(5):1142–1155.

80. Figueiredo MI, Cullen J, Hwang YT, Rowland JH, Mandelblatt JS. Breast cancer treatment in older women: Does getting what you want improve your long-term body image and mental health? *J Clin Oncol.* 2004;22(19):4002–4009.

81. Kane HL, Halpern MT, Squiers LB, Treiman KA, McCormack LA. Implementing and evaluating shared decision making in oncology practice. *CA Cancer J Clin.* 2014;64(6):377–388.

82. Andersen MR, Bowen DJ, Morea J, Stein KD, Baker F. Involvement in decision-making and breast cancer survivor quality of life. *Health Psychol.* 2009;28(1):29–37.

83. Recio-Saucedo A, Gerty S, Foster C, Eccles D, Cutress RI. Information requirements of young women with breast cancer treated with mastectomy or breast conserving surgery: a systematic review. *Breast.* 2016;25:1–13.

CHAPTER 17

CULTURAL CONSIDERATIONS IN BODY IMAGE AND CANCER

An Asian Cultural Perspective

Geok Ling Lee and Irene Teo

"When I was told that I had to undergo a total hysterectomy in order to save my life, I was conflicted about whether I should. I had sleepless nights and felt anguished. However I bottled it up and hid it so as to not worry my husband. I also felt that I couldn't turn to my own sisters although we are close; I did not want them to be burdened by my situation. I was unable to make a decision as I felt conflicted and guilty that my husband's family lineage will end with me. I have been married to my husband for three years. Because he is the only son, I knew my husband was facing pressure from his parents and elders to bear a son. I felt my worth as a woman was undermined by the impending possibility of infertility. Thus, I was worried that I might be asked for a divorce. I was also worried that I would look less attractive and less complete as a woman to my husband once my womb was removed. I have heard some friends mention that chemotherapy can lead to my long black hair falling out. How unpleasant will it be for those around me to witness such a thing happening; what will they say? I am devastated and cannot bear the shame I have brought to my husband and my family from this illness. I am so afraid to become a burden to the people around me. In the end, my husband initiated the talk. He told me that he would love to have a complete family, but he does not want to lose me more. He encouraged me to go ahead with the surgery and said we would learn to live as a family of two. That settled my anxiety slightly and gave me hope to continue on."

INTRODUCTION

What would the loss of childbearing ability mean to you? The loss of a breast? Inability to eat the food prepared at a family gathering? We make the case that body image is a social product, which is largely determined by the social experiences within a cultural context. The experience of body image changes conceptually transcends cultural boundaries, yet the standards by which a person's body image is perceived are undoubtedly colored by his or her cultural lens.

Our schemas of what "normal" is are fundamentally embedded in our cultural beliefs and thus cultural perspectives are important to consider in examining value-laden concepts such as body image, health, and illness.[1] Nevertheless, cultural perspectives are always difficult to study as it is hard to define any particular culture due to its evolving nature and the inherent subcultures within a larger cultural ecosystem. It is important to keep in mind, too, that with globalization and exchange of cultural ideas in recent times, cultural norms and perspectives have become more mixed and traditional beliefs and practices have become diluted. For instance, many Asian cultures are progressively influenced by Western norms that permeate mass and social media and that is without geographical boundaries.

In this chapter, we first define what is meant by the Asian cultural perspective, before discussing specific culturally bound concepts and how they relate to how the body is experienced for a cancer patient or survivor. We then synthesize research findings on body image in Asia by cancer site, before offering clinical considerations in working on body image issues in an Asian setting.

DEFINING ASIA AND AN ASIAN CULTURAL PERSPECTIVE

Asia constitutes a huge geographical area with a myriad of cultural and religious systems. China, the most populous country in Asia, alone consists of 56 ethnic groups. In addition, there are millions of overseas Chinese living in diverse regions of the world. It would thus be a mistake to assume that Asians are a homogeneous group and that Asians share a typical and unanimous set of beliefs, attitudes, and perspectives about body image and cancer. For this chapter, we decided to focus primarily on a discussion of body image and cancer in the context of the Asian cultural system that is rooted in Confucianism. The Asian cultural system we refer to encompasses countries like Japan, Korea, Taiwan, China, Hong Kong in East Asia, and subcultures in Southeast Asia that include Singapore and Malaysia. These countries share similar cultural values, although we expect nuances to exist amongst the different countries as well as their subcultures. It is important to keep in mind that the chapter describes Asian perspectives broadly and that the degree of adoption of the values discussed depends on many factors (such as religion, acculturation, education level) and thus vary from individual to individual.

CONFUCIAN CONCEPTS THAT ARE RELEVANT TO THE UNDERSTANDING OF BODY IMAGE IN CANCER

Family and cultural values, beliefs, and attitudes significantly influence how people perceive, behave, and respond to body image changes from cancer. Physical appearance and functional changes from cancer and its treatment not only affect an individual's intrapersonal well being; there are often consequent changes to the quality of an individual's social relationships. The Asian cultural perspective referred to in this chapter is deeply rooted in Confucianism, and a few key concepts are delineated next to help readers appreciate the context by which a person may view and experience his or her body.

RELATIONSHIP DOMINANCE

Confucianism is an ethic governing human relationships, and the five cardinal relationships are well discussed in the Analects (*Lun-yu*).[2] They are, namely, the relationship between ruler and minister, between father and son, between husband and wife, between brothers, and between friends.[2] The relationships are hierarchical in nature where the minister is expected to listen to the orders of the ruler, the son listens to the father, the wife to the husband, the younger brother to the elder brother, and someone who is more junior to someone who is more senior in age or status. The relationships are also patriarchal in nature, with deference to male opinion. Traditionally, when the husband passes away, the mother is expected to listen to the eldest son in the family. Essentially, one is expected to know how to behave and respond in relation to others. Ho termed it as "relationship dominance" to "capture the essence of social behavior in Confucian societies."[3(p. 116)]

Role dominance has implications on treatment decision-making, with deference to opinion given by the person in the more dominant role. This can have implication on the body image experience of patients as they experience physical changes from treatment for which they may not have been the main decision-maker. Alternatively, patients may experience heightened distress from having to be dependent on or appear vulnerable to others because of the more dominant role they have in the hierarchical relationship. For instance, a man who is considered the head and primary breadwinner of the family may experience exacerbated body image adjustment difficulty knowing he has to depend on the spouse and children to be dressed or fed. There are also clinical accounts of patients not wanting younger members of the family (especially children) to see them at deathbed, so as to preserve the image of dignity of the patient.

SELF AS LARGER THAN THE INDIVIDUAL

In Confucianism, a person's identity is embedded in relationships. The "self" is multilayered, consisting not only of "I" but also others who are socially connected. A person is a member of a family unit, of a particular ethnic group, and of a specific social status because of factors such as education, occupation, and family background. In a traditional self-introduction, it is common to hear a person introducing himself by first indicating what province and ethnic group he is from, his family surname, and who his father is before stating his name. In other words, a Confucian concept of identity must go with such social connectedness: it is relationship centered, in contrast to the Western concept of individual-centered identity or selfhood. This has very much to do with the fact that most Asian cultures are collectivistic in nature, emphasizing the importance of promoting and maintaining harmony within the family and even in the community. In such collectivistic cultures, members are expected not to behave in a manner that reflects poorly on the group.[4] Thus being diagnosed with cancer and experiencing physical appearance and functional changes can lead to a patient experiencing guilt for causing "trouble" or "disruption" to those around them. For instance, a patient who recently had a glossectomy and has not resumed eating solid food may report avoiding family gatherings because they would cause "trouble to others" by requiring a special diet and that their presence and "odd" speech would disrupt the "harmony" of the gathering.

RELATIONAL SELF

Selfhood, or one's formed identity, in Confucianism emerges in relation to the way one appears to others in the world. This includes considering one's position in society and membership in the social networks. Ho coined it "relational self," where one is intensely aware of the presence of other human beings and their experience.[3] Thus the self is perceived and experienced not only from one's own standpoint but also from the standpoint of others. For instance, a patient's sense of "self" may encompass herself, her spouse, and her children, a concept that may appear as an "enmeshed" or dependent relationship through a Western cultural lens but is perfectly normal given the Asian cultural context. Thus, cancer patients' preoccupation with what others think of them, or higher value placed on the perception of others on their changed appearance, in this context may not be pathological but a culturally influenced way of thinking about themselves. As an anecdotal example, we had a patient who refused to be discharged home with a nasogastric tube (NGT) and instead preferred insertion of a percutaneous endoscopic gastronomy (PEG) tube for feeding purposes. It later came to light that his request stemmed from the fear of the opinions of his neighbors if they saw him with the NGT, which is visible on his face. Although the PEG insertion is considered to be a more invasive procedure, the patient preferred to have it as he believed it will help him "keep up appearances" with those around him.

This is also well echoed in the vignette presented in the beginning of the chapter. The woman's view about herself includes how her husband and parents-in-law perceive and value her—physically and functionally—and these critically influence her final decision for treatment seeking. It is not a surprise that she might choose to preserve her womb if her husband insists on having a child of their own. This links to a related concept: *relational autonomy*.[5] In a Confucian society, there is no individual autonomy but relational autonomy. Decisions are made with family members' contributions and are intended to create the least possible burden to the family. Lee proposed a similar term, "ethical relational autonomy," which embraces moral consciousness for others in one's autonomy.[5] In a Confucian society, acting autonomously includes one's concern for the suffering, well-being, and happiness of others. Referring back to the opening vignette, the woman may minimize the consideration of her suffering to embrace the happiness and "face" of her husband and extended family.

SELF-CULTIVATION

Confucianism regards the ultimate purpose of life as achieving self-transcendence and transformation through self-cultivation, which is a process of suppressing one's personal desires and needs in accordance to the *li* (礼, meaning "doing what is proper and expected") to better one's self. *Li* denotes a set of prescriptive rules for proper conduct. From the sociological point of view, *li* serves to maintain hierarchical relationships. Self-cultivation is considered an essential condition for regulated and harmonious relationships, especially important for familial relationships.[3] As stated in the Analects, "To subdue one's self and return to propriety is perfect virtue." From the Asian cultural perspective, "to subdue one's self" denotes control of impulse and would be translated into behaviors through which one tries to temper strong emotions such as love and hate and to keep joy and anger in check. Inadvertently, this has led to some individuals being socialized to suppress emotional expression or to have low self-awareness of emotional states. A prime stereotype is the seemingly unfeeling Asian man who is not able to express emotion or recognize emotion-related social cues. This has broader implications for our patients with cancer seeking body image treatment, as some families may subscribe low value to the patient's emotional well-being, patients may not be able to identify body image disturbance for what it is, or patients who do seek treatment have difficulty expressing their emotions.

Another aspect of self-cultivation involves the idea that the opportunity for self-cultivation arises during times of hardship. Hardships and suffering are expected in life as test of the individual's ability to endure them for self-transcendence. Thus appearance and functional changes from the disease and treatment side effects may possibly be accepted as a test to endure and with a certain degree of pragmatism. An example would be a patient whose goal is to return back to work as quickly as possible with no room for self-pity, even if it would have been acceptable for the patient to take more time to adjust to his changed appearance or function. In the extreme form, the patient may not be willing to engage in a discussion of emotional adjustment (and body image adjustment), and instead only focus on practical matters. Another instance of self-cultivation is when patients consciously choose to make something positive of their situation, such as consciously choosing to be a positive role model by supporting and motivating fellow patients. This resolve may be driven by the belief that a person can only achieve "perfect virtue" or self-transcendence and transformation through abundance of "endurance" in daily life and suffering.

LEGACY AND CONTINUITY

From the Asian perspective, the concept of "self" extends beyond a person's lifetime and includes generation after generation. This explains why *xiao* (孝, meaning "filial piety") is the first of the eight virtues in Confucius' teachings (Table 17.1). The ability to father a

TABLE 17.1: Summary of Confucian Concepts and Their Relevance to Body Image and Cancer

Relationship dominance

Refers to the hierarchy in relationships, typically patriarchal and with deference to elders

- Patient may defer decision-making about treatments that lead to body image changes to person in dominant role
- Patients who are in the dominant role in their social relationships may have heightened body image distress from having to appear vulnerable or be dependent on others

Self as larger than the individual

Refers to a person's identity that centers around social connectedness

- Patients may express guilt for causing "disruption" or being a burden from perceived body image changes
- Patients may engage in behavior that they perceive to prioritize the well-being of others

Relational self

Refers to experiencing and seeing one's self through the eyes of other

- Patients may appear preoccupied with how they appear to others
- Patients may engage in behavior that they perceive to prioritize the well-being of others

Self-cultivation

Refers to the act of suppressing one's own selfish needs and doing what is proper and expected to achieve the ultimate goal of self-transcendence

- Patients may have been socialized to suppress emotional expression or have low awareness of emotional states
- Patients and their families may have low value for seeking help for body image disturbance
- Patients present as being especially pragmatic about their body image changes

Legacy and continuity

Refers to continuing the family name and legacy

- Patients may experience body image disturbance and guilt from fertility problems secondary to cancer and treatment

child, especially a male to continue the family surname or family line, is considered a son's most important duty to the family. Thus, for women, the cultural value of their bodies are intrinsically linked to their childbearing capabilities (Henson, 2002). This is well illustrated in the ancient Chinese character for the word "body" (身, *shēn*), which reflects that the body is not only a physical component but also has a functional purpose. The ancient Chinese character *shēn* shows a side view of a pregnant lady and the dot representing a fetus inside the body (Figure 17.1).[6] Thus, the original meaning of the Chinese character *shēn* is pregnancy.[6]

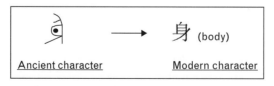

FIGURE 17.1: Ancient and modern Chinese character for body.

As such, the cultural implications of infertility can be significant for patients from traditional families. Cancers and treatments associated with reproductive organs or that can affect fertility such as gynecological, breast, penile, and testicular cancers can have especially significant connotations for the patient themselves in how they view their bodies as "failing" and their romantic partners in terms of family planning, marriage-ability, and future romantic prospects. The impaired body image has physical, emotional, social, and sociocultural connotations, as we have seen in the vignette, and as is further discussed later.

BODY IMAGE RESEARCH FINDINGS IN ASIA FROM A CULTURAL PERSPECTIVE

The following section discusses body image research findings from studies conducted in Asia that are presented by Confucian concepts outlined in the prior section. Based on our review of the current literature, cancer sites that have been most studied in the context of body image in Asia are breast cancer, gynecologic cancer, head and neck cancer, and gastrointestinal cancer. This section describes findings grouped by cancer sites, followed by findings of interventions conducted in Asia that were found to impact body image.

BREAST CANCER

A number of studies have examined body image in Asian women with breast cancer, specifically in the context of being a predictor of treatment decision-making and as an outcome of cancer treatment.[7–9] For example, Lam's group in Hong Kong reported that an emphasis on appearance and body image concerns predicted the decision to undergo breast-conserving therapy or mastectomy followed by reconstruction, compared to the decision for mastectomy without reconstruction.[8] Surgeon recommendation was also reported to significantly influence treatment choice.[8] Similar findings were reported in Adachi et al.'s and Zhang et al.'s studies, where greater investment in physical appearance by Japanese and Chinese women predicted choice for immediate breast reconstruction.[9] Interestingly, Zhang et al. even reported that one of the significant predictors of the decision included a positive recommendation from their husband, possibly related to the Confucian concepts of relational autonomy and role dominance.[7]

Body image was also examined as an outcome of breast cancer treatment. Sun et al. reported that Korean women who chose to undergo breast-conserving surgery ($n = 254$) reported higher body image satisfaction scores compared to those who underwent mastectomy with reconstruction ($n = 31$) and without reconstruction ($n = 122$).[10] Kim et al. further reported that worse body image was associated with depressive symptoms and poorer quality of life.[11] In samples of Taiwanese women, body image was found to be associated with receipt of mastectomy (in contrast to breast-conserving surgery) and younger age[12] as well as higher levels of objectified body consciousness.[13]

Overall, the literature emerging from Asia seem to be consistent with what has been reported in Western countries. It is worth noting that a couple of studies have reported partner approval and support as being important in facilitating body image satisfaction in women with breast cancer.[7,14] This is further underscored by Fang et al.'s report that perceived partner empathy moderated the relationship between body image and depression among Taiwanese breast cancer survivors; the greater the empathy, the lesser the depressive symptoms.[15] This aligns with the Confucian concept of *relational self* where the view and experience of one's body incorporates the perspectives of others. It is unclear whether the findings of the role of partner support are unique to the Asian setting or that discovery of these findings exists because researchers in this cultural context purposefully sought to examine their importance. Nevertheless, it is not surprising to see the significance of the reaction of the partner and his support for the breast cancer survivor, given that, from the Confucian perspective, the husband–wife relationship is a core relationship. The sense of self (which includes the corporeal self) is not simply captured by "I"; rather, there is a "we" consciousness.[16] The situation may be made more complex by the presence of the *relationship dominance* seen in Confucian societies.[3] It is argued that even appearance investment, which refers to the value one places in one's appearance, and body image acceptance incorporates the perspectives of one's partner. It is also possible the more passive roles of women in historically patriarchal societies have women seeking "approval" from their partners prior to making a decision about treatment.

GYNECOLOGIC CANCERS

Gynecologic cancers comprise cancers affecting a number of different sites in the female reproductive system, including the uterus/endometrium, ovaries, cervix, vagina, and vulva. A few studies have examined body image in Asian gynecologic cancer patients. One cross-sectional study conducted in Singapore with 104 gynecologic cancer patients found that approximately a quarter of patients reported feeling physically unattractive and dissatisfied with their body.[17] One large study in Korea compared 860 Korean women with cervical cancer to controls. Cervical cancer survivors reported worse body image and/or sexual functioning.[18] Another study based on the same sample reported that poor body image was associated with anxiety and depressive symptoms.[19] In another qualitative study of gynecologic cancer survivors' adaptation in Hong Kong,[20] a few issues that emerged include marital distress, concerns about sexuality and femininity, loss of fertility, and discomfort due to symptoms. There are certain cultural beliefs that are important to consider in understanding the body image experience of a patient with gynecologic cancer. For instance, the concept of legacy and continuity is traditionally important and can be an issue when fertility and reproductive ability is affected. Bearing children extends beyond the desire to expand the family tree; it is seen as a duty.[21] Infertility can be perceived as a disgrace to one's family and ancestors, and a woman would be considered unfilial to not produce an heir to the family.[22] In an Asian society where filial piety is foremost among the eight virtues from the perspective of Confucianism, the failure to bear a child is readily perceived as a major problem by the couple themselves, their extended family, and others within their social network and community. This remains true even in the new millennium when the power of decision-making on childbearing can often-times still involve the parents of the couple.[23] This aligns with the concept of "ethical relational autonomy," where the couple may be feeling guilty for not fulfilling their duty to the family and even causing the family to "lose face," which can be explained as losing social status or standing.

In one study, misconceptions about sexual functioning were reported to affect adaptation to illness.[20] This could potentially stem from the Confucian and Taoist beliefs that gynecologic cancers, under the larger umbrella of sexual disorders, are a result of imbalance of yin and yang elements, potentially from excessive sexual activity (Ngan et al., 1994). This has two implications: first, that gynecologic cancers are a result of excessive sexual activity or promiscuity and, second, that women who are diagnosed with gynecologic cancers should cease or reduce sexual activity as it will continue to "weaken" their body.

Asian cultures, in general, are also considered to be sexually conservative and ones in which discussion about the consequences of gynecologic cancer treatment on body image and sexual well-being may not be topics patients proactively report or seek help for. Reluctance to even complete assessments regarding sexual well-being indicates the extent to which gynecologic health and sexual well-being is a taboo topic.[24] This is one of the largest barriers to conducting research in this population, as data are usually collected from respondents who are able to overcome such conservative cultural beliefs, who tend to be younger and higher- or Western-educated women.

HEAD AND NECK CANCERS

Head and neck cancers refer to a group of cancers originating from the nasal cavity, oral cavity, tongue, salivary glands, larynx, and pharynx. The prevalence of head and neck cancers and their disease sites and etiology are different in Asia compared to Western and developed countries.[25] For instance, head and neck cancers are some of the most common cancers in South and Southeast Asia but only constitute 1% to 4% of cancers in Western nations. In Southeast China, Taiwan, and certain parts of Southeast Asia, nasopharyngeal cancer is the most common form of head and neck cancer and is linked to a genetic and lifestyle risk carried by those who originated, migrated, and descended from residents of China's Guangdong province.[26] More men than women are diagnosed with head and neck cancers, possibly due to lifestyle risk factors such as use of tobacco products, alcohol, and betel nuts. In the case of nasopharyngeal carcinoma, the consumption of certain foods such as salted fish, preserved vegetables, and cured meat is also linked to increased risk.[27] In Taiwan, oral cancer is the sixth leading cause of death, and betel nut is one of the leading causes of buccal cancer. The cultural practice of chewing betel nut is very common in Taiwan, particularly among the middle-aged male working group. Oral cancer and treatment can bring body image distress to a patient, particularly if he experiences changes in his appearance and the ability to form facial expressions (e.g., smiling) or has difficulty with speech/swallowing from surgical procedures such as mandibulectomies.[28]

Head and neck cancers affect patients' speech and ability to eat in a significant number of cases, with some of the impairment being temporary while others are permanent. The impairment or loss of the ability to eat is typically viewed as especially difficult to adjust to, as food is an important part of the Asian culture, reflecting identity and life quality.[29] Food is typically a focal point of family gatherings, and there exists psychological and social gratification that goes beyond nutritional nourishment from food. The Asian greeting of "have you eaten" is equivalent to the Western greeting of "how are you" or "hello," alluding to the importance of people not being in a state of hunger. Further, the concept of not being able to eat independently (e.g., being fed orally by someone else or tube-fed) creates anxiety in the form of being a "burden" to others.

Head and neck cancer is also unique compared to other cancers as there are often visible changes to a person's facial appearance as a result of treatment. This can take the form of, for instance, scarring and changes to the contour of the face or compromised symmetry of a smile. These changes can be difficult to conceal. The functional deficits associated with head and neck cancer treatment, both in appearance and function, is culturally viewed as a great test of endurance with fate. In an Asian cultural context, the ability to endure suffering and hardship is considered a process of self-cultivation toward self-transcendence.[30]

Despite the many cultural factors in considering head and neck cancer in Asian patients, limited research has been published on body image of these patients. It is possible that body image is not given due attention as a majority of patients are typically older men and it is assumed body image is not a relevant concern. Nevertheless, a recent study by Chen et al. reported from a cross-sectional study of Taiwanese head and neck cancer patients that patients who have visible disfigurement in the face or undergo reconstructive surgery are more likely to report worse body image.[31] Further, body image dissatisfaction is associated with negatively impacted ability to speak.[31]

GASTROINTESTINAL CANCERS

Gastrointestinal cancers consist of a group of cancers that affect the digestive system. This includes the esophagus, stomach, biliary system, pancreas, small intestine, large intestine, rectum, and anus. Commonly reported symptoms in long-term survivors include food sensitivities, diarrhea, and reflux. Further, adapting to use of ostomy bags as temporary or permanent is an issue that has been raised in the body image literature due to the difficulty of coming to terms with changed functioning of bowel movement, managing odor issues, and navigating the bag's use in social situations or intimate relationships.

In a prospective study following 254 Korean patients for five years after gastrectomy, body image was assessed as part of patients' quality of life.[32] Body image of patients was shown to worsen over time, with the biggest change within the first year of surgery, and although body image distress decreased in the span of five years, it did not return to pre-morbid levels. The authors concluded that addressing body image concerns is a consistent need of patients who underwent gastrectomy. In another study comparing Korean gastric cancer survivors to controls, body image was found to be significantly worse in the survivor group.[33] It may be worthwhile to note that based on clinical experiences, patients carrying ostomy bags began reducing their social outings or even became socially isolated because of the challenges in managing the bags. They were constantly worried about how they were perceived by others when they needed to frequent the washroom to clear the bags or about bringing inconvenience to the group because of their food restrictions.

INTERVENTION STUDIES

A search in the literature for interventions that have targeted body image of cancer patients brings to light the paucity of research in this area. Four studies detailing interventions were found, with the majority of interventions appearing to provide general therapy or counseling that had an effect on body image. Chujo et al. reported conducting group psychotherapy (six sessions) for Japanese breast cancer patients (19 intervention group vs. 9 control group) presenting with recurrence led by a psychiatrist.[34] Although the intervention did not specifically target body image issues, body image dissatisfaction scores were significantly decreased at postintervention and at three-month follow-up compared to pretreatment in the intervention group compared to controls. Hsu et al. also conducted a nurse-led, psycho-educational, face-to-face intervention that focused on general well-being of Taiwanese breast cancer patients.[35] Patients were assigned to two groups (32 intervention group vs. 31 control group) prior to undergoing modified radical mastectomy. The intervention consisted of two sessions; each lasted approximately two hours: Session 1 was conducted presurgery and provided information about treatment options using photos (e.g., reconstruction, use of breast prosthesis), expectations about appearance postmastectomy, and postsurgical care; Session 2 was implemented three days postsurgery and provided more information on breast prosthesis and support on how to rebuild self-confidence. The intervention had positive effects on body image two months after surgery. A study by Jun et al. in Korea described a group cognitive-behavioral therapy–based sexual life reframing program (six sessions) for breast cancer survivors who chose not to undergo breast reconstruction. The women were assigned to either the intervention group ($n = 22$) or control group ($n = 23$). Body image, marital satisfaction, and sexual interest improved in the intervention group, although the findings were not statistically significant.

Huang et al. in Taiwan conducted a cosmetic rehabilitation program for oral cancer patients to address changes in appearance and function.[36] The majority of patients enrolled (>90%) were middle-aged men with approximately 40% of the entire sample being diagnosed with buccal cancer, a cancer that is most common in Asia and associated with the practice of chewing betel nut. The intervention group ($n = 22$) received cosmetic rehabilitation with a focus on teaching cosmetic camouflage, whereas the control group ($n = 22$) received regular nursing care. The patients in the cosmetic rehabilitation program received cosmetic equipment, a manual with instructions to apply the cosmetic products, and visits with a trained facilitator. The intervention group reported decreased appearance evaluation scores (signifying body image distress) and increased satisfaction with their "face" at the end of the 12-week follow-up period. The authors advocated for cosmetic rehabilitation to be offered as part of nursing care for oral cancer patients.

CONSIDERATIONS IN INTERVENING ON BODY IMAGE ISSUES IN AN ASIAN SETTING

So far, information about Asian cultural values and "ways of thinking" as well as body image research findings and their interpretations have been discussed. They set the stage for understanding patient values, beliefs, and behaviors. In this section, we share some further considerations that healthcare professionals may want to take into account when conducting body image–related interventions with Asian patients.

COLLUSION ON DIVULGENCE OF DISEASE DIAGNOSIS OR PROGNOSIS

There are instances where patients (typically, elderly) are not told they have cancer as the family wants to protect them from being negatively affected by the news. This phenomenon, known as "collusion" or "keeping secrets" within the family, can place a lot of stress on the communication between healthcare providers and the patient; however, this continues to be practiced informally, with deference to the wishes of the family. The family is seen as an extension of the unit of the patient, and family members (typically children) are seen to "know what is best for the patient," which is that the patient, by being kept in the dark about his or her diagnosis, is better off than if he or she was told about the illness. Collusion tends to occur in situations where patients are elderly or lower educated, where the prognosis is poor, and in cultures where cancer is stigmatized. Although collusion is not encouraged and efforts are constantly made to educate both patients' families and healthcare providers who enable this practice, it is entrenched in the larger cultural system and continues to exist. Keeping secrets between patient and family caregivers has short-term functions. It maintains harmony in the family, protects the patient from unnecessary stress, and protects the hierarchical relationship structure of the Asian families. However, anxiety and guilt may arise from secrecy because of the conspiracy of silence over an extended period.

In such cases, engaging in body image work where appearance and functional changes of the disease are discussed in the context of a "tumor" or "illness" without the mention of "cancer" is possible, although it has its own limitations. The goal of body image therapy then is specific—to work on body image adjustment without the need to address or confront the actual "cancer" itself. For some, this may be viewed as impossible. This, at a fundamental level, highlights the level of public awareness and understanding of what cancer is and what it represents, and the stigma and fear surrounding the term. In such a case, helping patients to understand their diagnosis and what it represents is ideally the first step in the therapy session. The focus of intervention should be on strengthening the family's ability to share distressful information appropriately, where patient and family needs and changing information needs are met as part of the ongoing process of patient care. Whether this occurs or not, the point is that awareness (or lack thereof) of one's diagnosis due to cultural practices is a factor to consider.

MANAGING RELATIONSHIPS AND PERSPECTIVES OF OTHERS

It is common to have patients or clients constantly putting the welfare of others (family, friends, or even strangers) before themselves. For instance, it is normal for full-grown adults who have their own families and children to consider the welfare or perspective of their parents in their everyday cognitions. Thus, what may seem as a patient having dependent personality traits in defining life values or making treatment decisions is not necessarily that. Instead, this apparent inability to separate one's self from others stems from cultural importance placed on relationships as outlined in the earlier subsection of the cardinal Confucian concepts. In line with this idea, a lot of body image distress, in fact, can arise from managing perceived expectations and judgment of others. For instance, a cancer patient with a disfigurement may feel guilty for disrupting the "harmony" of a family gathering or social function. A thought they may present with is, "I will make people who I care about uncomfortable, and to save them the embarrassment or awkwardness, I should be considerate and not spoil their fun."

This constant consciousness of what other people think can lend itself to faulty assumptions. Culturally, there is great emphasis on presenting one's best self and the belief that a person not only represents himself or herself but his or her family and family name. Thus, a lot of choices and behaviors are usually in consideration of "saving face" or "not letting others know of our troubles." This can manifest itself through keeping knowledge of the disease away from others (for reasons of "saving face" rather than "protection of the person cared about"), going to great lengths to appear normal, and delaying seeking treatment. For such cases, there is a need for the therapist to be culturally sensitive and to work with the patient or even together with the spouse to help them achieve a new equilibrium as they adjust to the disease and treatment sequalae. One usual technique to engage patients and sometimes their spouses is an experiential and imagery exercise through which the therapist helps patients to get in touch with the personal aspects of their loss and grief and to help the marital couple to explore, understand, or even appreciate their differing views, if any.

MAINTENANCE OF HARMONY WITHIN SELF AND WITH OTHERS

Patients having cancer may experience intense anger, sadness, and even loss of hope when they feel that their life goals are unachievable. However, Asian cultural values and traditions do not typically encourage expression or open sharing of emotion. It is viewed as disruptive, not only to a person's internal equilibrium but to the harmony of relationships with others when a person shares intense emotions. Because the discussion of one's emotions is generally discouraged from a young age, the ability to identify and describe emotions in words can be challenging, even for adult patients who may be otherwise able to communicate their thoughts perfectly.

In such cases, use of expressive arts therapy, such as art making, may be one strategy to facilitate or promote expression of emotion for a psychosocial intervention. In the past few years, research has shown beneficial effects of art therapy in which art is used as a medium of expression and as a therapeutic process for patients who have difficulty expressing emotions verbally. One such study was done by Ho's group in Hong Kong with patients living with breast cancer.[37] The study reported changes in emotion as evidenced through art work expression, mainly toward a more peaceful and hopeful attitude, through the pre– and post–psychosocial intervention drawings.

CONCLUDING COMMENTS

Generally, we found significant paucity in the literature of body image in the context of oncology in Asia. In this chapter, we have attempted to explore the concept of body image through our professional experiences as both clinicians and researchers and our personal knowledge of the cultural landscape that is rooted in Confucianism. However, cultural perspectives are multifaceted and dynamic as our culture continually evolves. Furthermore, Asia encompasses many other countries and cultures that are not Confucian based. We noted several studies from the Middle East on body image that may have been considered Asia geographically; however, we did not feel competent to discuss them in this chapter. Theoretical or conceptual models of how culture interacts with body image that can be applied to many different cultures are needed. Subsequently, although research on body image is growing and there are a few notable studies that examine body image in cancer patients, further work needs to be done in the area of examining body image and cultural-specific themes such as the meaning of one's body and the expression of body image distress (e.g., guilt, shame). We encourage clinicians and researchers working with patients from diverse cultural backgrounds to continue considering how culture can interact with the body image experiences of patients with cancer.

REFERENCES

1. Marshall PA, Bennett LA. *Culture and Behavior in the AIDS Epidemic*. Arlington, VA: American Anthropological Association; 1990.

2. Nan H. *Lunyu BieZai*, 8th ed. Shanghai, China: Fudan University Press; 2005.

3. Ho DY. Selfhood and identity in Confucianism, Taoism, Buddhism, and Hinduism: contrasts with the West. *J Theory Soc Behav*. 1995;25(2):115–139.

4. Bond MH, Smith PB. *Social Psychology across Cultures: Analysis and Perspectives*. London: Harvester Wheatsheaf; 1993.

5. Lee SC. *The Family, Medical Decision-Making, and Biotechnology: Critical Reflections on Asian Moral Perspectives*. Vol. 91. Dordrecht: Springer Science & Business Media; 2007.

6. Lee GL, Chan CHY, Hui E, Chan CLW. Chinese traditional belief systems, livelihood and fertility. In: *Faith and Fertility: Attitudes towards Reproductive Practices in Different Religions from Ancient to Modern Times*. London: Jessica Kingsley; 2009:137–157.

7. Zhang Y, Xu H, Wang T, et al. Psychosocial predictors and outcomes of delayed breast reconstruction in mastectomized women in Mainland China: an observational study. *PLoS One*. 2015;10(12):15.

8. Lam WW, Fielding R, Ho EY, Chan M, Or A. Surgeon's recommendation, perceived operative efficacy and age dictate treatment choice by Chinese women facing breast cancer surgery. *Psychooncology*. 2005;14(7):585–593.

9. Adachi K, Ueno T, Fujioka T, Fujitomi Y, Ueo H. Psychosocial factors affecting the therapeutic decision-making and postoperative mood states in Japanese breast cancer patients who underwent various types of surgery: body image and sexuality. *Japan J Clin Oncol*. 2007;37(6):412–418.

10. Sun Y, Kim SW, Heo CY, et al. Comparison of quality of life based on surgical technique in patients with breast cancer. *Japan J Clin Oncol*. 2014;44(1):22–27.

11. Kim KR, Chung HC, Lee E, Kim SJ, Namkoong K. Body image, sexual function and depression in Korean patients with breast cancer: modification by 5-HTT polymorphism. *Support Care Cancer*. 2012;20(9):2177–2182.

12. Chen CL, Liao MN, Chen SC, Chan PL, Chen SC. Body image and its predictors in breast cancer patients receiving surgery. *Cancer Nurs*. 2012;35(5):E10–E16.

13. Fang S-Y, Chang H-T, Shu B-C. Objectified body consciousness, body image discomfort, and depressive symptoms among breast cancer survivors in Taiwan. *Psychol Women Q*. 2014;38(4):563–574.

14. Kwong A, Chu ATW. What made her give up her breasts: a qualitative study on decisional considerations for contralateral prophylactic mastectomy among breast cancer survivors undergoing BRCA1/2 genetic testing. *Asian Pac J Cancer Prev*. 2012;13(5):2241–2247.

15. Fang SY, Chang HT, Shu BC. The moderating effect of perceived partner empathy on body image and depression among breast cancer survivors. *Psychooncology*. 2015;24(12):1815–1822.

16. Hofstede G. *Cultures and Organizations: Intercultural Cooperation and Its Importance for Survival* (Software of the Mind). London: McGraw-Hill; 1991.

17. Teo I, Cheung YB, Lim YK, Padmavathi NR, Long V, Tewani K. The relationship between symptom prevalence, body image and quality of life in Asian gynecologic cancer patients. *Psychooncology*. 2017; 27: 69–74.

18. Park SY, Bae DS, Nam JH, et al. Quality of life and sexual problems in disease-free survivors of cervical cancer compared with the general population. *Cancer*. 2007;110(12):2716–2725.

19. Kim SH, Kang S, Kim YM, et al. Prevalence and predictors of anxiety and depression among cervical cancer survivors in Korea. *Int J Gynecol Cancer*. 2010;20(6):1017–1024.

20. Molassiotis A, Chan CW, Yam B, Chan ES, Lam CS. Life after cancer: adaptation issues faced by Chinese gynaecological cancer survivors in Hong Kong. *Psychooncology*. 2002;11(2):114–123.

21. Chan CL, Yip PS, Ng EH, Ho P, Chan CH, Au JS. Gender selection in China: its meanings and implications. *J Assist Reprod Genet*. 2002;19(9):426–430.

22. Ng E, Liu A, Chan C, Chan C. Hong Kong: a social, legal and clinical overview. In Eric Blyth and Ruth Landau (eds): *Third Party Assisted Conception across Cultures: Social, Legal and Ethical Perspectives*. London: Jessica Kingsley; 2007; 112–128.

23. Wong Y-k. [Stress and coping for women from infertility to assisted reproductive treatments]. 香港大學學位論文. 2000:1–0.

24. Molassiotis A, Chan C, Yam B, Chan S. Quality of life in Chinese women with gynaecological cancers. *Support Care Cancer*. 2000;8(5):414–422.

25. Joshi P, Dutta S, Chaturvedi P, Nair S. Head and neck cancers in developing countries. *Rambam Maimonides Med J*. 2014;5(2).

26. Titcomb CP. High incidence of nasopharyngeal carcinoma in Asia. *J Insur Med*. 2001;33(3):235–238.

27. Jia W-H, Luo X-Y, Feng B-J, et al. Traditional Cantonese diet and nasopharyngeal carcinoma risk: a large-scale case-control study in Guangdong, China. *BMC Cancer*. 2010;10(1):446.

28. Sui C, Lacey A. Asia's deadly secret: the scourge of the betel nut. BBC News; March 22, 2015.

29. Leung K, Tay M, Cheng S, Lin F. Hong Kong Chinese version, World Health Organization quality of life measure–abbreviated version. WHOQOL-BREF (HK). Geneva: World Health Organization; 1997.

30. Chan C, Leung P, Ho K. A culturally sensitive empowerment intervention for Chinese cancer patients in Hong Kong. *Asian Pac J Soc Work.* 1999;9:1–15.

31. Chen SC, Yu PJ, Hong MY, et al. Communication dysfunction, body image, and symptom severity in post-operative head and neck cancer patients: factors associated with the amount of speaking after treatment. *Support Care Cancer.* 2015;23(8):2375–2382.

32. Yu W, Park KB, Chung HY, Kwon OK, Lee SS. Chronological changes of quality of life in long-term survivors after gastrectomy for gastric cancer. *Cancer Res Treat.* 2016;48(3):1030–1036.

33. Lee SS, Chung HY, Yu W. Quality of life of long-term survivors after a distal subtotal gastrectomy. *Cancer Res Treat.* 2010;42(3):130–134.

34. Chujo M, Mikami I, Takashima S, et al. A feasibility study of psychosocial group intervention for breast cancer patients with first recurrence. *Support Care Cancer.* 2005;13(7):503–514.

35. Hsu SC, Wang HH, Chu SY, Yen HF. Effectiveness of informational and emotional consultation on the psychological impact on women with breast cancer who underwent modified radical mastectomy. *J Nurs Res.* 2010;18(3):215–226.

36. Huang S, Liu HE. Effectiveness of cosmetic rehabilitation on the body image of oral cancer patients in Taiwan. *Support CareCancer.* 2008;16(9):981–986.

37. Ho R, Potash J, Fu W, Wong K, Chan C. Changes in breast cancer patients after psychosocial intervention as indicated in drawings. *Psychooncology.* 2010;19(4):353–360.

CONCLUSION

CHAPTER 18

SYNTHESIS

Impressions and Future Directions

Michelle Cororve Fingeret and Irene Teo

When we initially set out inviting the chapter contributors to the book, we truthfully were not certain of the reactions and responses we would receive. However, to our delight, the authors were wholeheartedly enthusiastic in coming on board in our endeavor. It has been a privilege to bring together expert clinicians and researchers that are committed to this field that intersects body image and oncology and are dedicated to highlighting the importance and relevance of body image in the work with oncology patients and survivors. Indeed, the research literature indicates that interest in body image in the field of oncology is at its peak and will continue to grow as we see more survivors adjust to living with cancer. This chapter is dedicated to highlighting the take-away points from what we know so far based on the chapters in the book and offering suggestions for future directions of the field. Our goal is to emphasize broad ideas rather than to focus on specific points.

THEORETICAL FOUNDATIONS FOR THE FIELD

Although having roots in the field of body image, we see that the subspecialty of body image in cancer has emerged and grown in its own right, with theories being informed by clinical observations and research unique to the oncology population. Classical body image theorizing has typically been focused on appearance; however, body image frameworks within oncology have recognized the need to include function and somatosensory experiences in the conceptualization of body image experiences of the cancer survivor. The models developed thus far tend to be disease-specific, such as Rhoten's model for head and neck cancer and Fingeret's model for breast cancer patients undergoing reconstruction. We have also seen some existing frameworks that may be adapted for use in conceptualizing body image in oncology populations. Of particular interest are the Appearance Research Collaboration framework of adjusting to appearance changes discussed by Paraskeva, Clarke, and Harcourt and the World Health Organization's model of classifying function, disability, and health with integration of body image as offered by Henry and Alias. For the most part, most theoretical frameworks address body image as a *state* of body image satisfaction/dissatisfaction rather than a trait.

In our opinion, theoretical frameworks that take into account both demographic/background influences (such as gender, age/development stage, ethnicity/culture) as well as oncological clinical characteristics (status of disease, extent of disease and bodily changes, permanence of disease/treatment sequelae, time since diagnosis/treatment) offer distinct advantages. The conceptualization of body image may be further broadened to include physical competencies (e.g., fatigue and occupational loss) and cognitive impairment as changes in these domains can definitely affect the way individuals view their bodies and themselves. Other perspectives to consider include theories on body vulnerability and threat which have yet to be fully incorporated into the body image and cancer literature. Conceptual models may also greatly benefit from a focus on adaptive and positive body image (e.g., love and acceptance of one's body), rather than exclusive attention to maladaptive or negative body image outcomes.

BODY IMAGE ASSESSMENT WITHIN RESEARCH AND CLINICAL CONTEXTS

Most studies in the research literature have used quantitative measures of body image, although there are rich data to be acquired from qualitative interviews, as evident in shared excerpts in the chapter on older adults by Schuler, Roth, and Holland and in the chapter on men by Drummond and Gough. We see that many body image findings in the oncology literature relate to secondary aims/outcomes of studies. These findings are not always robust in nature especially when based on a single item embedded within a larger instrument of quality of life. There is an array of body image measures available for use in an oncology setting. Of the few specifically developed for cancer patients, the literature is concentrated overwhelmingly in the area of breast cancer. A welcome development is the translation of cancer-specific body image measures into other languages and validation of these measures in other cultures that have facilitated cross-cultural interest in the arena.

There are many opportunities for growth in the development of body image assessment tools, and the quality of the research in this field will be dependent on the quality of assessment instruments available for use. There needs to be a wider breadth of body image concepts measured beyond body image satisfaction, such as body image investment, body image coping behaviors, body integrity, and body stigma. In line with the conceptualization that body image includes somatosensory and functional competencies, measures should also incorporate items on perceived changes in these core domains. A critical objective is to strike a balance between developing generic body image measures that can be used with heterogeneous cancer populations versus those designed for a specific cancer type or treatment side effect. The benefit of broader-based measures that can be used across cancer types is that it would permit comparisons across different groups. It is vital to take into account the needs of subgroups such as younger and geriatric populations and to accommodate for reading level and complexity of the measure's items. In terms of assessment methodology, mixed methods that allow patients to quantify their experiences using scales but also give them the opportunity to report what they face in their own words can enrich our understanding of their lived experiences. This can only help with the refinement of our conceptual understanding and measurement of body image.

From a clinical standpoint, our general impression is that body image is not assessed as standard routine practice, both in psychosocial oncology and other subdisciplines within oncology. This is likely due to a lack of training and comfort of oncology healthcare professionals in addressing body image issues. In addition, most available body image tools have been developed for use in research, are relatively lengthy, and not necessarily sensible for clinical use. A major challenge is to find a way to balance psychometric validity/reliability of body image tools with practicality. An example of a brief and user-friendly screener that was developed for clinical use is the Body Image Screener for Cancer Reconstruction, although such a tool would need further validation and establishment of clinically relevant cut-off scores. We do believe there are ways to overcome the barrier posed by the absence of readily available body image–specific screening tools. We advocate for assessment of body image as routine care in clinics and have provided practical suggestions to aid healthcare practitioners within clinical assessment throughout the book, particularly in Chapters 3 (body image assessment), 12 (pediatrics), and 15 (couples).

INTERVENTIONS TO ADDRESS BODY IMAGE DISTRESS RESULTING FROM CANCER

Thus far, the most established interventions addressing body image are administered in an individual therapy format. A cognitive-behavioral framework is typically used focused on addressing maladaptive cognitions (e.g., unrealistic expectations) and using behavioral activation/skills training. Few interventions have been reported in the literature for patients with cancer where body image is the primary focus. Moreover, most studies investigating the effectiveness of interventions in this field have relied on small sample sizes. The stepped model of care for appearance-related interventions that is discussed by Lewis-Smith, Harcourt, and Clarke certainly captures the importance of matching patients' needs to appropriate level of resources; this model is currently being implemented in the UK.

Moving forward, implementing a stepped model of care should certainly be considered in countries beyond the UK, although planning is needed to determine how it can work within a country's unique health system. At the societal level, an important goal should be to raise public awareness regarding realistic standards for appearance and functional outcomes of cancer patients as many patients' expectations are set by what they see via mass or social media. For instance, hair loss is widely recognized as a symptom of oncologic treatment, but symptoms that are not as readily visible such as chronic cancer-related fatigue (which is one of the top symptoms across all cancers) is not commonly depicted. More work can also be done to celebrate positive images of body image in cancer survivors with the message of body and self-acceptance despite cancer. We personally facilitated an annual "Love Your Body Day Event" at the University of Texas MD Anderson Cancer Center, which was comprised of educational programs and public outreach to raise awareness about body image issues in cancer survivors. Each year this event differed in scope but included art classes where patients and families expressed their body image through artwork and educational sessions on topics such as "mindful-based eating and body image awareness" and "using make-up to restore balance." The centerpiece of this program was a Body Image Health Fair and Patient Fashion Show where cancer survivors served as fashion models, walked the runway, and shared meaningful stories about their survivorship experience with hundreds of people in the audience. For many, this offered an opportunity to gain greater confidence and comfort with their changed bodies. This program has received extremely positive feedback from participants and attendees and coincides with the Love Your Body Day Campaign from the National Organization for Women.

There is clearly much work to be done to educate healthcare providers and caregivers of cancer patients that most patients will struggle at some point and to some extent with body image changes as a result of their cancer and its treatment. Patients often feel too ashamed or guilty to mention their body image concerns because they feel they may perceived as "vain" or because it may make them seem ungrateful to their doctors or loved ones for surviving cancer. We believe it is important to educate those who are in contact with patients that body image is inherently subjective, so it is not the size, location, or type of bodily change which dictates extent of distress. Toward this end, it is vital that healthcare professionals within the oncology setting are aware of rudimentary assessment techniques to recognize body image concerns (e.g., the 3C's model) and route patients to appropriate resources. Vocabulary used to inquire/talk about body image issues with patients can set the stage for patients to feel comfortable enough to share and open up about their struggles. Particular care must be given in using words that are value laden such as "ugly," "pretty," "good," "bad," or "perfect." We caution specifically about well-meaning comments such as "You look so good!" or "We are going to be able to fix that," especially at the outset of a clinical encounter as this shuts down opportunities for patients to express their concerns and difficulties with adjusting to a changed body image. There is considerable room for formal training of body image assessment/intervention, such as training healthcare providers on how to best approach conversations about body image, training nurses in facilitating basic body image interventions, and developing formal coursework in body image and oncology at the graduate level.

Another important direction involves building further evidence for psychological-based interventions that has body image as the primary focus. It will be important to explore additional therapeutic frameworks, outside of cognitive-behavioral interventions, such as third wave, acceptance and commitment therapy, and other mindfulness-based therapies. Considering therapeutic delivery models that include participation of dyads/couples will be also be important, as is outlined by the chapter on couples by Hansen, Reese, and Grayer and the chapter on sexuality and fertility by Carpenter and Black. The ultimate goal is to not only establish the most effective therapeutic techniques but more specifically discover which techniques works best for a given population under a particular set of circumstances. Subsequently, we should be thinking about interventions that proactively promote positive body image adaption, instead of being disorder-focused, as every cancer patient and survivor experiences some level of change to his or her body. For instance, prevention programs that include work with a psychosocial specialist early in the treatment continuum can help set realistic expectations and incorporate tips on mirror-viewing assistance as routine care in acute postsurgical settings where appearance is impacted. The cost effectiveness of these relatively inexpensive interventions early in the treatment trajectory compared to intervening when the condition is debilitating will also be important to demonstrate. Lastly, what is most exciting to see is the potential for technology to break down geographical/logistical boundaries to offer resources and intervention access to survivors. There are, no doubt, ethical dilemmas to consider as we maneuver this frontier in relation to patient privacy issues.

CANCER-SPECIFIC BODY IMAGE SEQUELAE

There are a myriad of symptoms associated with cancer and its treatment that are pertinent to body image adjustment issues: hair loss, speech and swallowing difficulties, lymphedema, limb loss, stoma bag use, sexuality and fertility issues, and so on. Impairment in sexuality is intimately associated with body image yet continues to be underdiagnosed and undertreated, as discussed by Carpenter and Black. Secondary lymphedema is discussed by DeSnyder, Shaitelman, and Schaverien as affecting both appearance and functional aspects of body image and having an added layer of complexity due to the unpredictable nature of this sequelae. The vast majority of the body image research in this area has been with breast cancer patients. Speech and swallowing impairments are discussed by Lewin, Fingeret, and Hutcheson as having important implications on the resulting body image of cancer patients. Across all tumor types, the subjective experience of patients with cancer-specific sequelae may be conceptualized using models such as the visibility-stability continuum model offered by Lehmann and Tuinman or the noticeability-worry model presented by Paraskeva, Clarke, and Harcourt.

From a research perspective, there is room for growth in considering pain and cognitive impairment as cancer-specific body image sequelae. In addition, further attention needs to be paid to investigating survivors' body image experiences beyond one time point or only during the acute treatment stage. Whilst the longer-term impact of breast cancer on body image has been explored, the longer-term implications of body image outcomes related to other cancers still need to be investigated. Although there are studies that have examined body image in the context of cancer screening behaviors and in undergoing prophylactic treatment as covered by Sherman and Shaw, there remain many opportunities to further this line of inquiry.

SPECIAL POPULATIONS

We dedicated a number of chapters in this book to addressing cancer-related body image changes in pediatric and geriatric populations, in men, in couples, and from cross-cultural perspectives. We see that there is limited research on body image in cancer patients that take into account developmental or life stages, as is seen in the chapter on children and adolescents by Thompson and Wiener and the chapter on older adults by Schuler, Roth, and Holland There still is paucity in intervention research on children and adolescents, even though the existing data we have suggest that some of the most vulnerable patients are those who experience body image changes during their formative years. The data from survivors of childhood cancer suggest the effects can persist and be long term in nature. The literature on body image in male cancer patients and survivors is also observed to be lacking, as most of the literature tends to concentrate on female-specific cancers. However, it is important to consider perspectives of Drummond and Gough on how the male body is viewed in the context of masculinity and illness and how body image adjustment issues may present in men. In couples work, Hansen, Reese, and Grayer reported that the literature continues to be mixed on the extent to which body image adjustment difficulties are associated with poor romantic relationship outcomes. Research on couples-based interventions in patients with cancer usually includes body image as a secondary intervention target and outcome. It appears very promising to include romantic partners in interventions aimed at improving psychosexual adjustment to cancer and is especially interesting to consider that couple-based interventions have the potential to alter both patients' acceptance of their bodies and perceived partners' acceptance of their bodies. As with the other topics in the section, cultural differences in body image experiences of cancer patients is also not very well studied, even though body image as a construct is clearly a subjective evaluation that is shaped by internalized cultural standards. Cultural perspectives are indeed important to consider in any psychotherapeutic work, and this is no different with body image and cancer. According to Lee and Teo, although there are some good-quality long-term observational studies of body image changes in Asia, there are very few intervention studies, especially those that are counseling or therapy based.

In moving forward, it will be important to conceptually tease out how the characteristics of these special populations affect the body image experiences of the cancer survivor. More qualitative or mixed-method methodologies are needed to hear the voices of the unique subpopulations such as children and adolescents as well as individuals who are not from the mainstream culture. It will be important to understand how body image issues can present differently in these subpopulations such as men and older adults. We also need to consider how new interventions may be developed or ways existing therapies must be modified to meet the needs of these special populations, for instance by developmental age group or in a couples format. There certainly is need for more studies to be conducted in non-Western cultural settings.

CONCLUDING COMMENTS

It is our sincere hope that this book will be a useful handbook for clinicians and researchers who have interest in the field of body image and cancer and that the discussion points presented in this chapter inspire current and new researchers who will contribute to the growth of the field. Although there has been much interest and progress in body image work and cancer in the past decade, there is much more that needs to be done. As the world population is aging and the number of individuals living with cancer is expected to continue to rise, we are certain that survivorship issues involving body image adjustment will continue to be a topic of relevance and importance.

In an ideal envisioned future, an individual diagnosed with cancer would be assessed for body image distress as soon as he or she engages in treatment, as part of the standard routine of psychosocial care. The individual will be routed for further assessment and/or care that match his or her level of need (ranging from self-help to evidence-based intervention with a psychosocial specialist). Partners and/or families will be included in the intervention as needed. Individuals will be given information on how to seek further help if the need arises in the future. There will be ongoing communication between the specialist providing body image care and the individual's treatment team. Last but certainly not least, the individual's body image adjustment will continue to be monitored over time as part of ongoing psychosocial care.

INDEX

Tables, figures, and boxes are indicated by an italic *t, f,* and *b* following the page number.